STATISTICS FOR HEALTH CARE MANAGEMENT
AND ADMINISTRATION

STATISTICS FOR HEALTH CARE MANAGEMENT AND ADMINISTRATION

WORKING WITH EXCEL

Fourth Edition

David A. Rosenthal
John F. Kros

JB JOSSEY-BASS™
A Wiley Brand

For general information on our other products and services or for technical support, please contact our Customer Care Department within the United States at (800) 762-2974, outside the United States at (317) 572-3993 or fax (317) 572-4002.

Wiley also publishes its books in a variety of electronic formats. Some content that appears in print may not be available in electronic formats. For more information about Wiley products, visit our web site at www.wiley.com.

Library of Congress Cataloging-in-Publication Data applied for:

Paperback ISBN: 9781119901679

Cover image: © Table in Economic Writings (vol. 2) by William Petty (1899), djvu p. 121
Author Photos: Courtesy of the Authors
Cover design: Wiley

SKY10050353_070623

CONTENTS

David dedicates this edition to all those who have been called to a career in health care, and who serve others each day with passion, patience, and a commitment to excellence.

—David

John dedicates this edition to his entire family (grandmothers, grandfathers, mother, father, sisters, brother, wife, and children), who have always supported him in all he does, inspired him to always strive for excellence, and loved him all these years.

—John

The study and use of statistics have come a long way since the advent of computers. Particularly, computers have reduced both the effort and the time involved in the statistical analysis of data. But this ease of use has been accompanied by some difficulties. As computers became more and more proficient at carrying out statistical operations of increasing complexity, the actual operations—and what they actually meant and did—became more and more distant from the user. It became possible to do a wide variety of statistical operations with a few lines or words of commands to the computer. But the average student, even the average serious user of statistics, found the increasingly complex operations increasingly difficult to access and understand.

Introducing Excel

Sometime in the late 1980s, Microsoft Excel became available, and with it came the ability to carry out a wide range of statistical operations—and to understand the operations that were being carried out—in a spreadsheet format. John's first introduction to Excel was a revelation. It came during his MBA studies and continued through his doctoral studies and even in his first industry job. In fact, John quickly became somewhat indispensable in that first industry job for the plain fact that he was the most proficient of his peers at Excel. Through the years he found himself using Excel to complete all kinds of tasks (since he was too stubborn to learn to program properly). He discovered that Excel was not only a powerful statistical tool but also, more important, a powerful learning tool. When he began to teach the introductory course in business decision modeling to MBA students, Excel seemed to him to be the obvious medium for the course.

So How Did We Get to Here?

At the time John started using Excel in his teaching, there were a few textbooks devoted to statistics using Excel. However, none fit his needs very well, so he wrote *Spreadsheet Modeling for Business Decision Modeling*.

That was about the time John met David. David had earned his doctorate in technology management and had worked in the health care industry for more than 10 years (which ensures that the health care–specific examples and scenarios used in this book are appropriate). He discovered the power of Excel's statistical analysis functionality by using it to calculate the multiple regression and correlation analysis required for his doctoral dissertation.

Through his friend, Scott Bankard, John learned that the author of a successful text in the use of Excel to solve statistical problems in health care administration was looking for someone to revise that text. In turn, John and David became the coauthors of the revised text.

Intended Level of the Textbook

The original text was designed as an introductory statistics text for students at the advanced undergraduate level or for a first course in statistics at the master's degree level. It was intended to stand alone as the book for the only course a student might have in statistics. The same is true for the revised text, which includes some enhancements and updates that provide a good foundation for more advanced courses as well. Furthermore, since the book relies on Excel for all the calculations of the statistical applications, it was also designed to provide a statistical reference for people working in the health field who may have access to Excel but not to other dedicated statistical software. This is valuable in that a copy of Excel resides on the PC of almost every health care professional. Further, no additional appropriations would have to be made for proprietary software and there would be no wait for the "stat folks."

Textbook Organization

The revised edition of the text has been updated for use with the latest version of Microsoft Office Excel. It provides succinct instruction in the most commonly used techniques and shows how these tools can be implemented using the most current version of Excel for Windows. The revised text also focuses on developing both algebraic and spreadsheet modeling skills. Algebraic formulation and spreadsheets are juxtaposed to help develop conceptual thinking skills. Step-by-step instructions in Excel and numerous annotated screenshots make examples easy to follow and understand. Emphasis is placed on the model formulation and interpretation rather than on computer code or algorithms.

The book is organized into two major parts: Part 1, Chapters 1 through 6, presents Excel as a statistical tool and discusses hypothesis testing. Part 1 introduces the use of statistics in health policy and health administration–related fields, Excel as a statistical tool, data preparation and the data display capabilities of Excel, and probability, the foundation of statistical analysis. For students and other users of the book truly familiar with Excel, much of the material in Chapter 2, Chapter 3, and Chapter 4, particularly, could be covered very quickly.

Part 2, which includes Chapters 7 through 14, is devoted to the subject of hypothesis testing, the basic function of statistical analysis. Chapter 7 provides a general introduction to the concept of hypothesis testing. Each subsequent chapter provides a description of the major hypothesis testing tool for a specific type of data. Chapter 8 discusses the use of the chi-square statistic for assessing data for which both the independent and dependent variables are categorical. Chapter 9, on t tests, discusses the use of the t test for assessing data in which the independent variable is a two-level categorical variable and the dependent variable is a numerical variable. Chapter 10 is devoted to analysis of variance, which provides an analytical tool for a multilevel categorical independent variable and a numerical dependent variable. Chapters 11 through 13 are devoted to several aspects of regression analysis, which deals with numerical variables both as independent and dependent variables. Finally, Chapter 14 deals with numerical independent variables and dependent variables that are categorical and take on only two levels and introduces the use of Logit.

Leading by Example(s)

Each chapter of the book is structured around examples demonstrated extensively with the use of Excel displays. The chapters are divided into sections, most of which include step-by-step discussions of how statistical problems are solved using Excel, including the Excel formulae. Each section in a chapter is followed by exercises that address the material covered in that section. Most of these exercises include the replication of examples from that section. The purpose is to provide students an immediate reference with which to compare their work and determine whether they are able to correctly carry out the procedure involved. Additional exercises are provided on the same subjects for further practice and to reinforce the learning gained from the section. Data for all the exercises are included on the web at **www.wiley.com/go/kros4e**, and may be accessed by file references given in the examples themselves. Additional materials, such as videos, podcasts, and readings, can be found at www.josseybasspublichealth.com.

A supplemental package available to instructors includes all answers to the section exercises. In addition, the supplemental package will contain exam questions with answers and selected Excel spreadsheets that can be used for class presentations, along with suggestions for presenting these materials in a classroom. However, the book can be effectively used for teaching without the additional supplemental material.

Users who would like to provide feedback, suggestions, corrections, examples of applications, or whatever else can e-mail me at krosj@ecu.edu.

Please feel free to contact me and provide any comments you feel are appropriate.

ACKNOWLEDGMENTS

As always this newly revised version of the text would not have been possible without the support and guidance of numerous colleagues, friends, family, and all those poor souls who had to listen to us bounce ideas off of them, or for that matter anyone that just had to listen to us!

David thanks his wife Allyson and their entire extended family for their steadfast love and support. David also thanks his friend and colleague John for the years of collaboration and hard work pulling together the various editions of this textbook. It has been an honor and a privilege.

John thanks his wife, Novine, and his daughters, Samantha and Sabrina, for always being by his side and encouraging him in the special way they do when the light at the end of the tunnel starts to dim. Samantha always reminds her dad that she loves him, and maybe someday he will be cool again (no date has been set yet). Sabrina tells her dad that she expects great things from the East Carolina University Pirate football squad, the Texas Longhorn and Nebraska Cornhusker football teams, and the Virginia Cavaliers even if she is a Wolfpacker now. She also invites anyone interested to eat brunch on any given Sunday at her favorite establishment, the West End Dining Hall on East Carolina University's campus. John would like to say thank you to Novine, Samantha, and Sabrina and that he loves them very much. John also must thank his parents, Bernie and Kaye, who have always supported him, even when they didn't exactly know what he was writing about. Finally, John has to thank Scott Bankard for setting things in motion way back in 2007 and suggesting the project.

—*David A. Rosenthal, PhD, and John F. Kros, PhD*

THE AUTHORS

David A. Rosenthal is a Chief Information Officer with Campus Works, Inc., a higher education consulting firm that collaborates with colleges and universities to develop and implement insightful strategies that improve institutional effectiveness and enhance the student experience. He has over 20 years of health care industry experience in both academic and practitioner settings, having served in roles specific to hospital information technology leadership, multispecialty practice administration, and ambulatory services project management. Rosenthal earned a Master of Public Administration degree from Valdosta State University, and a PhD in Technology Management from Indiana State University. He is a proud veteran of the U.S. Air Force, and a Permanent Deacon in the Roman Catholic Church. David and his wife Allyson reside in Oakland, Tennessee.

John F. Kros is the Vincent K. McMahon Distinguished Professor in the Marketing and Supply Chain Management Department in the College of Business at East Carolina University, in Greenville, North Carolina. He teaches business decision modeling, statistics, operations and supply chain management, and purchasing and materials management courses. Kros was honored as the College of Business's Scholar/Teacher for 2004–2005, again in 2009–2010, was awarded the College of Business Commerce Club's highest honor, the Teaching Excellence Award, for 2006 and again in 2011, in 2013–2014 was awarded the East Carolina Alumni Association Outstanding Teaching Award, and in 2014–2015 was awarded the Board of Governors Distinguished Professor for Teaching Award. Kros earned his PhD in systems engineering from the University of Virginia, his MBA from Santa Clara University, and his BBA from the University of Texas at Austin. His research interests include health care operations, applied statistics, design of experiments, multi-objective decision making, Taguchi methods, and applied decision analysis. His textbook titled *Spreadsheet Modeling for Business Decisions* is in the fifth edition. He is also coauthor of *Health Care Operations and Supply Chain Management*. He enjoys spending his free time with his beautiful red-headed wife, Novine, and their two beautiful daughters, Samantha and Sabrina, traveling, snow skiing, vegetable gardening, spending time with his family and old fraternity brothers, watching college football, and attempting to locate establishments that provide quality food and liquid refreshment.

ABOUT THE COMPANION WEBSITE

This book is accompanied by a companion website:

www.wiley.com/go/kros4e

The website includes:

- Datasets
- PPTs
- Excel sheets
- Test banks

You will need a password to access the instructor material.

STATISTICS AND EXCEL

The statistics on sanity are that one out of every four Americans is suffering from some form of mental illness. Think of your three best friends. If they're okay, then it's you.

—Rita Mae Brown

Statistics is a subject that for many people is pure tedium. For others, it is more likely to be anathema. Still others find statistics interesting, even stimulating, but they are usually in the minority in any group.

This book is premised on the recognition that in the health care industry, as indeed among people in any industry or discipline, there are at least these three different views of statistics, and that any statistics class is likely to be made up more of the first two groups than the last one. This book provides an introduction to statistics in health policy and administration that is relevant, useful, challenging, and informative.

1.1 How This Book Differs from Other Statistics Texts

The primary difference between this statistics text and most others is that this text uses Microsoft Excel as the tool for carrying out statistical operations and understanding statistical concepts as they relate to health policy and health administration issues. This is not to say that no other statistics texts use Excel. Levine, Stephan, Szabat (2013) have produced a very usable text, *Statistics for Managers Using Microsoft Excel*. But their book focuses almost exclusively on non–health-related topics. We agree that the closer

LEARNING OBJECTIVES

- Understand how this book differs from other statistics texts

- Understand how knowledge of statistics may be beneficial to health policy or health administration professionals

- Understand the "big picture" with regard to the use of statistics for health policy and administration

- Understand the definitions of the following terms:
  - Populations and samples
  - Random and nonrandom samples
  - Types of random samples
  - Variables, independent and dependent

- Identify the five separate statistical tests: chi-square test, the *t* test, analysis of variance (ANOVA), regression analysis, and Logit the applications of statistics are to students' real-life interests and experiences, the more effective students will be in understanding and using statistics. Consequently, this book focuses its examples entirely on subjects that should be immediately familiar to people in the health care industry.

Excel, which most people know as a *spreadsheet* program for creating budgets, comparing budgeted and expended amounts, and generally fulfilling accounting needs, is also a very powerful statistical tool. Books that do not use Excel for teaching statistics generally leave the question of how to carry out the actual statistical operations in the hands of the student or the instructor. It is often assumed that relatively simple calculations, such as means, standard deviations, and *t* tests, will be carried out on paper or with a calculator. For more complicated calculations, the assumption is usually that a dedicated statistical package, such as SAS, SPSS, STATA, or SYSTAT, will be used. There are at least two problems with this approach that we hope to overcome in this book. First, calculations done on paper, or even those done with a calculator, can make even simple statistical operations overly tedious and prone to errors in arithmetic. Second, because dedicated statistical packages are designed for use rather than for teaching, they often obscure the actual process of calculating the statistical results, thereby hindering students' understanding of both how the statistic is calculated and what the statistic means.

In general, this is not true of Excel. It is true that when using this book, a certain amount of time must be devoted to the understanding of how to use Excel as a statistical tool. But once that has been done, Excel makes the process of carrying out the statistical procedures under consideration relatively clear and transparent. The student should end up with a better understanding of what the statistic means, through an understanding of how it is calculated, and not simply come away with the ability to get a result by entering a few commands into a statistical package. This is not to say that Excel cannot be used to eliminate many of the steps needed to get particular statistical results. A number of statistical tests and procedures are available as add-ins to Excel. However, using Excel as a relatively powerful—yet transparent—calculator can lead to a much clearer understanding of what a statistic means and how it may be used.

1.2   Statistical Applications in Health Policy and Health Administration

When teaching statistics to health policy and health administration students, we often encounter the same question: "All these statistics are fine, but how do they apply to anything I am concerned with?" The question not only is a reasonable one, but also points directly to one of the most important and difficult challenges for a statistics teacher, a statistics class, or a statistics text. How can it be demonstrated that these statistics have any real relevance to anything that the average person working in the health care industry ever needs to know or do?

To work toward a better understanding of why and when the knowledge of statistics may be useful to someone working in health policy or health administration, we've selected six examples of situations in which statistical applications can play a role. All six of these examples were inspired by real problems faced by students in statistics classes, and they represent real statistical challenges that students have faced and hoped to solve. In virtually every case, the person who presented the problem recognized it as one that could probably be dealt with using some statistical tool. But also in every case, the solution to the problem was not obvious in the absence of some understanding of statistics. Although these case examples are not likely to resonate with every reader, perhaps they will give many readers a little better insight into why knowledge of statistics can be useful.

Documentation of Medicare Reimbursement Claims

The Pentad Home Health Agency provides home health services in five counties of an eastern state. The agency must be certain that its *Medicare* reimbursement claims are appropriately and correctly documented in order to ensure that Medicare will process these claims and issue benefits in a timely manner. All physician orders, including medications, home visits for physical therapy, home visits of skilled nursing staff, and any other orders for service, must be correctly documented on a Form CMS-485. Poorly or otherwise inadequately prepared documentation can lead to rejection or delay in processing of the claim for reimbursement by the Centers for Medicare and Medicaid Services (CMS).

Pentad serves about 800 clients in the five-county region. In order to assure themselves that all records are properly documented, the administration runs a chart audit of 1 in 10 charts each quarter. The audit seeks to determine (1) whether all orders indicated in the chart have been carried out and (2) if the orders have been correctly documented in the Form CMS-485. Orders that have not been carried out, or orders incorrectly documented, lead to follow-up training and intervention to address these issues and ensure that the orders and documentation are properly prepared going forward.

Historically, the chart audit has been done by selecting each tenth chart, commencing at the beginning or at the end of the chart list. Typically, the chart audit determines that the majority of charts, usually 85 to 95 percent, have been correctly documented. But there are occasionally areas, such as in skilled nursing care, where the percentage of correct documentation may fall below that level. When this happens, the administration initiates appropriate corrective action.

Sampling, Data Display, and Probability

One of the questions of the audit has been the selection of the sample. Because the list of clients changes relatively slowly, the selection of every tenth chart often results in the same charts being selected for audit from one quarter to the next. That being the case, a different strategy for chart selection is desirable. It has been suggested by statisticians that using a strictly random sample of the charts might be a better way to select them for quarterly review, as this selection would have a lesser likelihood of resulting in a review of the same charts from quarter to quarter. But how does one go about drawing a strictly random sample from any population? Or, for that matter, what does "strictly random" actually mean and why is it important beyond the likelihood that the same files may not be picked from quarter to quarter? These questions are addressed by statistics, specifically the statistics associated with sample selection and data collection.

Another question related to the audit concerns when to initiate corrective action. Suppose a sample of 1 in 10 records is drawn (for 800 clients that would be 80 records) and it is discovered that 20 of the records have been incorrectly documented. Twenty of 80 records incorrectly documented would mean that only 75 percent of the records were correctly documented. This would suggest that an intervention should be initiated to correct the documentation problem. But it was a *sample* of the 800 records that was examined, not the entire 800. Suppose that the 20 incorrectly documented records were, by the luck of the draw, so to speak, the only incorrectly documented records in the entire 800. That would mean that only 2.5 percent of the cases were incorrectly documented.

If the required corrective action were an expensive five-day workshop on correct documentation, the agency might not want to incur that expense when 97.5 percent of all cases are correctly documented. But how would the agency know from a sample what proportion of the total 800 cases might be incorrectly documented, and how would they know the likelihood that fewer than, say, 85 percent of all cases were correctly documented if 75 percent of a sample were correctly documented? This, again, is a subject of statistics.

Emergency Trauma Color Code

The emergency department (ED) of a university hospital was the site of difficulties arising from poor response time to serious trauma. Guidelines indicate that a trauma surgeon must attend for a certain level of trauma severity within 20 minutes and that other trauma, still severe but less so, should be attended by a trauma nurse within a comparable time. In general, it had been found that the response time for the ED in the university hospital was more or less the same for all levels of severity of trauma—too long for severe cases and often quicker than necessary, given competing priorities, for less severe cases.

The ED director knew that when a trauma case was en route to the hospital, the ambulance attendants called the ED to advise that an emergency was on its way. Part of the problem as perceived by the director of the ED was that the call-in did not differentiate the trauma according to severity. The ED director decided to institute a system whereby the ambulance attendants would assign a code red to the most severe trauma cases, a code yellow to less severe trauma cases, and no color code to the least severe trauma cases. The color code of the trauma would be made known to the ED as the patient was being transported to the facility. The intent of this coding was to ensure that the most severe traumas were attended within the 20-minute window. This in turn was expected to reduce the overall time from admission to the ED to discharge of the patient to the appropriate hospital department. (All trauma cases at the red or yellow level of severity are transferred from the ED to a hospital department.)

Descriptive Statistics, Confidence Limits, and Categorical Data

A major concern of the director of the ED was whether the new system actually reduced the overall time between admission to the ED, treatment of the patient in the ED, and discharge to the appropriate hospital department. The director of the ED had considerable information about each ED admission going back a period of several months before the implementation of the new color-coding system and six months of experience with the system after it was implemented. This information includes the precise time that each trauma patient was admitted to the ED and the time that the patient was discharged to the appropriate hospital department.

The information also includes the severity of the trauma at admission to the ED on a scale of 0 to 75, as well as information related to gender, age, and whether the admission occurred before or after the color-coding system was implemented. The ED director also has information about the color code assigned after the system was initiated that can generally be equated to the severity score assigned at admission to the ED. Trauma scoring 20 or more on the scale would be assigned code red; below 20, code yellow; and not on the scale, no color.

Inferential Statistics, Analysis of Variance, and Regression

The question the ED director wishes to address is how she can use her data to determine whether the color-coding system has reduced the time that trauma victims spend in the ED before being discharged to the appropriate hospital department. At the simplest level, this is a question that can be addressed by using a statistic called the *t* test for comparing two different groups. At a more complex level, the ED director can address the question of whether any difference in waiting time in the ED can be seen as at all related to changes in severity levels of patients before or after the color-coding scheme was introduced. She can also examine whether other changes in the nature of the patients who arrived as trauma victims before and after the introduction of the color-coding scheme might be the cause of possible differences in waiting time. These questions can be addressed by using regression analysis.

Two Caveats of Statistics: Establishing a Significant Difference and Causality

Two caveats regarding the use of statistics apply directly to this example. The first is that no statistical analysis may be needed at all if the waiting time after the initiation of the color-coding scheme is clearly shorter than the waiting time before. Suppose, for example, that the average waiting time before the color-coding scheme was three hours from admission to the ED to discharge to hospital department, and that after the initiation of the scheme, the average waiting time was 45 minutes. In this scenario, no statistical significance tests would be required to show that the color-coding scheme was associated with a clear improvement in waiting time. Furthermore, it is likely that the color-coding scheme would not only become a permanent part of the ED armamentarium of the university hospital but also be adopted widely by other hospitals.

However, suppose that after the initiation of the color-coding scheme the average waiting time in the ED was reduced from 3 hours to 2 hours and 50 minutes. A statistical test (probably the *t* test) would show whether 170 minutes of waiting was actually less, statistically, than 180 minutes. Although such a small difference may seem to have little practical significance, it may represent a statistically significant difference. In such a case, the administrator would have to decide whether to retain an intervention (the color-coding scheme) that had a statistical, but not a practical, effect.

The second caveat to the use of statistics is the importance of understanding that a statistical test cannot establish causality. It might be possible, statistically, to show that the color-coding scheme was associated with a statistical reduction in waiting time. But in the absence of a more rigorous study design, it is not possible to say that the color-coding scheme actually *caused* the reduction in waiting time. In a setting such as this, where measurements are taken before and after some intervention (in this case, the color-coding scheme), a number of factors other than the color-coding scheme might have accounted for an improvement in waiting time.

The very recognition of the problem and consequent concern by ED physicians and nurses may have had more effect on waiting time than the color-coding scheme itself. But this is not a question that statistics, per se, can resolve. Such questions may be resolved in whole or in part by the nature of a study design. A double-blind, random clinical trial, for example, is a very powerful design for resolving the question of causality. But, in general, statistical analysis alone cannot determine whether an observed result has occurred *because of* a particular intervention. All that statistical analysis can do is establish whether two events (in this case, the color-coding scheme and the improvement in waiting time) are or are not independent of each other. This notion of independence will come up many more times, and, in many ways, it is the focus of much of this book.

Length of Stay, Readmission Rates, and Cost per Case in a Hospital Alliance

The ever-increasing costs of providing hospital services have sparked a keen interest on the part of hospital administrators in practical mechanisms that can account for—and control or mitigate—those costs. The administrators for the Sea Coast Alliance, a system of eight hospitals, want to be able to use the previous case data to provide guidance on how to control costs. Because Sea Coast is associated with eight hospitals, it has a substantial volume of case data that the administrators believe can be useful in achieving their goal.

There are, in particular, three measures of hospital performance related to costs that need to be evaluated in this case: length of stay (LOS), readmission rates, and cost per case. One of the initial questions is whether there are real differences among the eight hospitals in these three cost-related measures of hospital performance. The question of what is a real difference is, of course, paramount. If the average LOS in one of Sea Coast's hospitals is five days for all hospital stays over the past year while the average LOS for another Sea Coast hospital is six days, is this a real difference? Given certain assumptions about what the average LOS for a year in these two hospitals represents, this is a question that can be answered with statistics.

Establishing a Statistical Difference between Two Groups Using *t* Tests and Analysis of Variance

If the interest is in comparing two hospitals with each other, the statistic that could be used would be a *t* test. In general, though, the real interest would be in deciding if there was any difference among all eight hospitals, taken simultaneously. This question can be examined in a couple different ways. One would be to use analysis of variance (ANOVA). Another would be to use multiple regression. If by using any of these statistical techniques it is determined that LOS is different from hospital to hospital, efforts could be directed toward determining whether lessons could be learned from the better performers about how to control costs that might be applied to the poorer performers. The same approach could be applied to understanding readmission rates and cost per case.

One particular focus of the Sea Coast administrators is diagnostic-related groupings (DRG) that have especially high costs. In addition to looking at the performance across the eight hospitals on high-cost DRGs, Sea Coast would like to be able to examine the question of whether individual physicians seemed to stand out in LOS, readmission rates, or cost per case. Identification of individual physicians who have unusually high LOS, readmission rates, or cost per case can allow Sea Coast to engage in selective educational efforts toward reduced costs. But an important question in looking at individual physician differences is whether what may appear to be unusually high values for LOS, readmission rates, or cost per case actually are unusual. Again, this question can be answered with statistics. In particular, predicted values for LOS, readmission rates, and cost per case can be determined by using regression analysis.

Establishing a Statistical Difference between Two Groups Using Regression

Regression can also be used to assess whether the differences that may exist across hospitals or across individual physicians could be attributed to differences in the mix of cases or patients whom the hospitals accept or the physicians see. Such differences may be attributable statistically to such characteristics of patients as sex, age, and payer, which may differ across the eight hospitals or the numerous physicians. There might also be differences across cases related to severity or diagnoses. If these were differentially distributed among hospitals or physicians, they could account for visible differences. All of these questions can be addressed (although not necessarily answered in full) by using multiple regression analysis.

At the Carteret Falls regional hospital, the emergency department has instituted a major change in how physicians are contracted to provide services and consequently how services are billed in the ED. Prior to January 1 of a recent year, emergency department physicians were employed by the regional hospital, and the hospital billed for their services. Beginning January 1, the physicians became private contractors working within the emergency department, essentially working on their own time and billing for that time directly. Bills are submitted to Medicare under five different coding levels that correspond to the level of reimbursement Medicare provides. The higher the coding level, the more Medicare actually reimburses for the service.

The practice manager for the physicians is concerned that she will begin to see the billing level creep upward as physicians begin billing for their own services. As the distinction between levels is frequently a matter of judgment, the practice manager is concerned that physicians may begin, even unconsciously, upgrading the level of the coding because it is directly tied to their reimbursement. The question the practice manager faces is how to decide if the physicians are upgrading their codes, consciously or not, after the initiation of the new system. If they are, the practice needs to take steps, either to ensure that the coding remains constant before and after the change in billing, or to have very good justification for CMS as to why it should be different.

Establishing a Difference Using Statistical Tests

The first problem is to determine if the billing levels have changed from before the change in billing to after the change. But it is simply not enough to say that there is a change, if one is seen to have occurred. It is critical to be able to say that this change is or is not a change that would have been expected, given the pattern of billing in the past. In other words, is any change seen as large enough to be deemed a real change and not just a chance occurrence? If a change has occurred, and if it is large enough to be viewed as a real change, then the second problem arises: determining whether anything in the nature of the ED cases before and after the billing change might account for the difference and thus be the explanation of the difference that will satisfy the Medicare administration.

Both of these problems can be examined by using statistics. In regard to the first problem, a difference between the distribution of billings across the five categories before and after the change in billing source can be assessed by using the *chi-square statistic*. Or, because the amount of a bill is constant within the five categories, it is also possible to compare the two groups, before and after, using the t test. The second problem, of whether any difference can be attributed to changed characteristics of the cases seen in the ED, can be assessed by using regression—when the cost of the bills before and after is the measure of change.

A Study of the Effectiveness of Breast Cancer Education

A resident at a local hospital has been asked by the senior physician to develop a pilot study on the effectiveness of two alternative approaches to breast cancer education, both aimed at women coming to a women's health center. The first alternative is the distribution of a brochure on breast cancer to the women when they arrive at the clinic. The second alternative is time specifically allocated during a clinic visit wherein the physician spends 5 to 10 minutes with each woman, giving direct information and answering questions on the same topics covered in the brochure.

The resident recognizes that a study can be designed in which one group of women would receive the brochure and a second group would participate in a session with a physician. She also believes that a questionnaire can be developed to measure the knowledge women have about breast cancer before the distribution of the brochure or session with the physician and after either event, to assess any difference in knowledge. She also is concerned about possibly needing a control group of women to determine whether either method of information dissemination is better than no intervention at all. And perhaps she is interested in whether the brochure and discussion with the physician together would be better than either alternative singly.

Although she has been asked to design a pilot study only, the student-resident wishes to be as careful and as thoughtful as possible in developing her study. She might consider a number of different alternatives. One would be a simple t test of the difference between a group of women who received the brochure and a group of women who participated in the sessions with a physician. The measurement for this comparison could be the knowledge assessment administered either after the distribution of the brochure or after the physician encounter.

Using Analysis of Variance versus t Tests

But the resident may very well be dissatisfied with the simple t test. One problem is that she wants to include a control group of women who received no intervention at all. She may also wish to include another group of women—those who received the brochure *and* spoke to a physician. Again, the effect of any intervention (or of none) could be measured using her previously developed knowledge assessment, administered after the fact. This assessment could be carried out using a one-way analysis of variance.

Again, however, the resident may not be entirely satisfied with either the t test or the one-way analysis of variance. She might wish to be sure that in her comparison she is not simply measuring a difference between women that existed prior to the receipt of the brochures or the physician sessions. To ensure this, she might wish to measure women's knowledge both before and after the interventions, at both times using her knowledge assessment questionnaire. This assessment could be carried out using a two-way analysis of variance.

Regardless of whether the resident decides to go with a t test, a one-way ANOVA, or a two-way ANOVA, one of the more important aspects of the study will be to randomly allocate women to the experimental or control group. When measuring knowledge only after the intervention, the resident will be able to ensure that prior knowledge is not responsible for any differences she might find only if she is certain that there is only a small chance that the groups of women receiving different interventions were not different to begin with. The only effective way to ensure this is through random assignment to the groups.

Calculating a Standard Hourly Rate for Health Care Personnel

In an article published in *Healthcare Financial Management*, Richard McDermott (2001) discusses the problem and importance of establishing standard hourly labor rates for employee reimbursement. He points out that many compensation systems have been worked out over a number of years by different human resources directors, each with his own compensation philosophy. As a result, these systems may fail to reflect market conditions and may be inconsistent in their treatment of differing categories of labor. McDermott suggests a regression approach to calculating labor rates that have both internal consistency and external validity.

The approach McDermott suggests for establishing labor rates is based on an example in which he provides data for 10 different positions. Each position is assigned a score from 0 to 5 based on the degree of complexity in the job in five separate categories, such as level of decision making, amount of planning required, educational requirements, and so on. He does not indicate specifically which five characteristics are employed in the example. The assigned scores in each category would have been developed through an examination of the requirements of the job by a compensation consultant after interviews with the incumbent of each position. Each of the 10 positions also includes an actual hourly wage.

Relating Variables via Regression Analysis: Some Issues

Regression analysis was used by McDermott to assess the relationship between each of the five characteristics of the job and the actual hourly compensation. The regression analysis indicates both the relationship between any one of the five characteristics (when all characteristics are considered simultaneously) and hourly compensation, and it provides a set of coefficients by which to translate assigned values on any set of characteristics into a predicted hourly compensation. This, then, becomes a relatively objective means of determining hourly compensation for a person in any position.

There are purely statistical problems in using this regression approach, at least as discussed by McDermott, to propose hourly compensation. Particularly, 10 observations (the jobs assessed) are rarely considered by statisticians to be an adequate number with which to assess the relationship between five predictor variables (the characteristics) and a sixth predicted variable (the hourly compensation). While there are no absolute rules for the number of observations needed relative to the number of variables assessed, it is often accepted that there should be at least three times as many observations as variables, and some statisticians suggest a ratio of as many as 10 observations to each variable.

A second problem with this approach to assigning hourly compensation is inherent in the fact that many jobs are essentially the same, with similar job titles and expectations. If such jobs are included in an analysis of the type discussed here, one of the basic premises of regression analysis, that there is no correlation between observations, will be violated. This can be overcome, in part, by the use of *dummy variables*.

EXERCISES FOR SECTION 1.2

1. Look online, and in magazines or journals that might deal with subjects relevant to your current work situation or your planned area of work. Can you find discussions that involve statistics? If so, briefly describe these and how the statistics are applied.

2. Consider experience you have had or a situation that you are familiar with in your work or planned area of work. Can you imagine any way that this experience or situation could benefit from the application of statistics? Briefly describe this experience or situation.

1.3   What Is the "Big Picture"?

Having discussed several specific examples of why a health care worker might be interested in knowing statistics, and having suggested some ways in which this book can provide that knowledge, we now want to step back and ask, what are we actually trying to do? To put it another way, what is the "big picture"? The big picture is basically this: In any situation in which statistics may be applicable and useful, the beginning is the question for which an answer is sought. Are our Medicare claims properly completed? Does a color-coding scheme for emergencies reduce emergency room time? Do the hospitals in a region differ in terms of costs? Will an education strategy work?

In attempting to answer any of these questions, it is generally true that not all the data that might bear on the answer will ever be available. In some cases, though it might be possible to access all the relevant data, it might just be too costly to do so. This would be true, for example, with regard to Medicare claims in a home health agency. Because it would be very costly to examine every claim, the answer must rely on a subset of the claims. In other cases, it might never be possible to access all records or all people who might be necessary to provide a definitive answer. With regard to the question of whether an education intervention will increase the knowledge women have of breast cancer, it would be physically impossible to assess all women who might ever be potential subjects of such an education effort.

The consequence of this inability to access all the data that may be relevant to a decision means that it will be necessary, generally, to rely on only a subset of the data—a *sample*—to make whatever decision is called for. Statistics is about the rules and procedures for using a subset of the data to make the decisions desired. In learning statistics, one learns these rules and procedures, when and what types of data to apply, and the confidence that one can have in using the results of the sample data to make inferences about the total population. This is the basic function of statistics.

In considering the function of statistics as the process of using a sample to make inferences about a larger population, it is important to point out that in many cases this is the only way, and often the best way, to reach decisions. In the case of the acceptability of Medicare claims, for example, it is highly likely that if the staff of a home health agency were required to review every one of the files, they would become tired, bored, and generally unhappy with the process. They might make mistakes or errors in judgment that they would perhaps not make if they were working with only a sample of records. When they had finished their audit of the entire population of claims, they could very well have less useful information than they would have had under the limitations of a sample. And, in any case, the cost would be prohibitive.

1.4   Some Initial Definitions

Before proceeding much further in this discussion, it is essential to make certain that everyone is clear about a number of terms that will crop up again and again in this text.

Populations and Samples

Populations are those groups of entities about which there is an interest. Populations may be made up of people—for example, all citizens of the United States or all patients who have shown up or ever will show up at a specific emergency room clinic. Populations may be made up of organizations—for example, all hospitals in the United States, or all long-term care facilities in New York state. Populations may be made up of political entities—for example, all the countries in the world or all the counties in California. All the persons who might ever receive a particular type of assessment are a population, and all people who ever will have an magnetic resonance imaging (MRI) could be considered another population, or these two groups together could be considered a population.

Populations tend to be large groups of individual persons, objects, or items from which samples can be taken.

In general, we are interested in characteristics of populations as opposed to characteristics of samples. We might wish to know the average cholesterol level of all persons age 55 or older (a population). We might wish to know the daily bed occupancy rate for hospitals in the United States (a population). Or we might wish to know the effect of a specific drug on cholesterol levels of some group of people (a population). If we knew these specific pieces of information, we would know a *parameter*. Parameters are information about populations. In general, except for some data collected by a complete census of the population (even most complete censuses are not complete), we do not know parameters. The best we can usually do is estimate parameters based on a subset of observations taken from populations.

Samples are subsets of populations.

Samples are subsets of populations. If a population of interest consists of all patients who have shown up or ever will show up at a specific emergency room clinic, a sample from that population could be all the patients who are there on a specific afternoon. If a population of interest consists of all long-term care facilities in New York state, a sample from that population might be all these facilities in Buffalo, Syracuse, and Albany. If a population of interest is all persons who have used or ever will use a cholesterol-reducing drug, a sample from that population might be all persons who received prescriptions for such a drug from a specific physician. An individual member of a sample might be referred to as an element of the sample or, more commonly, as an observation.

Information from samples can be used to make estimates of information about populations (parameters). When a specific value from a sample is used to make an estimate of the same value for a population, the sample value is known as a statistic. Statistics are to samples what parameters are to populations. If the parameter of interest is, for example, waiting time in emergency rooms, an estimate of that parameter could be the average waiting time for a small, carefully selected group of emergency rooms. The estimate would be a statistic. In general, we can know values of statistics but not parameters, even though we would wish to know the values of parameters.

Random and Nonrandom Samples

The samples, or subsets of a population, may be selected in a random manner or in a nonrandom manner. All patients in an emergency room on a specific afternoon would probably not constitute a *random sample* of all people who have used or will use an emergency room. All the hospitals in Buffalo, Syracuse, and Albany might be a random sample of all hospitals in New York state, but they probably would not be. All persons who received prescriptions for a cholesterol-reducing drug from a specific physician would, in general, not be a random sample of all persons who take such drugs. All of these examples would probably be considered nonrandom samples. Nonrandom samples may be drawn in many ways. In general, however, we are not interested in nonrandom samples. The study of statistics is based on and assumes the presence of random samples. This requires some discussion of what constitutes a random sample.

Random samples are drawn in a manner whereby every member of the population has a known probability of being selected.

A random sample is a sample drawn in a manner whereby every member of the population has a known probability of being selected. At a minimum, this means that all members of the population must be identifiable. Frequently, there is a gap between the population of interest and the population from which the sample is actually drawn. For example, suppose a health department wished to draw a random sample of all families in its area of responsibility to determine what proportion believed that the health department was a possible source of any type of health services—prevention, treatment, advice—for members of the family.

The *target population* is all families in the area of responsibility. If we assume that this is a county health department, a random sample would assign a known probability of selection to each family in the county. In general, this would mean that each family in the county would have an equal probability of selection. If there were, for example, 30,000 families in the county, each one would have a probability of 1/30,000 of being selected as a member of the sample.

But, in general, it would be very difficult to be certain that every family in the county had exactly a 1/30,000 probability of being selected for the sample. The difficulty arises from the problem of devising an economically feasible mechanism of identifying and contacting every possible family in the county. For example, one relatively inexpensive way of collecting the information desired would be to contact a sample of families by telephone and ask them questions. But some families do not have phones, making their probability of selection into the sample not 1/30,000 but simply zero. Other families may have more than one phone, and if care is not taken to ensure that the family is not contacted twice, some families might have twice the chance (or more) of being selected into the sample. Still other families—especially in the present age of telemarketing—would decline to participate, which would make their probability of being included zero as well.

Other mechanisms of identifying all families in a county or other area have equal difficulties. Voter rolls list only registered voters. Tax rolls list only persons who pay taxes. Both of these rolls also contain single persons. A decision would have to be made about whether a single person constitutes a family. In summary, then, it is very often nearly impossible, or at least very expensive, to draw a truly random sample from a target population. What often happens instead is that the sample drawn is actually from a population very close to the target population but not the target population exactly. Instead of all the families in the county being the population from which the sample is drawn, the population may be all families with telephones.

> The sampled population is the population from which the sample is actually drawn.

The population from which the sample is actually drawn is known as the *sampled population*. Inferences from the sample to the population are always to the sampled population; one hopes that these inferences hold for the target population as well. Given that the population sampled may not be exactly the target population desired, there still needs to be a mechanism for assuring that each member of the population to be sampled has a known probability generally equal of being selected. There are lots of ways of assuring randomness in specific settings. Shuffling cards is a way of assuring that each person has an equal chance of getting the good cards and the bad cards during the deal—essentially a random distribution of the cards. Rolling dice is a way of ensuring a random distribution of the faces of a die. Flipping a coin is a way of ensuring the random appearance of a head or a tail.

But sampling from a population of all families served by a health department is more complicated. One workable mechanism might be to put every family's name on equal-sized slips of paper, put all the slips of paper in a box, shake the box, and without looking at the slips of paper, draw out the number of slips desired. But this approach, although it would produce a random sample of families, would be both cumbersome and time consuming. Excel provides several mechanisms that can be used to draw random samples.

There are basically four different types of random samples: systematic samples, simple random samples, stratified samples, and cluster samples.

Systematic Samples

Systematic samples are samples drawn by first dividing the population into subsets equal to the number of observations ultimately desired in the sample and then drawing a specific observation from each subset. If the total population of interest consisted of 30,000 families and the sample to be drawn was to consist of 100 families, the first step in drawing a systematic sample would be to divide the total population into 100 subsets. Suppose we have the 30,000 families on a list in alphabetical order. The common way to divide the families into 100 subsets would be to take the first 300 families as the first subset, the second 300 as the second subset, and so on to the end of the list.

A systematic sample is drawn from equally divided subsets of a population.

The next step in drawing a systematic sample would be to select randomly one family from the first subset of 300. Then the corresponding family from each of the other 99 subsets would be selected to fill out the sample. For example, if the family in position 137 in the alphabetical list were selected at random, then family number 437 (the 137th family in the second subset of 300) would be taken as the next member of the sample, and family number 737 would be selected as the third member, all the way to family number 39,837. This would produce a sample of 100 families, all of which are spaced 300 families apart in the alphabetically sorted list.

A systematic sample actually represents a single observation in statistical terms. This is because once the selection is made from the first subset, all other observations are fixed. If a sample of 100 is to be selected systematically from a population of 30,000, 300 different samples can be selected. These 300 samples correspond to each of the 300 families that can be selected as the first element of the sample. Because systematic samples are samples made up from a single random selection, the results expected from statistics do not actually apply to systematic samples. Nevertheless, systematic samples are often treated as if statistics do apply appropriately to them. This is generally considered acceptable for drawing inferences about populations.

Simple Random Samples

Simple random samples are samples drawn in such a way that every possible sample of a given size has an equal likelihood of being selected for the sample. If the total population of interest consisted of 30,000 families and the sample to be drawn was to consist of 100 families, every possible sample of 100 families would have an equal likelihood of being drawn in a simple random sample. Before the widespread availability of computers, simple random samples were typically drawn by associating each element of the population with a number from a random number table. If the number in the random number table was in a certain range, the element was included in the sample; if not, the element was not included in the sample. The advent of personal computers, and especially such programs as Excel, has eliminated the need for random number tables. Excel can generate lists of random numbers that can be used to select simple random samples.

Simple random samples assume that each sample has an equal likelihood of being selected.

Whereas only 300 different systematic samples of size 100 could be drawn from a population of 30,000 families, there are far more simple random samples of size 100. The number of different simple random samples of 100 families that can be taken from a population of 30,000 families is so large that it would take several lines of text to write it out completely. It is approximately the number 46,815 followed by 285 zeros. And each one of this very large number of samples has an equal likelihood of being selected as the one simple random sample taken.

Stratified Samples

Stratified samples are samples drawn by dividing the total population into two or more groups, or strata, and then drawing a specified proportion of each stratum for the sample. The specified portion might be proportional to the stratum size, or it might be equal to the number drawn from other strata, regardless of whether the stratum sizes are equal. Within each stratum, the sample may be drawn by simple random sampling or by systematic sampling. The sample is typically drawn by simple random sampling.

A stratified sample is drawn by dividing the population into strata and then drawing a specified proportion from each stratum.

Consider how a stratified sample might apply to our sample of 100 families from a population of 30,000 families. Suppose we know that within our population of 30,000 families, 3,000 have Hispanic surnames. If we want to draw a stratified sample that would guarantee that it had proportional representation of families with Hispanic surnames, we could first divide the total population into two strata: those with Hispanic surnames and those with other surnames. Then we could take a sample of 10 families from among those with Hispanic surnames and a sample of 90 families from among those who do not have Hispanic surnames.

In general, stratified samples are drawn for two reasons:

1. The researcher wishes to ensure that the groups represented by the strata are appropriately represented in the final sample.

2. There is reason to believe that the subject of interest to the study is closely related to the characteristics upon which the strata are based.

In the latter case, for example, if a health care professional wished to estimate average height among teenagers 17 to 19 years of age, it would probably be useful to stratify on sex. As teenagers, males are likely to be taller than females. At preadolescence, it might be useful to stratify on sex because females are likely to be taller than males.

Cluster Samples

Cluster samples are samples drawn by first dividing the sample into several groups, or clusters. The sampling then proceeds in two or more stages. This discussion is of a two-stage cluster sample only. In the first stage, a set of the clusters is drawn using either systematic or simple random sampling, although simple random is most commonly employed. In the second stage, either all members of the cluster or a sample of members of the cluster are selected to be included in the final sample.

Cluster samples are drawn via two stages: Groups are drawn first using random or systematic sampling techniques, and then samples are drawn from those groups.

In the case of our sample of 100 families from among 30,000, the families to be selected could be divided into ZIP code areas first. The sample of ZIP code areas randomly selected is the first stage. In the second stage, families could be selected randomly from those ZIP code groups selected to fill out the sample of 100. Typically, cluster samples are used when the collection of data from a simple random sample would involve a great deal of travel time. The use of clusters limits the travel required for data collection to only those clusters selected. A major drawback of cluster sampling is that it is likely to increase the variability of those statistics about which estimates are to be made.

Cluster Samples versus Stratified Samples

Cluster samples and stratified samples differ from one another. In using cluster samples, only a few of the groups or clusters actually have members represented in the final sample. When using stratified samples, all groups, or strata, have members represented in the final sample. For the material presented in this book, it is assumed that the data were drawn in what would be considered either a simple random method or a stratified method with the number of observations drawn from each stratum proportional to stratum size.

Variables, Independent and Dependent

Throughout this book there are frequent references to the term "variable."
A *variable* is a characteristic of an observation or element of the sample
that is assessed or measured. A value for a variable across all members of a
sample (e.g., the average height of preadolescent teens) is typically referred
to as a *statistic*. The comparable value for the population is a parameter.
Most statistical activities are an attempt either to determine a value for
a variable from a sample (and thus to be able to estimate the population
value) or to determine whether there is a relationship between two or
more variables.

> A variable is a characteristic of an observation or an element of the sample that is assessed or measured.

In order to show a relationship between two or more variables, the
variables must vary. That is to say that they must take on more than one
value. Any characteristic of a population that does not vary is a constant.
There can be no relationship between a constant and a variable. This
is equivalent to saying that there can be no way of accounting for the
value of any variable by referring to a constant. For example, if we wished
to describe variations in adult-onset diabetes rates among persons with
Hispanic surnames, it would be useless to employ Hispanic surname as an
explanation, because it is constant for all these people. It cannot explain
differences. But if we wished to describe differences in adult-onset diabetes
among all the people living in, say, New Mexico, Hispanic surname or
non-Hispanic surname might be a useful variable to employ.

Variables, Categorical and Numerical

Variables are typically classified as either of two types: categorical or
numerical. Numerical variables are further classified as either discrete or
continuous. These distinctions are important for the type of statistic that
may effectively be employed with them.

> Categorical variables are distinguished simply by name.

Categorical variables are variables whose levels are distinguished simply
by names. Hispanic and non-Hispanic surname is a two-level categorical

variable that roughly distinguishes whether a person is of Hispanic ancestry. Sex is a two-level categorical variable that in general divides all persons into male or female. Categorical variables can take on more levels as well. Type of insurance coverage, for example, is a multilevel categorical variable that may take on the values Medicare, Medicaid, voluntary not-for-profit, for-profit, self-pay, and other. Other categorical variables may take on many levels.

Although a variable may be represented by a set of numbers, such a representation does not automatically mean that it is not a categorical variable. The International Classification of Disease (ICD)-11 -CM (Clinical Modification) code is a categorical variable, even though the codes are represented as numbers. The numbers simply classify diagnoses into numerical codes that have no actual numerical meaning. Another type of categorical variable that is assigned a number is the dummy variable. The dummy variable is a two-level categorical variable (e.g., sex) that is assigned a numerical value, usually the values 1 and 0. The value 1 might be assigned to female and 0 assigned to male, or vice versa. Although this type of variable remains a categorical variable, it can be treated as a numerical variable in some statistical applications that require numerical variables. However, a categorical variable with more than two levels, such as the ICD-9-CM code, can be treated as a numerical variable in analysis only by dividing the multilevel categorical variable into a number of two-level categorical variables that can be treated as dummy variables.

Numerical variables are distinguished by number.

Numerical variables are, as the name implies, variables whose values are designated by numbers. But unlike ICD-9-CM codes, the numbers have some meaning relative to one another. At the very minimum, a numerical variable whose value is, for example, 23 is presumed to be larger than a numerical variable whose value is 17. Numerical variables may be measured on three scales: the ordinal scale, the interval scale, and the ratio scale.

Ordinal Scale

The ordinal scale is a scale in which the values assigned to the levels of a variable simply indicate that the levels are in order of magnitude. A common ordinal scale is the *Likert scale*, which requests a response to one of usually five alternatives: strongly agree, agree, undecided, disagree, or strongly disagree. These responses are then assigned values of 1 to 5, or 5 to 1, and treated as values of a numerical variable. Treating Likert scale responses like numerical variables assumes that the conceptual difference between strongly agree and agree is exactly the same, for example, as the conceptual difference between undecided and disagree. If that cannot be assumed, then ordered variables, such as Likert scale variables, even if assigned numerical values, should not be treated as numerical variables in analysis but must be treated as categorical variables.

Interval Scale

The *interval scale* is a scale in which the values assigned to the levels of a variable indicate the order of magnitude in equal intervals. The commonly employed measures of temperature, Fahrenheit and Celsius, are interval scales. For Celsius, for example, the value of 0 refers not to the complete absence of heat but simply to the temperature at which water freezes. One hundred on the Celsius scale refers to the temperature at which water boils at sea level. The distance between these two has been divided into 100 equal intervals. Because this is an interval scale measurement, it is accurate to say that the difference between 10 degrees Celsius and 15 degrees Celsius is the same as the distance between 20 degrees Celsius and 25 degrees Celsius. But it is not accurate to say that 20 degrees Celsius is twice as warm as 10 degrees Celsius.

Ratio Scale

The ratio scale is a scale in which the values assigned to the levels of a variable indicate both the order of magnitude and equal intervals but, in addition, assumes a real zero. The real zero represents the complete absence of the trait that is being measured. Temperature measured on the Kelvin scale has a real zero, which represents the complete absence of heat. At a more prosaic level, the number of patients in an emergency room is measured on a ratio scale. There can be zero patients in the emergency room, representing the complete absence of patients, or there can be any number of patients. Each new patient adds an equal increment to the number of patients in the emergency room. In general, any variable that is treated as numeric for statistical analysis is assumed to be measured on at least an interval scale and most commonly on a ratio scale.

Discrete and Continuous Numerical Variables

Discrete numerical variables are variables that can take on only whole number values. Discrete numerical variables are typically the result of the counting of things, persons, events, activities, and organizations. The number of persons in an emergency room is a discrete numerical variable.

There must always be a whole number of persons in the room—for example, 23. There can never be 23.7 persons in an emergency room. The number of children born to an unmarried woman, the number of organizations that are accredited by a national accrediting body, the number of physicians on a hospital staff, the number of health departments in a state—these are all discrete numerical variables.

Continuous numerical variables are variables that can take on any value whatsoever. They can be whole numbers, such as 47, or they can be numbers to any number of decimal places, such as one-third (which is 0.33333 ... and so on forever). The amount of time that a person spends in an emergency room is a continuous variable that can be stated to any level of precision (in terms of minutes, seconds, parts of seconds) that we have the ability and interest to measure. Body temperature, pulse rate, height, weight, and age are all continuous numerical variables. Measures that are created as the ratio of one variable to another, such as cost per hospital admission or cost per day or proportion of children fully immunized, are also continuous numerical variables.

Probabilities of occurrence of discrete or continuous numerical variables cannot be found in the same ways. In general, it is possible to find the exact probability of the occurrence of a discrete outcome based either on an a priori distribution or on empirical information. Probabilities of outcomes for continuous numerical variables, however, can only be approximated. Despite this, the distribution of continuous numerical variables has been extensively researched and in the form of the normal distribution: Particularly, it forms the basis of most statistical analyses for numerical variables, whether the variables are measured as discrete or continuous.

EXERCISES FOR SECTION 1.4

1. For each of the following sets of entities, decide whether you think the set is more likely to be a population or a sample, and explain why.

   a. All hospitals in the United States

   b. All patients in the emergency room of a given hospital on a given day

   c. One hospital from each of the 50 largest cities in the United States

   d. All health departments in a given state

   e. The patients who visit a single physician

   f. Operating room procedures for February 11 in a single hospital

2. What mechanisms might you use to obtain a list of all members of the following target populations, and how successful might you be?

   a. Emergency room visitors for the past six months at a single hospital emergency room

   b. Hospitals in the United States

   c. Patients visiting a single health department

   d. All food service facilities in a health department catchment area

   e. All people in a single hospital catchment area

   f. People who will dial 911 in the next six months in a given municipality

3. Determine whether each of the following is a systematic sample, a simple random sample, a stratified sample, a cluster sample, or a nonrandom sample, and indicate why.

   a. A sample drawn by randomly selecting 50 pages from a telephone book and taking the fifth name on each page

   b. A sample drawn by dividing all persons visiting an emergency room in the past six months into male and female and randomly selecting 100 from each group

   c. A sample drawn by selecting the person who arrives at a doctor's office at a time closest to a randomly selected time of day (say, 9:10 A.M.) and each person coming closest to that time on 40 subsequent days

   d. Any five cards drawn from a well-shuffled deck

   e. A sample drawn by randomly selecting six health departments from among those in a state and then randomly selecting six staff members from each of the six health departments

   f. A sample taken by selecting 20 hospitals in such a way as to ensure that they are representative of the types of hospitals in the United States

4. For each of the following random variables, determine whether the variable is categorical or numerical. If the variable is numerical, determine whether the phenomenon of interest is discrete or continuous.

   a. The number of clients at a health department Maternal and Child Health (MCH) clinic

   b. The primary reason for an MCH clinic visit

   c. The length of time in minutes spent by a client waiting to be seen at the clinic

   d. Whether children at the clinic have the recommended immunizations

   e. The weight of children seen at the clinic

   f. The income of families of clients seen at the clinic

5. Determine whether each of the following scales is nominal, ordinal, interval, or ratio and indicate why.

   a. The classification of patients into male and female

   b. The designation of male patients as 0 and female patients as 1

   c. The number of live births to a woman coded 0, 1, 2, 3, or more

   d. The measured pulse rate

   e. The number of staff members in a health department

1.5   Five Statistical Tests

This book consists of two sections. The first section, which comprises the first six chapters, is essentially preparatory material designed to equip the user of the book for the second section. The first section includes this introduction, a chapter on the use of Excel for statistical analysis, a chapter on data acquisition and preparation for statistical analysis, a chapter on descriptive presentation of data and Excel's graphing capability, a chapter on probability, and a chapter on the examination of data distributions.

The second section of the book, which comprises Chapters 7 through 14, is concerned with hypothesis testing. Hypothesis testing is essentially the act of determining whether data from a sample can be seen to support or not support a belief in independence between two or more variables in a population; one is commonly considered a *dependent variable* and the other or others are thought of as *independent variables*.

Five separate statistical tests that address this question of independence are discussed in this book. They are the chi-square test, the *t* test, *analysis of variance (ANOVA)*, regression analysis, and *Logit*. In practical terms, each of these tests can be thought of as testing whether sample values for two or more variables could have been drawn from a population in which the variables are independent of one another. Without considering specifically what independence means in regard to any one of these tests, it is possible to distinguish between these five tests on the basis of the type of data for which they are able to assess independence.

Chi-Square Test

The chi-square test can be used to assess the independence of two variables, both of which are categorical. Either of the two variables may take on two or more levels or categories, but the data itself are measured simply as named categories. For example, the chi-square can be used to determine whether coming to an emergency clinic for a true emergency or for a visit that is not an emergency (a two-level categorical variable) is independent of whether one comes during the day or during the night (another two-level categorical variable). Or a chi-square test could be used to determine whether the desire of women for an additional child (a two-level, yes–no variable) is independent of the number of children she already has in the three categories—for example, one, two or three, and four or more. The chi-square can be used on variables that take on larger numbers of values as well, but in practical terms, it is unusual to see a chi-square that involves variables having more than three or four levels.

t Test

The *t* test can be used to assess the independence of two variables. The *t* test assumes that one variable is a numerical variable measured in either discrete or continuous units and the other is a categorical variable taking on only two values. For example, the *t* test can be used to determine whether the score people receive on a test of knowledge about breast cancer measured on a 20-point scale (a numerical variable) is independent of whether those people were specifically and consciously exposed to knowledge about breast cancer or were not (a two-value categorical variable). Or a *t* test could be used to determine whether the cost of a hospital stay (a numerical variable) was independent of whether the patient was a member of an HMO or was not (a two-level categorical variable).

Analysis of Variance

Analysis of variance, or ANOVA, an extension of the *t* test, can be used to assess the independence of two or more variables. ANOVA assumes that one variable is a numerical variable measured in either discrete or continuous units and the others are categorical variables that may take on any number of values rather than only two. ANOVA, for example, could be used to assess not only whether a knowledge score about breast cancer was independent of exposure to knowledge about breast cancer but also whether the score might be independent of several different types of exposure. Exposure could be the reading of a brochure, a one-on-one discussion with a physician, both, or neither. Analysis of variance could also be used to determine whether the length of a hospital stay (a numerical variable) was independent of the hospital in which the stay took place over five separate hospitals (a categorical variable taking on five values).

Regression

Regression, a logical last stage in this progression, is a technique that can test the independence of two or more numerical variables measured in either discrete or continuous units. Regression may also include one or more categorical variables, any one of which can take on only two values (in which case, it is often referred to as analysis of covariance). Regression, then, could test the independence, for example, of the cost of a hospital stay (a numerical variable) and the length of a hospital stay (a second numerical variable) across an essentially unlimited number of hospitals. Or it could assess the independence of the dollar value of all hospital billings (a numerical variable) and the number of patients admitted (a second numerical variable) for a sample of for-profit and not-for-profit hospitals (a categorical variable taking on two values).

Logit

Logit, an extension of regression, can examine the independence of two or more variables where the dependent variable is a dichotomous categorical variable and the independent variable or variable set may be categorical (taking on only two values) or numerical—either discrete or continuous. Logit could be used, for example, to assess the independence of the outcome of an emergency surgical procedure (measured as successful or unsuccessful) and such variables as the degree of presurgery trauma, the length of time between the emergency and the surgical procedure, the age of the patient, and so on.

EXERCISES FOR SECTION 1.5

1. Consider which type of analysis could be used to assess independence for each of the following sets of data and state why this would be so (the dependent variable is given first).

    a. Hospital length of stay per admission and insurance type, including Medicare, Medicaid, private not-for-profit, private for-profit, and self-pay

    b. Cost per hospital stay and sex, age, and whether medical or surgical

    c. Whether a woman desires an additional child and the number of children now living categorized as none, one or two, and three or more

    d. Blood pressure readings for a group of people before and after the initiation of a six-week exercise and diet regimen

    e. Hospital length of stay per admission for the first digit of the ICD-9/ICD-10 code

    f. Birth weight for newborns measured as low or normal and gestational age, mother's age, and whether she is a smoker or a nonsmoker

2. Suggest a dependent variable and at least one independent variable for a question that could be analyzed using each of the following:

    a. Chi-square analysis

    b. A *t* test

    c. Analysis of variance

    d. Regression

    e. Logit

KEY TERMS

analysis of variance (ANOVA)	parameter
categorical variable	population
chi-square statistic	random sample
cluster sample	sample
continuous numerical variable	sampled population
dependent variable	simple random sample
discrete numerical variable	spreadsheet
dummy variable	statistic
independent variable	stratified sample
interval scale	systematic sample
Likert scale	*t* test
Logit	target population
Medicare	variable
numerical variable	

CHAPTER 2

EXCEL AS A STATISTICAL TOOL

Facts are stubborn, but statistics are more pliable.

—Mark Twain

Many people have used Microsoft Excel spreadsheets for financial management, for budget keeping, or for maintaining lists, but not as a statistical tool. Excel has powerful statistical capabilities, and this book uses these statistical capabilities for examples and for problem sets. But to ensure that the user will have some facility with Excel from the outset, this chapter provides a basic introduction to most of what Excel can and will do as a statistical tool. Readers who are already comfortable with the use of Excel might skip Sections 2.1 and 2.2. However, anyone not currently carrying out statistical applications with Excel is likely to benefit from the material in the later sections of the chapter.

2.1 The Basics

Excel is a spreadsheet application. This means that it is made up of columns that are designated by letters (A through XFD) and of rows that are designated by numbers (1 through 1,048,576). There are 16,384 columns and 1,048,576 rows in Excel. Figure 2.1 shows the initial view of an Excel spreadsheet. The intersection of each row and column (e.g., column C and row 12, designated C12 in Excel) is a cell in which, generally, one piece of information can be stored, viewed, and manipulated. This means that there are potentially more than 17 billion data cells available on a single spreadsheet. In practical terms,

LEARNING OBJECTIVES

- Understand and use the basic functions of an Excel spreadsheet

- Understand and create a graph in Excel

- Understand and perform data and data string sorting and frequency calculation functions

- Understand the functions associated with Excel's Data Analysis Pack and understand when the Data Analysis Pack should be "added in"

- Understand Excel's dollar sign ($) convention and its use

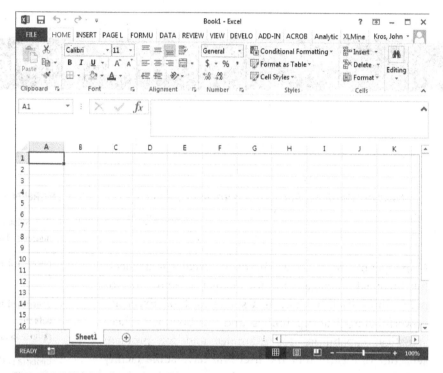

Figure 2.1   Initial view of an Excel spreadsheet

though, it is unlikely that any statistical application will use all the available space on a single spreadsheet. In fact, it is not clear that Excel would function within a reasonable amount of time if it had to manipulate data in a completely full spreadsheet. However, in the vast majority of statistical applications using Excel, it is likely that only a small fraction of the spreadsheet, probably less than 5 percent, will actually be used.

Spreadsheets as Workbooks

Spreadsheets can be grouped in what Excel calls *workbooks*. Any actual application might consist of a workbook of several worksheets. For example, one spreadsheet might contain an explanation of the application, a second sheet might contain the data, and a third sheet or additional sheets might contain the statistical analyses conducted using the data. If a large amount of data—say, 2,000 or 3,000 observations—is subjected to analysis using several spreadsheets, the resulting data file may become quite large. For most statistical applications, however, this will not be the case.

As shown in Figure 2.1, the Excel spreadsheet includes a ribbon (called the menu bar in earlier versions of Excel) across the top (with the words Home, Insert, Page Layout, and so on representing task-specific ribbons—click a name to display each ribbon). Three icons that are particularly useful

	A	B	C	D	E	F
1						
2	Addition	5	2	=B2+C2	=5+2	7
3	Subtraction	5	2	=B3-C3	=5-2	3
4	Multiplication	5	2	=B4*C4	=5*2	10
5	Division	5	2	=B5/C5	=5/2	2.5
6	Raise to power	5	2	=B6^C6	=5^2	25
7						

Figure 2.2 Excel arithmetical conventions

to statistical applications are the icon Σ, the icon f_x, and the Charts groups icon. The Home ribbon contains the Σ icon, the function of which is to automatically provide the sum of the values in a set of contiguous cells. The f_x icon resides in the Formulas ribbon and calls up an extensive menu of special *Excel functions*, including statistical and mathematical functions. The Charts group can be found on the Insert ribbon; it allows the user to create a wide variety of charts from one or a number of data entities.

Carrying Out Mathematical Operations

Excel enables the user to carry out all mathematical operations within cells. In carrying out the operations, Excel can refer to other cells for values needed for the arithmetical operations, or actual values (numbers) can be included in cells. Figure 2.2 shows all the important arithmetical operations that will be considered in this book. Row 2 shows the addition of the numbers 5 and 2. As shown in columns D and E, this can be done in two different ways. The addition can be carried out by referencing the cells B2 and C2, in which the values of 5 and 2, respectively, are found (cell D2) or it can be carried out by simply putting the numbers 5 and 2 into the addition equation (cell E2). It should also be noted that Excel arithmetical operations must always begin with the equal sign (=) in order for Excel to recognize that an arithmetical result is desired. Addition and subtraction use the plus sign (+) and minus sign (−), respectively. Multiplication uses the asterisk (*), which appears above the number eight on most keyboards. Division uses the right-leaning slash (/), which is the last key on the right in the bottom row on most keyboards. Raising a number to a power uses the caret (^), which is found above the number six on most keyboards. (The caret, incidentally, is almost universally called "hat" by statisticians.)

EXERCISES FOR SECTION 2.1

1. Carry out the following arithmetical operations in an Excel spreadsheet:

   a. $= 6 + 6$

   b. $= 22 - 16$

   c. $= 11 \times 5$

   d. $= 14/7$

   e. $= 4\char94 3$

2. Enter the following numbers into the indicated cells and carry out the operations given by referencing the cells:

   a.   A1, 11; B1, 13: add

   b.   A2, 16; B2, 5: subtract B2 from A2

   c.   A3, 21; B3, 15: multiply

   d.   A4, 36; B4, 4: divide

   e.   A5, 16; B5, 2: raise A5 to the power in B5

2.2   Working and Moving Around in a Spreadsheet

One difficulty faced by most novice users of Excel is not knowing how to move around in a spreadsheet and select specific cell references for operations. A second difficulty most new users face is not knowing how to let Excel do the work. This includes allowing Excel to correct mistakes, allowing Excel to enter formulas in multiple cells, and knowing the easy ways to move data around in a spreadsheet. There is absolutely no substitute for actual hands-on experience in learning what the capabilities of Excel are, but some initial hints should be helpful.

Consider the spreadsheet in Figure 2.3, which shows a small data set of 15 records for people who had used a service—for example, that of an ambulatory clinic. The variables shown are an ID or identifier, age of the patient, number of visits to the clinic, total cost of all clinic visits, and average cost per visit. This section also shows three different types of moves that can easily be made within a data set. Assuming a starting point at cell A2, hold down the Ctrl and Shift keys and press the right arrow to highlight the entire row 2 to the first blank column. This also works with Ctrl+Shift+Down arrow, Ctrl+Shift+Left arrow, and Ctrl+Shift+Up arrow. Again, assuming a starting point in cell A2, hold down Ctrl alone and press the down arrow to move the cursor from cell A2 to the last cell in column A that contains data, cell A16. This also works with Ctrl+Right arrow, Ctrl+Left arrow, and Ctrl+Up arrow. Figure 2.3 illustrates that both the current cell and the one next to it are highlighted. Hold down Shift and press the down arrow to highlight both the initial cell (A2) and cell A3.

Figure 2.3 Moving around a data set

This, too, works with Shift+Left arrow, Shift+Right arrow, and Shift+Up arrow. These operations can also be combined in virtually any order; for example, from a starting point of cell A2, Ctrl+Shift+Right arrow followed by Shift+Down arrow+Down arrow would highlight cells A2 to E4. Or, as a further example, from a starting point in cell A2, Ctrl+Shift+Right arrow followed by Ctrl+Shift+Down arrow would highlight cells A2 to E16.

Highlighting Cells

Any contiguous group of cells can be highlighted by left-clicking in any corner cell of the area to be highlighted and dragging the cursor to include all the cells that are to be highlighted. Two shortcuts when highlighting cells can make this task much easier. The first of these is Ctrl+Shift+Arrow (right arrow, left arrow, down arrow, up arrow), which will highlight every cell from the selected cell to the last contiguous cell containing data. For example, Figure 2.4 shows the result of the use of Ctrl+Shift+Right arrow when the cursor starts in cell A5. At this point, it is possible to highlight cells A5 to E16 with the use of Ctrl+Shift+Down arrow. The value of this capability is, perhaps, not evident when the data set consists of only 15 rows and 5 columns. But when the data comprises, for example, 357 rows and 42 columns, it is much easier to use Ctrl+Shift+Arrow to highlight all of a row or all of a column than to drag the cursor to highlight all those cells.

The second shortcut that is useful in highlighting is the ability to highlight an entire row (16,384 cells) or an entire column (1,048,576 cells). Clicking either the letter that represents the column or the number that represents the row will highlight the entire column or the entire row. For example, Figure 2.5 shows only the first 18 rows of column B, but clicking the B at the head of the column has highlighted the entire column, from

Figure 2.4   Result of Ctrl+Shift+Right arrow

Figure 2.5   Highlighting an entire column

cell 1 to cell 65,536. It is also useful to know that the entire worksheet can be highlighted at one time by clicking in the empty cell at the top of the row-number column (or to the left of the column-letter column).

Copying a Cell to a Range of Cells

Another useful capability of Excel is its ability to copy one cell to a range of other cells. For example, Figure 2.6 shows the data from Figure 2.3, but before the E column was completely filled in. While the actual spreadsheet from which both Figure 2.3 and Figure 2.6 were taken has numbers in columns A through D (entered manually), cell E2 represents a simple formula (shown in the formula line above the spreadsheet) that simply

	E2		= =D2/C2				
	A	B	C	D	E	D	E
1	ID	Age	Visits	Total Cost	Cost/Visit	Cost	Cost/Visit
2	1	30	1	$ 59.77	$ 59.77	59.77	$ 59.77
3	2	69	3	$ 323.02		323.02	$ 107.67
4	3	73	1	$ 92.82		92.82	$ 92.82
5	4	22	5	$ 589.40		589.40	$ 117.88
6	5	15	4	$ 530.60		530.60	$ 132.65
7	6	29	2	$ 170.31		170.31	$ 85.16
8	7	50	3	$ 386.58		386.58	$ 128.86
9	8	47	1	$ 117.03		117.03	$ 117.03
10	9	17	8	$1,078.59		,078.59	$ 134.82
11	10	63	2	$ 143.70		143.70	$ 71.85
12	11	48	2	$ 77.92		77.92	$ 38.96
13	12	70	6	$ 175.55		175.55	$ 29.26
14	13	8	1	$ 135.68		135.68	$ 135.68
15	14	38	8	$ 213.42		213.42	$ 26.68
16	15	41	5	$ 637.49		637.49	$ 127.50
17							

Figure 2.6 Copying a formula to several cells

divides cell D2 (Total Cost) by cell C2 (Visits). The result is the average cost per visit. Rather than typing the same formula in each cell from E3 to E16, or even copying and pasting the formula in each cell, it is possible either to drag or to double-click the formula in cell E2 to all the cells from E3 to E16. To do either, it is necessary to put the cursor on the lower right-hand corner of cell E2, as shown in Figure 2.6. Doing this turns the cursor into a small black cross. With the cursor as a small black cross, dragging with the mouse will copy the formula to each successive cell down the E column. Or, still with the cursor as a small black cross, double-left-clicking with the mouse will fill the entire E column to the last occupied cell in the D column.

The double-left-click on the lower right corner can be used to copy a formula down a column as far as the last filled cell in a column on either the right or the left of the column to be filled. But if there is a blank cell on the left of a column, even with a filled column on the right, it is necessary to drag the formula to the end of the data set, because the double-click will go only to the first empty cell on the left. Also, if you wish to copy a formula or other data across columns, or up columns, you can do so only with the drag on the lower right corner of the master cell.

Moving Data with Drag and Drop

Moving data around in Excel is made easy with the use of drag and drop. A highlighted area (see cells B1:B16 in Figure 2.7) can be moved anywhere in the spreadsheet simply by placing the cursor on the highlight outline and dragging it to the spot where it is to be placed. This process is illustrated in Figure 2.7. The highlighted area, cells B1:B16, is moved to cells G1:G16.

	A	B	C	D	E	F	G
1	ID	Age	Visits	Total Cost	Cost/Visit		Age
2	1	30	1	$ 59.77	$ 59.77		30
3	2	69	3	$	Age 107.67		69
4	3	73	1	$	30 92.82		73
5	4	22	5	$	69 17.88		22
6	5	16	4	$	73 32.65		15
7	6	29	2	$	22 85.16		29
8	7	50	3	$	16 28.86		50
9	8	47	1	$	29 17.03		47
10	9	17	8	$1	50 34.82		17
11	10	63	2	$	47 71.85		63
12	11	48	2	$	17 38.96		48
13	12	70	6	$	63 29.26		70
14	13	8	1	$	48 35.68		8
15	14	38	6	$	70 26.68		38
16	15	41	5	$	8 27.50		41
17					38		
18					41		
19							

Figure 2.7 Moving a data range with drag and drop

When the drag and drop is completed, the data will no longer be in cells B1:B16. If a drag and drop is executed, any formulas that either referenced or were referenced by the data when the data was in column B will now reference the data correctly in column G.

Undoing Changes

A very useful tool is the Undo command. Suppose you have a large spreadsheet in which a great amount of data has been entered and on which, perhaps, a number of complex operations have been carried out. Just as you are about to save the entire spreadsheet, you somehow inadvertently erase the whole thing. Is this the appropriate time to slit your wrists? No. You can recover the spreadsheet exactly by going to the Quick Access Toolbar, where you will find an arrow, shown in Figure 2.8, that points to the left or, more intuitively, counterclockwise. Clicking this arrow allows you to back up through a series of up to 16 operations and "undo" them. So if you inadvertently cleared an entire data sheet, you could just click the Undo button and your most recent action—the deletion of the spreadsheet's content—would be reversed.

Figure 2.8 The Undo button

EXERCISES FOR SECTION 2.2

1. Enter the identifiers for each column and the data for columns A through D, as shown in Figure 2.3 (or use the data in the file Chpt 2-1.xls) and do the following:

   a. Start in cell A2 and press Ctrl+Shift+Down arrow.

   b. Start in D3 and press Ctrl+Shift+Left arrow.

   c. Start in C1 and press Ctrl+Down arrow.

   d. Start in A1 and press Shift+Right arrow.

   e. Start in A1 and press Shift+Right arrow, followed by Ctrl+Shift+Down arrow.

   f. Left-click the A column head; the 2 row head.

2. Using the data from Exercise 1 of this section, do the following:

   a. Type the label Cost/Visit in cell E1. Type the formula = D2/C2 in cell E2 and press Enter.

   b. Put the cursor in the lower right-hand corner of cell E2 (the cursor will become a black cross) and double-left-click.

   c. Confirm that the resulting data are the same as given in column E of Figure 2.3.

   d. Highlight column E by clicking the E above the column and, with the cursor on the edge of the highlighted area, drag it to column G.

   e. Confirm that the formulas in the cells still refer to columns D and C.

   f. Click the Undo button in the Standard toolbar.

2.3 Excel Functions

Clicking the f_x icon in the Formulas ribbon displays the Insert Function dialog box, shown in Figure 2.9. At the top of the dialog box is the Search for a function field, and directly below is the drop-down list from which to select a function by category. When a function is selected (such as the AVERAGE function in Figure 2.9), the bottom of the dialog box shows the name of the selected function and a brief description of what it does. To use a particular function, select it and click OK. Excel will then lead you through a short sequence of steps that designate the cells in which the numbers are found for the calculation for the selected function. As an example, the =AVERAGE() function will produce the average value for a series of numbers contained in several cells.

Figure 2.9 Insert Function dialog box

=AVERAGE() Function

Let's take a look at the working of the =AVERAGE() function. Suppose the spreadsheet contains a column of five numbers in cells B4 through B8 and you wish to calculate the average of those five numbers in cell B9. When you click OK in the Insert Function dialog box (see Figure 2.9), the Function Arguments dialog box, shown in Figure 2.10, will be displayed. Several things about this dialog box, with the =AVERAGE() function already selected, are worth discussing. First, the highlighted field designated Number1 shows the five cells—B4 to B9—that are being averaged. These cells are shown by using the standard Excel convention for designating a set of contiguous cells, which is to display them as B4:B9. To the right of this field is an equal sign and the actual numbers that are in the cells. (If there had been, say, 20 cells being averaged, only the first few would have been displayed.) The field marked Number2 can be ignored in this calculation. Below the areas designated Number1 and Number2 is some additional information. The number 31.4 is the actual value of the average that will be put into cell B9 when the calculation is completed. The absence of a number there means

Figure 2.10 Function Arguments dialog box

that Excel does not have the information needed from you, the user, to calculate a result. Below the result is a brief statement of what the function actually does. Clicking OK will dismiss the dialog box and put the result of the formula into the selected cell (in this case B9).

Figure 2.11 shows a portion of the spreadsheet in which the =AVERAGE() function has been employed. The representation is a record of total clinic visits for a single outpatient clinic for a five-day period. The purpose is to determine the average number of persons coming to the clinic over these five days. In cell B9 is shown the actual function being calculated. When you click OK in the Function Arguments dialog box

Figure 2.11 Calculation of average

(see Figure 2.10), the function statement is replaced by the value 31.4. The average function being shown in cell B9 is also shown in the line just above the spreadsheet area, to the right of the f_x icon. This area is known as the *formula line* or *formula bar*. In general, if you wish to know if a value in a particular cell is a number or a formula, click the cell to find the answer in the formula line. If it is a formula, the formula for the cell will be displayed in terms of cell references, as shown in Figure 2.11.

Number of Arguments and Excel Functions

It should be noted that the numbers actually being averaged in cell B9 in Figure 2.11 are represented by cell references within the parentheses following the name of the function. This indication of cell references is called an *argument* of the function. The =AVERAGE() function takes only one argument: the reference to the cells in which the data to be averaged are found. Other Excel functions may take more than one argument, and some functions—for example, =RAND(), which returns a random number between 0 and 1, and =PI(), which returns the value of pi to 14 decimal positions—take none. If a function takes more than one argument, commas separate the arguments when they are given within the parentheses.

Eighty separate statistical functions are built into Excel. Excel also has several mathematical and trigonometric functions that are useful in doing statistical analyses. It may be helpful to look at the various Excel statistical and math and trig functions (click f_x and scroll through the functions in the Select a function window) as a means of getting a preview of what the functions do. It is likely that right now most of them will be obscure, but as you work through this book you will become increasingly familiar with many of the functions.

Direct Input of Excel Function

Functions can be invoked in Excel without using the f_x icon. If you know the precise spelling and *syntax* of the function name, you can type it directly into the cell in which it is to be applied. For example, to enter the =AVERAGE() function directly into a spreadsheet, it is necessary to begin with an equal sign (=). This informs Excel that you are going to enter a formula, and it is why functions are referred to throughout this text by the = prefix. (The same convention holds if you want to carry out any mathematical operation, such as adding the numbers in two cells; the addition command must begin with an equal sign for Excel to recognize the input as a mathematical formula.) The equal sign is followed immediately (no spaces) by AVERAGE (it does not have to be in caps), which is followed by (again, no spaces) a left parenthesis. At this point, you can directly type the cell references in which the numbers to be averaged are found, or you can highlight the cells with your cursor. A right parenthesis completes the formula, and pressing Enter calculates the result of the formula, which appears in the selected cell. If the function name is misspelled or the syntax is incorrect, Excel will let you know by showing #NAME? in the cell where the function was to be calculated.

Contiguous and Noncontiguous Cells

In general, any of the Excel functions will operate on any contiguous set of cells. For some functions, such as the =AVERAGE function already discussed, the =SUM function (activated by clicking the $\sum$ icon on the Formulas ribbon), and a number of others, the numbers do not have to be in contiguous cells. However, if noncontiguous cells are to be the subject of the operation, it is necessary to use the Excel convention of pressing the Ctrl key before highlighting any second or subsequent set of noncontiguous cells that are part of the operation. For example, take a look at the spreadsheet shown in Figure 2.12. The two columns B and D, representing the clinic visits for the five days of two different weeks, could be summed with the =SUM() command, as shown in the formula line. Entering the actual cell references directly into the cell from the keyboard, rather than highlighting the areas with the help of the Ctrl key, will also produce this result. If the cell references were entered from the keyboard, a comma would be used to separate the two different sets of cell references.

AVERAGE	▼ ✕ ✓ _fx_	=SUM(B4:B8,D4:D8)		
A	B	C	D	E
1				
2	Week 1		Week 2	
3 Day	Clinic Visits	Day	Clinic Visits	
4 Day 1	23	Day 1	23	
5 Day 2	47	Day 2	47	
6 Day 3	19	Day 3	19	
7 Day 4	37	Day 4	37	
8 Day 5	31	Day 5	31	
9			=SUM(B4:B8,D4:D8)	
10				

Figure 2.12 Summing two noncontiguous areas

EXERCISES FOR SECTION 2.3

1. A well-baby clinic recorded the weight for the infants receiving services during one workday. The weight of the infants is given here in pounds (lbs.). Enter the data into a spreadsheet (or take it from the file Chpt 2-2.xls, worksheet Infants) and do the following:

10.7	18.2	17.8	16.0	17.8	15.9	21.5
17.1	20.6	18.8	15.4	20.8	19.8	18.3
17.2	15.8	10.8	19.6	17.9	17.8	14.5

 a. Use the =COUNT () function to confirm that there are 21 infants.

 b. Use the $\sum$ function to obtain the total weight of all infants coming to the clinic on the given day.

 c. Use the =AVERAGE () function to determine the average weight of infants coming to the clinic.

 d. Use the =MAX () function to determine the weight of the heaviest child coming to the clinic on the given day.

 e. Use the =MIN () function to determine the weight of the lightest child coming to the clinic on the given day.

2. Over the course of several days, the number of inpatients in Mercy Hospital was recorded in the business office. The inpatient totals for those days are given here. Enter the data into a spreadsheet (or use Chpt 2-2.xls, worksheet Days) and do the following:

89	92	93	93	92	100	97
100	102	95	91	103		

 a. Use the =COUNT () function to confirm that there are records for 12 days.

 b. Use the $\sum$ function to obtain the cumulative total of inpatient days represented by the data.

 c. Use the =AVERAGE () function to determine the average inpatient census for the 12 days.

 d. Use the =MAX () function to determine the highest inpatient census for the 12 days.

 e. Use the =MIN () function to determine the lowest inpatient census for the 12 days.

3. A dentist kept track of the time he spent with each patient in a single morning of visits. The total time in minutes that he spent with each is given here. Enter the data into a spreadsheet (or use the file Chpt 2-2.xls, worksheet Time) and do the following:

9	18	9	13	11	5	7
13	15	10	10	18	13	16
9	14	5				

a. Use the =COUNT () function to confirm that there are records for 17 patients.

b. Use the $\sum$ function to obtain the cumulative total of minutes the dentist spent with patients during this morning.

c. Use the =AVERAGE () function to determine the average time in minutes the dentist spent with each patient.

d. Use the =MAX () function to determine the most time the dentist spent with a patient.

e. Use the =MIN () function to determine the least time the dentist spent with a patient.

2.4   The =IF () Function

The =IF () function is a particularly useful function that provides a way to make decisions within a spreadsheet. The =IF () function tests a condition and produces one result if the condition is true and a different result if the condition is false. For example, suppose that we have the data shown in Figure 2.13. We have 12 patients identified by the numbers 1 through 12 in column A and the minutes they spend waiting in the emergency room identified in column B. In column C, we want to assign a 1 or a 0, depending on whether each patient spent more or less than the average time patients typically spend waiting. Excel allows us to do this with the =IF () function. Column C in Figure 2.13 already has the values of 1 or 0 assigned, using the =IF () function.

The syntax of the function for cell C2 is shown in the formula line. As you can see there, the =IF () function is written with three arguments. The first of the arguments is the decision. In this case, Excel is asked to decide whether the value in cell B2 is greater than (>) the value in $B$15 (the average for all 12 values in column B). The $ convention is used for cell B15 because we want to compare each of the 12 values in column B

C2			f_x	=IF(B2>$B$15,1,0)	
	A	B	C	D	E	F
1	Patients	Minutes (x)				
2	1	2	0			
3	2	8	0			
4	3	11	1			
5	4	12	1			
6	5	6	0			
7	6	10	1			
8	7	7	0			
9	8	8	0			
10	9	14	1			
11	10	8	0			
12	11	7	0			
13	12	14	1			
14						
15	Mean(x)	8.92				
16						

Figure 2.13 Use of the =IF () function

to the same value, the average for all 12, which is found only in cell B15 (see Section 2.9). The second argument, always separated from the first by a comma, is a 1, and the third argument, again separated by a comma, is a 0. The =IF () function operates by evaluating the relationship in the first argument. If that relationship is true, it assigns the value of the second argument to the cell in which the function is being invoked. If it is false, the =IF () function assigns the value of the third argument to the cell in which the function is being invoked. The way the function works can be stated as follows: If the value in cell B2 is greater than the value in cell B15, put a 1 in cell C2; otherwise, put a 0 in cell C2. This same function is copied to all cells C2 through C13 and automatically produces the desired results.

Nested =IF () Functions

In the example in Figure 2.13, the =IF () function is used to make only a single decision. Nested =IF () functions can be used to make more complex decisions. For example, instead of assigning a 1 or a 0, depending on whether the waiting time was above or below the average, suppose we wished to determine whether the waiting time was short, long, or medium. For the sake of the example, let us say that a short waiting time is anything under 5 minutes and a long waiting time is anything more than 10 minutes. That would leave any waiting time from 5 to 10 minutes as medium.

	C2		▼	fₓ	=IF(B2>10,"Long",IF(B2<5,"Short","Medium"))			
	A	B	C	D	E	F	G	H
1	Patients	Minutes (x)						
2	1	2	Short					
3	2	8	Medium					
4	3	11	Long					
5	4	12	Long					
6	5	6	Medium					
7	6	10	Medium					
8	7	7	Medium					
9	8	8	Medium					
10	9	14	Long					
11	10	8	Medium					
12	11	7	Medium					
13	12	14	Long					
14								

Figure 2.14 Nested =IF () functions

Figure 2.14 shows one =IF () function nested within another so that Excel can make both decisions simultaneously. What the decision statement (shown in the formula line for cell C2) does is the following: If the value in cell B2 is greater than 10 (shown now as the actual value of 10, and not as a cell reference), the =IF () function assigns the word "Long" to cell C2. If the value in cell B2 is not greater than 10, a second =IF () function asks if the value in cell B2 is less than 5, and if so, it assigns the word "Short" to cell C2 (which is what it actually assigned). If the value in cell B2 is not less than 5, the =IF statement assigns the word "Medium" to cell C2. Excel will operate on up to 64 nested =IF () statements. It is also useful to mention that the exact way in which the nested =IF () function is developed in Figure 2.14 is not the only possible way such a function could be expressed to assign the appropriate term to each waiting time. An alternative nested =IF () function, such as =IF (B2>5, IF (B2>10, "Long", "Medium"), "Short"), will produce exactly the same result as produced by the statement actually used in the figure.

Figure 2.14 also shows one additional important point: It is possible to produce a number as the result of a decision or it is possible to produce an alphabetic character (or, for that matter, any printable character). But if the result to be produced is not a number, it must be contained in quotation marks in order for the function to work. The function =IF (B2>10, Long, IF (B2<5, Short, Medium)) would result in an Excel error message, which in this case would be to display #NAME? in the cell in which the function was invoked.

EXERCISES FOR SECTION 2.4

1. Use the data from Exercise 1 of Section 2.3 and do the following:

   a. Create an =IF() statement that determines whether the infant is greater or less in weight than the overall average, and assign a 1 to those greater and a 0 to those less.

   b. Create an =IF() statement that determines whether the infant is less than 15 lbs., greater than 20 lbs., or between the two extremes, and assign a "low" to the lightest group, a "high" to the heaviest group, and a "medium" to the middle group.

   c. Create an =IF() statement that determines whether the infant is the lowest weight or the highest weight in the group, and assign a 1 to the lowest and highest and a 0 to all others.

   d. Create an =IF() statement that divides the infants into 4-lb. age groups (beginning at 10 lbs.), and assign a 1 to the lowest group, a 2 to the second, and so on.

2. Use the data from Exercise 2 of Section 2.3 and do the following:

   a. Create an =IF() statement that determines whether the day has more or fewer inpatients than the overall average and assign a 1 to days with more and a 0 to days with fewer.

   b. Create an =IF() statement that determines whether the day has fewer than 90 inpatients or more than 100 inpatients or is between the two extremes, and assign a "low" to the days with fewest patients, a "high" to the days with most patients, and a "medium" to the middle group of days.

   c. Create an =IF() statement that determines whether the day had the fewest inpatients or the most, and assign a 1 to the lowest and highest and a 0 to all others.

   d. Create an =IF() statement that divides the days into four patient groups (beginning at 88 patients), and assign a 1 to the lowest group, a 2 to the second, and so on.

3. Use the data from Exercise 3 of Section 2.3 and do the following:

   a. Create an =IF() statement that determines whether the dentist spent more or less time with a patient than the overall average, and assign a 1 to patients with whom the dentist spent more time and a 0 to patients with whom the dentist spent less time.

   b. Create an =IF() statement that determines whether the dentist spent less than 9 minutes or more than 15 minutes with a patient or was between the two extremes, and assign a "low" to the patients with whom the dentist spent the least time, a "high" to patients with whom the dentist spent the most time, and a "medium" to the middle group of patients.

    c. Create an $=\texttt{IF()}$ statement that determines whether a patient had the fewest minutes of the dentist's time or the most, and assign a 1 to the patients with the fewest and most minutes and 0 to all others.

    d. Create an $=\texttt{IF()}$ statement that divides the patients into three-minute groups (beginning at five minutes), and assign a 1 to the lowest group, a 2 to the second, and so on.

2.5   Excel Graphs

The Excel Charts function is exceedingly valuable for an understanding of how data actually look. This can be useful to gain a better understanding of the data, or for helping to ensure that the data conform to the assumptions of particular statistical operations. You invoke the Charts function by selecting the Insert ribbon and then clicking one of the options in the Charts menu or clicking the small arrow in the bottom right corner of the Charts menu.

Insert Chart Menu in Excel

Figure 2.15 shows the Insert Chart dialog box, about which several things should be noted. For example, there are 11 types of standard charts (shown on the left). Several different chart subtypes within the standard types exist for each of these 11 standard types. These are shown on the right. Highlighting the chart type of interest on the left shows (on the right) the subtype of charts that can be produced within that chart type option. When you have selected the appropriate chart type, click OK.

Identifying and Formatting Chart Data

To begin the charting process, first highlight (select) the data of interest, and then choose a chart style. When you click OK, the chosen type of chart appears in the active spreadsheet. Figure 2.16 displays a basic bar graph for the clinic visit data. You now have many options to choose from. One of the most important is to identify the data shown in the chart. The data making up this chart are the same data that were used to find the average in Figure 2.11. To identify where the data making up the bar graph are coming from, right-click a bar in the bar graph itself. Once you right-click,

Figure 2.15   Insert Chart dialog box

Figure 2.16   A basic bar graph

Figure 2.17 Excel's chart pop-up menu

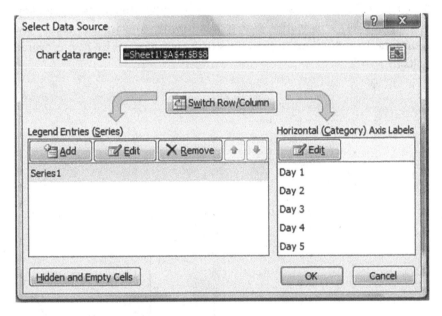

Figure 2.18 Select Data Source dialog box

a pop-up menu will appear, as shown in Figure 2.17. Choose the Select Data option in the menu, and the Select Data Source dialog box, shown in Figure 2.18, appears.

The Select Data Source Dialog Box

The Select Data Source dialog box has four distinct areas. The first area is the Chart data range area, at the top. The Chart data range area identifies where the data for the graph are located. As shown in Figure 2.18, the location is =Sheet1!$A$4:$B$8. Sheet1! identifies the data in the table as coming from sheet number 1 of the workbook. This is useful because not only is it possible to use data from a sheet different from the one that may be active at the time the charting process is begun, but also it is possible to use data from more than a single worksheet. The meaning and use of the dollar signs that appear before both the alphabetic column references and the numerical row references are discussed in detail in Section 2.9.

The second area to take a look at is the Switch Row/Column button, which changes the view of the graph. Currently days are listed in the Horizontal (Category) Axis Labels area (area three of interest) and Series 1 is listed in the Legend Entries (Series) area (area four of interest). When you click the Switch Row/Column button, Excel literally switches what is in the Horizontal (Category) Axis Labels area with what is in the Legend Entries (Series) area. If you click the Switch Row/Column, a chart will appear (see Figure 2.19). As noted earlier, this is a different view of the same data. Figure 2.19 now has all days bunched together under one legend key, literally Week1. This feature is very handy when you wish to cross-view your data from different perspectives (e.g., overall visits by day or overall visits by week).

Figure 2.19   A different view of the same data

Formatting the Finished Graph

You can format a graph in Excel in two main ways. One way is to select the Design ribbon and then choose from the groups in the ribbon depending on what type of modification you wish to make. The Chart Layouts group is most likely the first that you should choose; it allows for various chart layout types and provides a quick and easy method for formatting your graph. The Chart Styles group contains many chart styles to choose from if you are interested in changing colors and/or data point/bar configuration.

Another way to format your graph is by right-clicking the graph itself. After you do so, you'll see the pop-up menu shown in Figure 2.20. This menu contains options that allow you to change the chart type, move the chart, format the chart area, and so on.

What we've discussed so far with respect to graphs is only a beginning. A number of exercises in the book will employ Excel's graph capabilities,

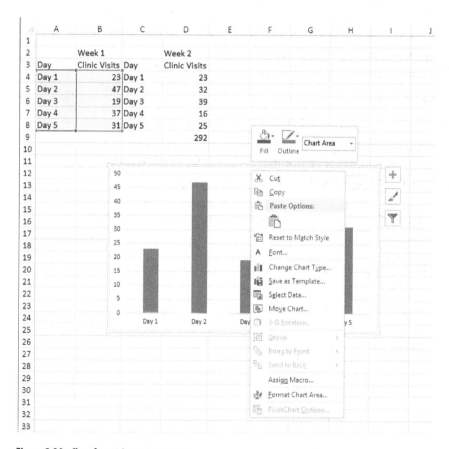

Figure 2.20 Chart formatting pop-up menu

and further detail on the use of graphs will be given as specific uses of the graph capability are introduced. Some introductory exercises in creating graphs follow.

EXERCISES FOR SECTION 2.5

1. At the well-baby clinic referred to in Exercise 1 of Section 2.3, a clerk tallied the number of infants who received care for the day into four weight categories. The weight categories and the number of infants in each are given here. Enter the data into a spreadsheet and do the following:

Weight (lbs.)	Number
<=12	2
>12<16	5
>16<20	11
>20<24	3

    a. Use Excel to construct a histogram (chart with vertical bars) of the number of infants in each weight category.

    b. Insert the weight categories as labels for the x-axis.

    c. Give the chart an appropriate title.

    d. Use Excel to indicate that the chart should go on a new worksheet.

2. The Mercy Hospital Health Information Management (HIM) Department has produced the following average daily inpatient census data for each day of the week for a one-year period. Enter the data into a spreadsheet and do the following:

Day of Week	Inpatient Average
Monday	98.6
Tuesday	107.5
Wednesday	102.2
Thursday	96.4
Friday	90.7
Saturday	89.1
Sunday	93.4

a. Use Excel to construct a histogram (chart with vertical bars) of the average inpatient census for each day of the week.

b. Insert the days as labels for the *x*-axis.

c. Use Excel to give the chart an appropriate title.

d. Use Excel to indicate that the chart should go on a new worksheet.

e. Interpret the chart and suggest any kind of pattern in inpatient census for Mercy Hospital.

3. A dentist kept track of the time he spent with each patient over the course of six months, according to the major purpose of the visit. Here is the average time of each visit by purpose. Enter the data into a spreadsheet and do the following:

Purpose	Time
Orthodontic	25.2
Gum-Related Problems	14.5
Filling/Crown	12.2
Extraction	10.1
Routine Checkup	4.3

a. Use Excel to construct a histogram (chart with vertical bars) of the time spent by the dentist during each type of visit.

b. Insert the purpose of the visit as labels for the *x*-axis.

c. Use Excel to give the chart an appropriate title.

d. Use Excel to indicate that the chart should go on a new worksheet.

e. Interpret the chart. What does it say about the dentist's time distribution?

2.6 Sorting a String of Data

A very useful Excel capability, especially with regard to sample selection (discussed in detail in Chapter 3), is the ability to sort a data set. The entire data set is going to be sorted on two variables, Sex and Age. The first step is to click the Data label to display the Data ribbon. On the Data ribbon, click the Sort icon to display the Sort dialog box (see Figure 2.21). This is the first step in a data sort. This example will be using the small data set introduced in Figure 2.3 with the addition of a column representing Sex

Figure 2.21   Sort dialog box

	A	B	C	D	E	F	G	H
1	ID	Age	Sex	Visits	Total Cost	Cost/Visit		
2	1	30	Male	1	$ 59.77	$ 59.77		
3	2	69	Male	3	$ 323.02	$ 107.67		
4	3	73	Female	1	$ 92.82	$ 92.82		
5	4	22	Male	5	$ 589.40	$ 117.88		
6	5	15	Female	4	$ 530.60	$ 132.65		
7	6	29	Female	2	$ 170.31	$ 85.16		
8	7	50	Female	3	$ 386.58	$ 128.86		
9	8	47	Male	1	$ 117.03	$ 117.03		
10	9	17	Female	8	$ 1,078.59	$ 134.82		
11	10	63	Male	2	$ 143.70	$ 71.85		
12	11	48	Male	2	$ 77.92	$ 38.96		
13	12	70	Female	6	$ 175.55	$ 29.26		
14	13	8	Female	1	$ 135.68	$ 135.68		
15	14	38	Male	8	$ 213.42	$ 26.68		
16	15	41	Female	5	$ 637.49	$ 127.50		
17								
18								
19								
20								
21								
22								
23								
24								
25								
26								
27								
28								

Figure 2.22   Sort dialog box and data to be sorted

(column C). It should be noted that the cursor has been positioned in cell A2 (see Figure 2.22). It doesn't matter in what cell in the data set the cursor is positioned, but it is important to have it inside the boundaries of the contiguous data set that is to be sorted.

The Sort Dialog Box

When you click the Sort icon, two things happen. The entire data set to be sorted is highlighted, and the Sort dialog box appears (see Figure 2.22). We want to sort the data on Sex and Age. To sort data, we use the first drop-down list in the Sort dialog box, Sort by. The options displayed in the list match our column headers because the option My data has headers, located in the upper right of the Sort dialog box, is checked. When this option is checked, the top row is designated as the *header row*. If you uncheck the box, you can see that the first row in the spreadsheet is then included in the data.

When we click the drop-down list, we can pick Sex as a column to sort on. However, we also wish to sort on Age, and there isn't another drop-down list from which to choose Age. To create another drop-down list under the Column header, click the Add Level button at the top left of the Sort dialog box. Figure 2.23 displays the Sort dialog box with a Column sort option of Sex and another sort option of Age. It is also possible to sort text values in ascending (A to Z) or descending (Z to A) order and to sort numbers from smallest to largest or largest to smallest. We will leave the defaults, which are A to Z for the Sex variable and Smallest

Figure 2.23 Sort dialog box with two-column sort options

	C2		▼		f_x	Female		
	A	B	C	D	E		F	G
1	ID	Age	Sex	Visits	Total Cost		Cost/Visit	
2	13	8	Female	1	$	135.68	$ 135.68	
3	5	15	Female	4	$	530.60	$ 132.65	
4	9	17	Female	8	$ 1,078.59		$ 134.82	
5	6	29	Female	2	$	170.31	$ 85.16	
6	15	41	Female	5	$	637.49	$ 127.50	
7	7	50	Female	3	$	386.58	$ 128.86	
8	12	70	Female	6	$	175.55	$ 29.26	
9	3	73	Female	1	$	92.82	$ 92.82	
10	4	22	Male	5	$	589.40	$ 117.88	
11	1	30	Male	1	$	59.77	$ 59.77	
12	14	38	Male	8	$	213.42	$ 26.68	
13	8	47	Male	1	$	117.03	$ 117.03	
14	11	48	Male	2	$	77.92	$ 38.96	
15	10	63	Male	2	$	143.70	$ 71.85	
16	2	69	Male	3	$	323.02	$ 107.67	
17								

Figure 2.24 Result of data sort on two variables

to Largest for the Age variable. You can see these options in the Order drop-down list on the right side of the Sort dialog box. Another drop-down list within the Sort dialog box is that for Sort On. The default for the Sort On drop-down menu is Values, and we will leave the default because we wish to sort on values and not another aspect of the data (e.g., cell color or font color).

If we click OK, the data will be sorted by both Sex and Age in that order, and you can see the resulting data set in Figure 2.24. Looking at this figure, you can see that the data are ordered first into those who are female and those who are male, and within these two groupings by age from youngest to oldest.

EXERCISE FOR SECTION 2.6

1. Use the data for the exercises for Section 2.2 (data from Figure 2.3 or Chpt 2-1.xls) and do the following:

   a. Sort the data on the variable Age.

   b. Sort the data on the variable Visits.

   c. Sort the data on Visits first and Age second.

   d. Return the data to the original configuration by sorting on ID.

2.7   The Data Analysis Pack

Excel comes with a set of statistical analysis tools in addition to the functions available with the f_x icon. These are contained in what Excel calls the Analysis Tools. The Analysis Tools menu is found on the Data ribbon and is labeled Data Analysis (see Figure 2.25).

Figure 2.25 Data Analysis option

Installing the Data Analysis Pack

Frequently, the Data Analysis option will not be shown, and if that is the case, it means that the Analysis ToolPak has not been "added in" to your version of Excel. To add the Analysis ToolPak, click the File button (at the upper left) and then click the Excel Options button at the bottom left of the drop-down menu (see Figure 2.26). This brings up the Excel Options

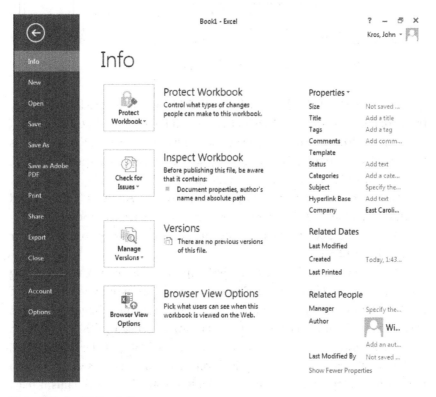

Figure 2.26 Excel Options button

Figure 2.27 Excel Options dialog box with add-ins screen displayed

dialog box. In the dialog box, click the Add-Ins option on the left to display the available add-ins, as shown on the right in Figure 2.27. In this area click the Manage drop-down list at the bottom of the figure, select Excel Add-Ins from the list (in the figure it is already selected), and click the Go button. The Add-Ins dialog box (Figure 2.28) appears.

Two of the items in the Add-Ins window are Analysis ToolPak and Analysis ToolPak—VBA. Once these have been checked and you've dismissed the dialog box by clicking OK, the Data Analysis option will appear on the Data ribbon.

When you click the Data Analysis option, the Data Analysis dialog box appears (see Figure 2.29). Shown in the figure is only a sampling of the 19 different analysis options available through the Analysis ToolPak. Selecting a specific analysis (e.g., Correlation) and clicking OK brings up an analysis window that will be tailored to the particular analysis requested. Specific analyses using the Analysis ToolPak are discussed as we move into the various categories of analysis available through this mechanism (e.g., correlation, ANOVA, regression).

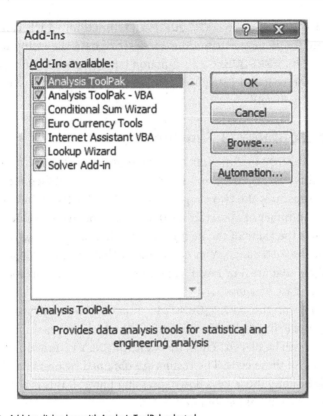

Figure 2.28   Add-Ins dialog box with Analysis ToolPak selected

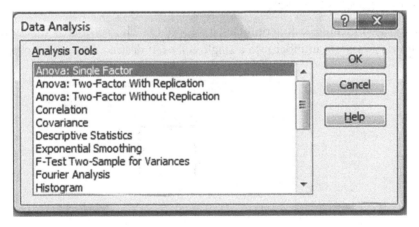

Figure 2.29   Data Analysis dialog box

2.8   Functions That Give Results in More than One Cell

Excel incorporates several functions useful for statistical applications that produce results in more than one cell of the worksheet. One of the most important of these is the =FREQUENCY() function, which can be used to calculate frequency distributions for a set of data according to a set of categories. The =FREQUENCY() function takes two arguments—the data range and the range of categories into which the data are to be counted (called bins by Excel).

The =FREQUENCY() Function

The =FREQUENCY() function has two arguments. These are the DATA range (in this case, B2:B13) and the BIN range (C2:C4) (see Figure 2.30). A comma separates the two ranges. The =FREQUENCY() function accumulates the number of observations that lie at or below the value of the bin but lie above the value of the next lower bin. So the bin values are actually the top of the BIN range. You can confirm that the data range contains two numbers that are 3 or lower, six numbers that are 6 or lower, and four numbers that are 9 or lower.

In order for the =FREQUENCY() function to work properly, it is necessary first to highlight the entire area into which the resulting frequency distribution will be placed. Then, the =FREQUENCY() function is entered into the first of these cells. The results are obtained by pressing Ctrl+Shift and, while holding those keys down, pressing Enter. If this is not done, the correct results will not be obtained.

The =RAND() Function

Excel also includes a function called =RAND(). The =RAND() function inserts a random number into a single cell or, if desired, into any number

D2			f_x {=FREQUENCY(B2:B13,C2:C4)}		
	A	B	C	D	E	F
1		Data	Bins	Frequency		
2		2	3	2		
3		8	6	6		
4		4	9	4		
5		7				
6		9				
7		4				
8		3				
9		6				
10		5				
11		7				
12		5				
13		4				

Figure 2.30 Frequency calculation

of cells. As mentioned earlier, =RAND() has no arguments. It is possible to highlight, for example, 20 cells in four rows and five columns. If the =RAND() function is then used, Ctrl+Shift and then Enter will put a random number between 0 and 1 into each of the 20 cells.

> To complete functions in Excel that put results into a single cell, it is necessary only to type the function into the appropriately highlighted cell and press Enter. To complete a function that puts a result into more than one cell, it is necessary, first, to highlight all the cells into which the results are to go, enter the formula according to the convention for that formula, and then simultaneously press Ctrl+Shift and then Enter. If Ctrl+Shift+Enter is not used, the right answer will not be obtained.

Matrix Math Functions

Excel also incorporates several functions with the ability to perform matrix math operations directly in the spreadsheet. Most statistical analyses can be carried out without any reference to matrix math. However, such statistical operations as multiple regression are more easily understood by using matrix math. Three matrix math capabilities of Excel are most useful in statistical applications. These are =MMULT(), which multiplies two matrices together; =MINVERSE(), which inverts a matrix; and =TRANSPOSE(), which changes a vertical range of cells into a horizontal range and vice versa. =MMULT() and =MINVERSE() are found in the Math and Trig function category in the Insert Function dialog box (see Figure 2.9); the =TRANSPOSE() function is found in the Lookup and Reference function category.

The =MMULT() Function

The matrix capabilities of Excel are demonstrated partially in Figure 2.31, which shows an example of matrix multiplication (=MMULT()). On the formula bar it is possible to see that the =MMULT() function is multiplying the matrix in A2:D3 times the matrix in F2:G5. The result, for those who are familiar with matrix math, will be a two-by-two matrix (because matrix 1 has two rows and matrix 2 has two columns). In order to complete a matrix operation with Excel, it is necessary to know the dimensions of the resulting matrix. The area of the resulting matrix is highlighted, and the =MMULT() formula is entered into the upper left-hand cell of the highlighted area. The cell references of the two matrices to be multiplied are then typed within the parentheses, or the cell ranges are highlighted, always with a comma separating them. To complete the matrix multiplication operation, it is necessary to use the convention Ctrl+Shift+Enter.

Figure 2.31 Matrix math example

EXERCISES FOR SECTION 2.8

1. Use the data for the well-baby clinic from Exercise 1 of Section 2.3 (or data from Chpt 2-2.xls, worksheet Infants). Create a frequency distribution with Excel using 14, 18, and 22 as the top of the BIN ranges. Remember that you must highlight three contiguous cells in a column, enter =FREQUENCY() into the first of the cells, and press Ctrl+Shift+Enter in order to produce the frequency distribution.

2. Use the data from Figure 2.3 (Chpt 2-1.xls).

   a. Create a frequency distribution for Total Cost using $400 as the first BIN range and $400 increments thereafter.

   b. Create a frequency distribution for Age in 10-year age intervals.

3. Use the =RAND() function to fill the cells A2:B12 with random numbers. (Make sure that you first highlight the area A2:B12, enter =RAND() in cell A2, and press Ctrl+Shift and then Enter.)

4. Enter the following data for matrix A and matrix B into a spreadsheet, and carry out the =MMULT() function. Confirm that the result is as given in matrix C.

Matrix A

2	3	5
3	3	4
5	4	5

Matrix B

2	3
4	2
3	4

Matrix C	
31	32
30	31
41	43

2.9   The Dollar Sign ($) Convention for Cell References

An understanding of the dollar sign ($) convention for handling data in a spreadsheet is critical to the maximum effectiveness of Excel operations. The $ symbol in any particular row or column reference indicates that the row or column designation preceded by the $ symbol is fixed.

Absolute and Relative Cell References

In general, Excel uses what are known as absolute and relative cell references. For example, if you wished to average the clinic visits for Week1 in Figure 2.12 (those in column B), the formula would be =AVERAGE (B4:B8). If this operation were carried out, the result would be the average of the five clinic visit totals for Week1. To get the average for the clinic visit totals for Week2, it is possible to copy the result in B9 and paste it into D9. If this is done, the formula in D9 will read =AVERAGE(D4:D8). This is what is meant by relative cell reference. When a formula is copied from one cell in a spreadsheet to another cell, the cell references change to make the formula refer to the same relative area rather than to the same actual area.

The $ Symbol and Absolute References

A $ symbol before any column or row reference means that the particular row or column is fixed (absolute). If the formula in cell B9 discussed earlier had been =AVERAGE($B4:$B9) and that formula had been copied into cell D9, the result would have been that the formula in D9 would still read =AVERAGE($B4:$B9). The value that appeared in cell D9 would be the average of the number of clinic visits in Week1. For example, suppose you wished to know what proportion of all visits occurred on each day of Week1. There are 157 visits to the clinic in Week1. This is shown in cell B9

C4			f_x	=B4/$B$9	
	A	B	C		D
1					
2					
3	**Day**	**Clinic Visits**	**Percent**		
4	Day 1	23	15%		
5	Day 2	47	30%		
6	Day 3	19	12%		
7	Day 4	37	24%		
8	Day 5	31	20%		
9		157			
10					

Figure 2.32 Calculations of percentages

of Figure 2.32, which now contains the sum of clinic visits for Week1. Column C shows the percentage of visits that took place in each day.

In the formula line, it is also possible to see that the formula for the percentage in cell C4 is calculated as =B4/$B$9. The cell reference to B9 in the formula is absolute. This means that it is possible to copy the formula in cell C4 to each of the cells in C5 through C8, and the proper formula will be calculated for each of the cells in the C column. The numerator, being a relative reference, changes for each cell in the C column, whereas the denominator, which is an absolute reference, remains the same for each cell in the C column. For example, the formula in cell C5 is actually =B5/$B$9. Because the percentage values are always in the C column, it would have been equally feasible to use the formula =B4/B$9 to calculate the first percentage and then to copy that formula to each cell in column C. The results would have been the same.

Absolute References and the F4 Function Key

Rather than go through the somewhat tedious process of putting $ symbols in front of each row and column reference when they are needed, you can use the F4 function key to select $ symbol status. It is possible to toggle through all four possible combinations of $ symbols for any cell reference. For example, if the cell reference B9 is entered into a formula, pressing F4 once will change that cell reference to $B$9. Pressing F4 a second time will change the cell reference to B$9. A third press will change the cell reference to $B9, and a fourth press will change it back to B9. The importance and versatility of the dollar sign convention—and the F4 function key—should become clearer as you proceed through the book.

KEY TERMS

#NAME?	formula bar
=AVERAGE()	formula line
=COUNT()	header row
=IF()	syntax
argument	workbook
Excel function	

Table 2.1 displays a glossary of key Excel terms that are used throughout the text. The terms definition and chapter location are included in the table.

Table 2.1 Glossary of Key Excel Terms Used throughout Text

Excel Term	Definition	Chapter Reference
#DIV/0!	Excel error message caused by trying to divide by 0.	2
#NAME?	Excel error message generally denoting the misspelling of an Excel function name.	2
#NUM!	Excel error message generally caused by trying to perform an undefined mathematical procedure, such as taking the square root of a negative number, or by requesting a result that exceeds Excel's limits, such as =FACT(171).	8, 12, 14
#VALUE!	Excel error message generally caused by including a nonnumerical value in a mathematical operation.	2
=AND()	Excel function that returns the result of two comparisons, TRUE if both comparisons are true and FALSE if either comparison is false.	7
=AVERAGE()	Excel function that returns the mean of a series of data.	2, 6
=BINOMDIST()	Excel function that returns the probability for the appearance of any value from a binomial distribution, given the number of trials and the outcome probability for a single trial.	5
=CHIDIST()	Excel function that returns the probability of a chi-square value, given degrees of freedom.	8, 10
=CHIINV()	Excel function that returns the chi-square value, given the probability of the chi-square value and degrees of freedom.	8
=CHITEST()	Excel function that returns the probability of a chi-square value, given the observed and expected values.	8
=COUNT()	Excel function that returns the number of values in a series of numerical data.	2
=COUNTIF()	Excel function that returns the number of times a given value appears in a series of data.	7
=EXP()	Excel function that returns the value of e (approximately 2.718282) raised to the power of the number in the parentheses.	5
=FACT()	Excel function that returns the factorial of the number in parentheses. Limited to numbers less than 171.	5
=FDIST()	Excel function that returns the probability of an F value, given degrees of freedom.	10, 11

(continued)

Table 2.1   (*Continued*)

Excel Term	Definition	Chapter Reference
=FINV()	Excel function that returns the *F* value, given the probability of the *F* value and degrees of freedom.	10
=FREQUENCY()	Excel function that returns a frequency distribution for a series of data in terms of a series of categories.	4, 6, 9
=IF()	Excel function that returns the result of an if–then decision.	2
=MAX()	Excel function that returns the maximum value in a series of data.	4
=MDETERM()	Excel function that returns the determinant for a square matrix.	12
=MEDIAN()	Excel function that returns the median value for a series of data.	6
=MIN()	Excel function that returns the minimum value in a series of data.	4
=MINVERSE()	Excel function that returns the inverse of a matrix (array).	12, 14
=MMULT()	Excel function that returns the product of two matrices (arrays).	2, 12, 14
=MODE()	Excel function that returns the modal value for a series of data. If the data have more than one mode, =MODE() will return the value of the numerically smallest mode.	6
=NORMDIST()	Excel function that returns probability for any value from a normal distribution, given the mean and standard deviation of the distribution.	6
=OR()	Excel function that returns TRUE if either or both of two comparisons are true and FALSE if both comparisons are false.	3
=POISSON()	Excel function that returns the probability of an appearance of any value from a Poisson distribution, given the mean of the distribution.	5
=RAND()	Excel function that returns a uniform random number between 0 and 1.	3, 6
=RANDBETWEEN()	Excel function that returns a uniform random number between two selected numbers.	3
=ROUND()	Excel function that returns the selected number rounded to the number of decimal places specified.	3
=SQRT()	Excel function that returns the square root of a number.	6
=STDEV()	Excel function that returns the standard deviation of a series of data assumed to represent a sample.	6
=SUM()	Excel function that returns the sum of a series of data.	2
=SUMPRODUCT()	Excel function that returns the sum of the product of the values of two series of data.	11, 12
=SUMSQ()	Excel function that returns the sum of the squares of a series of data.	11, 12
=TDIST()	Excel function that returns the probability of a *t* value, given degrees of freedom and a one- or two-tailed test.	6, 7, 9, 11, 12
=TINV()	Excel function that returns the *t* value, given the probability of the *t* value and degrees of freedom.	6, 7
=TRANSPOSE()	Excel function that returns the transpose of a matrix (array).	12, 14
=TRUNC()	Excel function that returns the integer portion of a number.	3
=TTEST()	Excel function that returns the probability of a *t* value, given a data set with a numerical dependent variable and a two-level categorical independent variable.	6, 7
=VAR()	Excel function that returns the variance of a series of data assumed to represent a sample.	6
=VARP()	Excel function that returns the variance of a series of data assumed to represent a population.	6
=YEARFRAC	Excel function that returns the number of years between two calendar dates.	3

CHAPTER 3

DATA ACQUISITION: SAMPLING AND DATA PREPARATION

Statistics is the grammar of science.

—Karl Pearson

Most statistics texts take the facile approach to data, which is to assume that the data were all successfully collected and made ready for analysis before anyone with an interest in statistical analysis came along. The happy result of this view is that the statistics text can usually ignore the thorny issues of where the data come from, how good they are, how they were collected, and how much confidence one can have in them. This text departs from that paradigm, to the extent of talking a little about where data come from, how to get data, and what to do with data before analysis begins. This chapter is devoted to the acquisition of data: sampling and data collection.

3.1 The Nature of Data

The first thing to be discussed in this chapter is simply the nature of data. Data are the fodder, the raw material of statistical analysis. It is essential to understand two aspects of data in any analysis setting. First, data are recorded in regard to or about cases or observations. Each case or observation represents a record in the data file. Second, data are made up of variables. Each case or observation— each data record—includes one or more measures of the case or record. These are the components of data that are subjected to analysis. For example, Figure 3.1 shows the

LEARNING OBJECTIVES

- Identify and distinguish between variable types

- Compare and contrast the scales of the measurement process

- Classify variables to the scales of measurement

- Understand sampling and sample selection with specific reference to simple random sampling

- Understand random number generation

- Understand how to access and prepare data

- Understand what missing data are and what impact they may have on your data set

	A	B	C	D	E	F
1	ID	Age	Sex	Visits	Total Cost	Cost/Visit
2	1	30	Male	1	$ 59.77	$ 59.77
3	2	69	Male	3	$ 323.02	$ 107.67
4	3	73	Female	1	$ 92.82	$ 92.82
5	4	22	Male	5	$ 589.40	$ 117.88
6	5	15	Female	4	$ 530.60	$ 132.65
7	6	29	Female	2	$ 170.31	$ 85.16
8	7	50	Female	3	$ 386.58	$ 128.86
9	8	47	Male	1	$ 117.03	$ 117.03
10	9	17	Female	8	$ 1,078.59	$ 134.82
11	10	63	Male	2	$ 143.70	$ 71.85
12	11	48	Male	2	$ 77.92	$ 38.96
13	12	70	Female	6	$ 175.55	$ 29.26
14	13	8	Female	1	$ 135.68	$ 135.68
15	14	38	Male	8	$ 213.42	$ 26.68
16	15	41	Female	5	$ 637.49	$ 127.50
17						

Figure 3.1   A small data set

Excel spreadsheet that was discussed in various ways in Chapter 2. This spreadsheet represents a small data set of 15 observations and 6 variables.

The observations in Figure 3.1 represent 15 people who may have come to an ambulatory clinic. Each observation appears on a different row of the spreadsheet. The variables in Figure 3.1 are in columns A through F. They include a unique identifier for each observation (ID in column A), the age of the person (Age), the sex of the person (Sex), the number of visits the person has made to the clinic (Visits), a total cost for visits to the clinic for each person (Total Cost), and an average cost per visit (Cost/Visit).

Data are usually displayed and conceived of in the way that is depicted in Figure 3.1. That is, the observations are perceived as occupying rows and the variables are perceived as occupying columns. Observations, it should be pointed out, do not need to be persons. They could be organizations, such as hospitals, health departments, or well-baby clinics. They could be political or geographic entities, such as states, counties, or hospital service areas. But variables always represent some attribute of the observation.

Types of Variables

A general characteristic of variables—at least as far as statistical analysis is concerned—is that they vary. In looking at the data set shown in Figure 3.1, it is easy to see that every variable takes on at least two values (e.g., Sex takes on two), and most take on a different value for each observation. In the unusual event that a variable does not vary—that is, it is a constant—it is useless for statistical analysis. Statistical analysis is almost universally about relating one variable to another. If a variable takes on only one value, it cannot statistically be related to other variables. This idea was discussed in some detail in Chapter 1.

Categorical and Numerical Variables

As also indicated in Chapter 1, variables may be characterized as being two basic types—categorical and numerical. Sex in Figure 3.1 is a categorical variable, classifying each person in the file as male or female. ID is also a categorical variable, classifying each person in the file as a separate entity. Other types of categorical variables could include membership in an HMO; a coding for the seriousness of an emergency, such as yellow and red; the source of coverage for a hospital charge; or blood type.

The remaining variables in the file in Figure 3.1 are numerical data. Again, as introduced in Chapter 1, there are two types of numerical data: discrete and continuous. Discrete numerical data are produced by a counting action and represent measures that can be made in discrete individual units only—never fractions of units. The number of visits to the clinic shown in Figure 3.1 is an example of discrete numerical data. Visits must always be in terms of whole units. Other discrete variables would include the number of persons in an emergency room, the number of unpaid accounts, and the number of immunizations received by a child.

Continuous Numerical Variables

Continuous numerical data are the result of a measurement or a mathematical operation. Age (a measure of the length of time from birth to the present moment) and cost per visit (the result of the division of total cost by the number of visits) are both continuous numerical variables. Other continuous numerical variables include waiting time in an ER or average waiting time, blood pressure, height, temperature, and drug dosage.

The total cost of all visits to the clinic is a little more difficult to classify. When cost is measured in dollars, fractions of dollars (e.g., pennies) might be considered to produce a continuous variable. When measured in pennies, however, each cost is a discrete measure—a result of counting—and cannot be expressed as fractions of pennies. But it is possible, as with height or age, to think of cost as an abstract notion that is approximated (as are height and age) by our measuring tool—in this case, dollars. From this perspective, cost is definitely a continuous variable. But, at the same time, it is possible to say that cost in the abstract is a meaningless concept, and that it becomes meaningful only when measured in some currency; thus, it is a discrete variable. Happily, although we may never resolve this issue, the type of statistics that applies to numerical variables tends to apply equally well to either discrete or continuous variables.

Distinguishing Variables as a Scale

There is a second way, introduced in Chapter 1, of distinguishing variables that refers to the scale upon which they are measured. Scale of measurement is classified as nominal, ordinal, interval, or ratio. The categorical variable Sex in Figure 3.1 is a nominal variable. It names each observation, each person in the file, as male or female. All nominal variables are categorical variables, but not all categorical variables are necessarily nominal variables. They may be ordinal variables or even, possibly, interval variables.

Scale variables can be classified as nominal, ordinal, interval, or ratio.

Ordinal Variables

Ordinal variables are nominal variables, the values of which establish some logical order. For example, young, middle-aged, and old, assigned to three age groups based on the data in Age in Figure 3.1, could be an ordinal variable. An assignment to the young age group might include all three people under 20 (persons with ID 5, 9, and 13). The middle-aged group might include all eight persons from 20 to 50 (persons with ID 1, 4, 6, 7, 8, 11, 15, and 16). Finally, the old group might include the remaining four persons (ID 2, 3, 10, and 12). This variable would be ordered in the sense that there is a logical order assumed by the young, middle-aged, and old. However, there is no assumption that the intervals are equal in any way.

The variable ID in Figure 3.1 is not an ordinal variable. There is no underlying logic to the assignment of 1 to the first person, 2 to the second, and so on. To distinguish one person from another, it would be equally possible to assign C to the first person, 231 to the second, Ralph to the third, and 17 to the fourth. As long as we assign a different code to each, we can keep them separated in our analysis, which is the primary function of an ID. ID, whether it is a number, a letter, or a sequence of nonsense syllables, is a nominal variable.

Interval Variables

Interval variables are ordinal variables that have equal intervals. The categories young, middle-aged, and old are ordinal variables without equal intervals. It would, however, be feasible to create a set of age groupings that contained equal intervals. Suppose we were concerned with a population of Medicare patients and divided their ages into five-year categories, beginning at age 65. If we assign 1 to the first group (ages 65 to 69), 2 to the second group (ages 70 to 74), and so on, we will have created an interval variable.

Ratio variables are interval variables with a true zero point. In the interval measure assigned to the ages of Medicare patients mentioned earlier, there is no true zero point. A 0 would simply mean the age group 60 to 64. It would be possible to create a ratio variable for age in five-year age intervals by beginning with 1 as the ages birth to four. Of course, age measured in one-year intervals is a ratio measure. In Figure 3.1, in addition to Age, the other variables—Visits, Total Cost, and Cost/Visit—are all ratio variables. Each of these variables has equal intervals, and each has a true zero point.

Independent and Dependent Variables

In most statistical analysis, there is a basic assumption that variables are either independent or dependent. Independent variables may often be termed causal variables, whereas dependent variables are considered caused variables. The term "causal variable" is quite commonly employed in statistics and research, but the term "caused variable" is rarely used. Independent variables are typically perceived as variables that are not affected or changed by the other variables under analysis, whereas dependent variables are, as the name implies, assumed to be dependent on or affected by the other variables in the analysis. Independent variables may also be termed predictor variables, because they are perceived to predict the performance of the dependent variables.

> Independent variables may be termed causal variables, whereas dependent variables are considered caused variables.

The distinction between independent and dependent variables is not always completely black and white, but with regard to data that are of interest to the health care world, there are some clear types. For example, Figure 3.1 includes two variables—Age and Sex—that are always considered independent variables. It is generally true that age and sex are determined (rather, predetermined) independent of any other variables in a data set. They are also generally perceived as independent of each other.

Conversely, the number of visits to the clinic (Visits) might be determined by age or sex or both. In this context, visits would be a dependent variable. Total cost might also be seen as dependent on age or sex or both, but it is also likely to be dependent on visits. So visits may be dependent relative to age or sex, but they may also be independent relative to total cost. Cost per visit (Cost/Visit) might be seen as dependent on age or sex, but not on visits or total cost. A statistical analysis might show that there is a relationship between either visits or total cost and cost per visit. However, because cost per visit is a composite of visits and total cost (in fact dependent on both because it was created from both), there is no appropriate way to apply statistics to the relationship.

In Chapter 1, we suggested that the "big picture" was that statistics were used to determine whether a value found in a sample could be assumed to have come from a population with certain characteristics. Another way of viewing statistical analysis is to think of it as a means of establishing whether a variable assumed to be dependent on another (assumed independent) can be shown from the data to be so. These two views may seem incompatible, or at least not obviously compatible. However, our discussion of various statistical analyses will attempt to show how the analysis addresses both questions.

Statistics That Apply to Different Types of Variables

As indicated in Chapter 1, this book includes sections on five different basic types of statistical analysis: chi-square statistics, t tests, the analysis of variance (ANOVA), regression, and Logit. The chi-square statistic is designed specifically for data analysis that is limited to categorical data. A chi-square could be used in the case of the data shown in Figure 3.1 to determine, for example, whether there was a relationship, for this data set, between age and sex. However, in order to do this, age would have to be collapsed into two or a few categories. The categories young, middle-aged, and old that were discussed earlier in this chapter could be an example of such an operation. This would result in a new variable that could be used for the chi-square analysis.

The t test can be thought of as a special case of a single dependent variable and a single independent variable. The dependent variable must be numerical and can be measured either on an interval or a ratio scale. The single independent variable can take on only two values and must be categorical. It can be either nominal or ordinal. Thus, a t test could compare, for example, cost per visit for males and females. In this case, cost per visit is the dependent, continuous numerical ratio variable, whereas sex is the single two-value independent variable.

Analysis of variance can be thought of as a direct extension of the t test to a single categorical, either nominal or ordinal independent variable, that may take on several different values, as opposed to simply two. But analysis of variance may also be extended to include more than one independent variable. In general, however, all independent variables would be categorical and measured either on nominal or ordinal scales. Again, as with the t test, the dependent variable must be numerical—either discrete or continuous—and hence must be measured either on an interval or a ratio scale.

Regression analysis may be thought of as an extension of analysis of variance to numerical independent variables. At the same time, regression analysis does allow the inclusion of categorical variables that take on only two values. The ability to code categorical variables with more than two values as multiple two-value categorical variables extends the utility of regression to encompass almost the entire range of capabilities of analysis of variance. But as with the t test and with analysis of variance, the dependent variable in regression must remain a numerical (discrete or continuous) variable.

Finally, Logit analysis is one of a family of techniques designed specifically to analyze data where the dependent variable is a two-level categorical variable (e.g., the presence or absence of health insurance coverage), whereas the independent variable may be either categorical or numerical.

Much of what has been discussed in the preceding paragraphs will probably not be clear at this time. One of the things this book tries to do is to make these points clear and show how they are important in the use of statistics.

Figure 3.2 represents constructed data (made-up data) for an imaginary clinic. There is an ID for each of the 20 people who are included in the data set, along with nine variables. The variable Age is coded as expected,

	A	B	C	D	E	F	G	H	I
1	ID	Age	Sex	Opinion 1	Opinion 2	Charges	Visit Time	Insurance	Prior
2	1	33	F	5	3	$ 58.00	40	Self Pay	5
3	2	21	F	2	3	$ 59.00	44	Medicaid	1
4	3	56	F	1	3	$ 78.00	51	Medicaid	5
5	4	53	M	2	4	$ 24.00	36	BCBS	2
6	5	51	F	5	4	$ 46.00	55	Private	5
7	6	22	F	1	5	$ 30.00	21	BCBS	2
8	7	62	F	4	1	$114.00	33	BCBS	0
9	8	39	F	1	2	$ 51.00	43	BCBS	4
10	9	60	F	5	5	$100.00	34	Private	4
11	10	61	F	3	4	$ 45.00	59	Private	6
12	11	65	M	1	3	$ 55.00	24	Private	2
13	12	60	F	1	2	$ 36.00	53	Medicaid	6
14	13	61	M	3	2	$ 62.00	31	Self Pay	4
15	14	28	F	4	3	$100.00	25	Self Pay	3
16	15	54	F	4	3	$111.00	48	Self Pay	3
17	16	64	F	2	4	$ 59.00	44	Medicaid	3
18	17	44	F	3	2	$ 45.00	57	BCBS	4
19	18	25	F	2	3	$ 58.00	43	Private	1
20	19	35	M	1	1	$ 95.00	45	Private	3
21	20	32	F	5	3	$ 92.00	33	Private	4

Figure 3.2 Constructed data for an imaginary clinic

in years of life. Sex is coded as F or M for female or male. The variable Opinion 1 is the answer to the question (asked on a patient questionnaire) "Do you feel this clinic meets your medical service needs: all the time, most of the time, about as often as not, some of the time, never?" An answer of never was coded 1, some of the time was coded 2, and so on. Opinion 2 is the response to the statement "The service here is better than I would get at a hospital emergency room." The answers were Strongly agree (coded 5), Agree (coded 4), Undecided (coded 3), Disagree (coded 2), and Strongly disagree (coded 1). The variable Charges represents the charge for the most recent clinic visit for each person. Visit Time represents the amount of time the person was at the clinic, from sign-in to departure. Insurance represents the type of insurance held by the patient, and Prior represents the number of previous times the patient has come to the clinic.

EXERCISES FOR SECTION 3.1

1. Using the data given in Figure 3.2 (or the data in Chpt 3-1.xls), indicate whether each of the variables in the figure is categorical or numerical, and if numerical, whether continuous or discrete, and give your reason(s) for saying so.

2. Using the data given in Figure 3.2, do the following:

   a. Using =IF (), transform Sex into a 1 if Sex is F and a 0 if Sex is M. Call this Sex1. Show the results in an Excel spreadsheet. What type of variable is the resulting variable, and why?

   b. Using nested =IF (), transform Age to another variable that combines Age into 10-year age groups, beginning with the youngest age among the patients listed. Assign 1 to the youngest group. Call this Age1. Show the results in an Excel spreadsheet. What type of variable is the resulting variable, and why?

   c. Using nested =IF (), transform Age to another variable that combines Age into 10-year age groups, beginning at birth. Assign 1 to the youngest age group. Call this Age2. Show the results in an Excel spreadsheet. What type of variable is the resulting variable, and why?

   d. Using nested =IF (), transform the variable Insurance into a new variable called Insurance1—that is, 1 if the insurance type is Medicaid, 2 if the insurance type is Blue Cross Blue Shield, 3 if the insurance type is private, and 4 for self-pay. Show the results in an Excel spreadsheet. What type of variable is the resulting variable, and why?

   e. Using nested =IF (), transform the variable Prior into a variable called Prior1, where no prior visits is coded None, 1 to 2 prior visits is coded Low, 3 to 4 prior visits is coded Medium, and 5 or 6 prior visits is coded High. Show the results in an Excel spreadsheet. What type of variable is the resulting variable, and why?

3.2   Sampling

All statistical analysis assumes that a sample of some type is under study. Thus the subject of sampling is central to the study of statistics.

Samples and Populations

The term "statistics" is generally used to refer to the subject of this book—that is, the set of calculations that can be used to draw inferences about the relationships between variables and make inferences about populations from samples. "Statistics" is also frequently used as simply the plural of "statistic." The affinity between these two meanings should be made clear. Statistics is the study of samples, characteristics of samples, and the ways in which inferences about populations may be drawn from those samples. A statistic is a value derived from a sample that can be used to infer something about a population.

Imagine that the data shown in Figure 3.1 represent a 15-person sample. This sample is from some much larger population of all persons who have come to the health center or clinic from which the data had been taken. We can calculate the mean or average of, for example, the number of visits to the clinic. For this sample, the mean comes out to about 3.47 visits per person. This number is a statistic because it came from a sample. We would designate the number $\bar{x}$ pronounced x-bar, because it was a statistic. The corresponding mean or average for the population from which the sample came would not be called a statistic; it would be a parameter, and it would be designated μ, which is pronounced "mu" and is the lowercase Greek letter μ. This leads to a generally applicable statement: Statistics refer to samples and are designated by lowercase Roman letters; parameters refer to populations and are designated by lowercase Greek letters. As you proceed through this book, you will encounter other measures for both samples and populations that have similar distinctions.

Parameters refer to populations, whereas statistics refer to samples.

The one important contradiction to this general statement about the designation of sample and population values is the designation of size. Sample sizes are universally designated n for number. Population sizes are universally designated N for number. So in the case of the data in Figure 3.1, n is 15, but because we have no information about the size of the population from which the data were drawn, N is unknown.

Drawing a Random Sample from a Population

There are entire books devoted to the subject of sampling, so this treatment will necessarily be only an introduction. But all of the statistics discussed in this text assume at some point that a sample has been taken. Furthermore, as was suggested in Chapter 1, the statistics discussed in this book also assume that the sample selected was either a simple random sample or a systematic sample. This section discusses sampling and sample selection with specific reference to simple random sampling.

It is generally accepted that a person, without some resources other than his or her own intellect, cannot draw a true random sample. No matter how hard we might try, any sample we might draw would be very likely nonrandom. For example, suppose we wish to draw a random sample of 5 persons from a group of 20 people. Suppose further that we also wish to have the sample equally divided into four groups by gender and age at, for example, age 30. This would allow us to have within the overall group a group of five young men, five young women, five older men, and five older women. The basic premise of a simple random sample is that each possible sample that may be selected must have an equal probability of selection as the actual sample.

If we were to try to draw a simple random sample of 5 from this group of 20, we would almost unconsciously end up with a sample that included two men and two women and two older persons and two younger persons. Filling out the five-person sample would be a problem for us because we would be concerned that adding a fifth person would make the sample unrepresentative of the entire group. And herein lies the problem of trying to draw a random sample with no form of external aid. Random samples are not representative; they are random.

Human beings seek to be representative when they try to extract a smaller group from a larger. This inevitably results in the exclusion of many possible combinations of samples that a truly random selection would allow. For example, a person would be very likely not to select five young men as the sample, because the sample would not be perceived as representative of the group of 20 as a whole. But random sampling allows for the selection of the five young men. It is unlikely that it would occur in a random sample, but all statistical analysis is based on the premise that it might happen.

Because the basic assumption of statistics is that a random sample has been selected (and, for the purposes of this book, a simple random sample), it is essential to have some mechanism for making this sample selection. One way to do this would be to assign a number to each member of a population from which a sample is to be drawn. Write each number on a slip of paper. Then put each slip of paper into a large box, shake the box well, and draw out (without looking at the numbers on the paper slips) the number needed. However, this could be both time-consuming and very boring.

Random Number Tables

For years, prior to the common availability of computers, statisticians used a modification of this slip-of-paper technique to draw random samples. They did this by using tables of random numbers, which were published in book form for the specific purpose of drawing random samples. Excerpts from these tables of random numbers are often reproduced in the back of statistics texts, occasionally with instructions on how to use the tables to draw true random samples. Typically, the use of these tables involved the time-consuming task of associating each observation in the population with an entry in the random number table. If that entry was smaller than some predetermined value, the observation in the population would become a member of the sample. For example, if the random number table were divided into three-digit sequences and the population consisted of a thousand observations, to select a 5 percent sample, any observation in the population associated with a three-digit sequence less than 050 would be included in the sample. If the observation were associated with a three-digit sequence larger than 050—for example, 274—that population observation would not be included in the sample.

Random Number Generation via a Spreadsheet: The =RAND () Function

The advent of computers made tables of random numbers obsolete. Even though tables of random numbers continue to be published, it is now many years since anyone has used them to draw random samples. The computer can generate sequences of random numbers and associate them with population observations far faster than we could from a random number table. Excel, as a computer program, is able to generate random numbers in a variety of different ways. This capability allows the Excel user to draw random samples in a variety of different ways, with a great deal of ease and efficiency. Perhaps the simplest of these mechanisms is the =RAND() function.

To employ the =RAND() method of selecting a random sample, it is necessary to have a worksheet reference for each observation in the population. If a researcher desired to draw a random sample from among all the people who work for a state department of health, for example, it would be necessary to have some reference to each of these persons in a spreadsheet. This might be each employee's name on the spreadsheet or, at a very minimum, a number associated with each employee. To continue with the example, suppose names were not on a spreadsheet but were only in an alphabetical hard copy list. Suppose that there are 3,427 employees on the list and we wish to draw a random sample of 100. To draw this sample, we can begin by listing the numbers 1 through 3,427 in column A of a spreadsheet. Do not type each number into 3,427 subsequent cells in column A. Listing the numbers might be done in a couple different ways, but the simplest procedure is probably to put 1 in cell A1 and 2 in cell A2. Then highlight both cells, A1 and A2, and, with the cursor on the lower right corner of the highlighted area (the cursor should appear as a small black cross rather than a large white cross), drag the cursor down to cell A3427. This will probably take 30 seconds or less.

Using the =RAND ( ) Function

Now go back to the top of the spreadsheet and type =RAND ( ) in cell B1. (As was indicated in Chapter 2, it is not necessary to type an Excel function such as =RAND ( ) in caps; lowercase will work just as well.) With =RAND ( ) in cell B1, put the cursor on the lower right corner of the cell (the cursor becomes a small black cross) and double-click. This will fill cells B1 to B3427 with random numbers in the range 0 to 1. Figure 3.3 shows the appearance of the spreadsheet just prior to the double-click that fills column B with random numbers. Column A in Figure 3.3 is the first approximately nine entries in a list that runs to 3,427. When cell B1 is double-clicked with the small black cross on the lower right corner of the cell, the random number represented by the entry in B1 will be copied to the first 3,427 cells in column B.

Now we have a random number associated with each entry in cells A1 through A3427. We could now go down the list of random numbers and include in the sample any entry in column A associated with a random number equal to or less than 0.02918 (100/3427 = 0.02918). But this has two disadvantages.

Figure 3.3 Beginning of random number generation

First, it is still quite time-consuming to review all 3,427 entries. Second, because the generated numbers are random, it is likely that there will be more or fewer than exactly 100 random numbers with values of 0.02918 or less. A more efficient strategy would be to sort the data in column A and column B (the first 3,427 cells in each column) by column B. This will order the data in column A by column B, after which the first 100 cases (or any 100 cases determined a priori) can be selected as the sample. This will not only make the sample selection fast and efficient but also ensure for us a sample of exactly 100 observations.

Working with the =RAND () Function: Random Number Regeneration

One important additional piece of information is needed before you can proceed, however. When the =RAND () function is used to enter values in cells B1 through B3427, what is actually entered into the cells is not a random number but, rather, the random number function. The random number function is regenerated every time the worksheet recalculates. The function also regenerates if an operation, such as sorting, is applied to the worksheet. Consequently, if you sort the data on the column containing the =RAND () function, you will have the unsatisfying result of not seeing the entries in column B appear ordered from lowest to highest, or in any other apparent order, because as soon as the sort occurs, the random number function is regenerated. Hence, the sequence in B will never appear ordered.

Working with the =RAND () Function: Copying the Random Numbers

There is an easy way to get around the problem of recalculation, however, and to feel a little more secure in the result of the sort. After the random numbers have been copied to the first 3,427 cells in column B, while the entire 3,427 cells are still highlighted, select Edit ➤ Copy, followed by Edit ➤ Paste Special. In the Paste Special dialog box, click the radio button marked Values. Figure 3.4 shows the Paste Special window with the Values radio button checked. When you click OK and dismiss the dialog box, the formulas in column B, which to this point all show =RAND () in the formula line if you highlight them, will change to the actual numbers shown in the cell. Now both columns A and B can be sorted on column B.

Excel's Sort Routine

The Excel Sort routine is found on the Data Ribbon in the Sort & Filter group. When you invoke the Sort command, you will see the Sort dialog box, shown in Figure 3.5. The Sort command allows for sorting on numerous

Figure 3.4 Paste Special dialog box

Figure 3.5 Sort dialog box

columns at a time. As shown in Figure 3.5, the sort will be on only one column (column B), and it will be in ascending order. Because there is no label on either column A or column B, the checkbox in front of "My data has headers" is not checked. When you click OK and dismiss the Sort dialog box, the 3,427 numbers in column A will be sorted by column B. The result of this sort is shown in Figure 3.6. Figure 3.6 shows the first 14 rows of the spreadsheet that contain the 3,427 numbers in column A, now sorted on column B. The entry in row 1 of column A is observation 777. This is associated with the smallest random number in column B—0.000152—and

	B1	▼	=	0.000151695338435953	
	A	B	C	D	E
1	777	0.000152			
2	1966	0.000288			
3	1415	0.000802			
4	953	0.001047			
5	2063	0.001391			
6	190	0.001846			
7	1999	0.00198			
8	878	0.002364			
9	3378	0.003274			
10	2976	0.004237			
11	616	0.004636			
12	1513	0.005061			
13	13	0.005577			
14	2648	0.005616			

Figure 3.6 Result of sort operation

is the first observation to be included in the sample of 100. The second observation included is number 1,966, which is associated with the next smallest random number, 0.000288. The last observation in the sample (not shown in the figure) is the observation numbered 3,066, which is associated with the random number 0.030386.

Now that you've carried out the steps previously discussed, a random set of 100 observations has been selected from among the original 3,427 observations. It remains to the researcher to go to the files and select the employee records corresponding to each of the first 100 numbers in the sample. But the task of selecting the random sample has been completed. This random sample of employees can now be used to calculate any estimates of the total population of employees that one would normally calculate from a random sample.

A Random Sample of Home Health Agency Records

Chapter 1 introduced the problem of the home health agency that wished to do an audit of 10 percent of its 800 records each quarter. The agency had been selecting the records for audit by taking the first record and every tenth record thereafter. It was suggested that perhaps a better way would be to select a simple random sample of records for review. A simple random sample can be selected easily by following the process described previously, in the second subsection of Section 3.2. The records can be put into a consecutive list. Each record can then be given a number from 1 to 800, with this number listed in column A of the spreadsheet. Once the numbers have been listed, each can be assigned a randomly generated number between 0 and 1 using =RAND(). The list can then be sorted on the random number, and the first 80 records can be selected for audit.

Selecting a Sample of Women to Receive a Cancer Education Intervention

Chapter 1 also introduced an example of the use of statistics in which a resident was expected to develop a study in which a sample of women received one type of breast cancer education—a pamphlet. Another sample of women experienced a short talk on breast cancer from a physician and received the pamphlet as well. The question was whether the women who had experienced the talk would show greater knowledge of breast cancer on a brief questionnaire administered after the fact.

For such a study to be effective, it is essential that the women who receive the two different interventions be randomly assigned to the two groups. Suppose the resident hopes to have 30 women in each of the two groups at the completion of the study. However, she does not know who these 60 women are because they are women who will be coming to the clinic in the future.

The easiest way to assign the 60 women randomly to either of the two interventions would be to begin by listing the numbers 1 through 60 in column A of a spreadsheet. Then each of the 60 numbers is assigned a random number using =RAND ( ) in column B. After the Edit ➢ Copy and Edit ➢ Paste Special ➢ Values option is used, the 60 numbers can be sorted by the random numbers. Now the first 30 numbers in the list (those in cells A1 to A30) represent the women who will receive one intervention (e.g., the pamphlet only). In turn, the second 30 numbers (those in cells A31 to A60) represent the women who receive the other intervention (both the pamphlet and the talk).

After the numbers 1 through 60 have been randomly assigned to two groups, the list of those assigned to each group can now be sorted so that they are easier to track. The results of such a sort might be as those shown in Figure 3.7. The figure shows the first 15 women in each of the two groups—those receiving the pamphlet only and those receiving the pamphlet plus the talk. As the figure shows, at the initiation of the study, the first two women seen in the clinic will receive both the pamphlet and the talk. The third woman will receive only the pamphlet, the fourth and fifth women will receive both interventions, and so on. This assignment can be used for the next 60 women coming to the clinic who meet the other study criteria.

There is an important point to be made from Figure 3.7 beyond that of a way of displaying the women who will be selected for each group. It might be noted that the sixth through the eleventh woman arriving at the clinic will be given only the pamphlet. Readers might be tempted to ask how this can be a random ordering if six people in a row are assigned to

	A	B	
1	**Pamphlet**	**Talk**	
2	3	1	
3	6	2	
4	7	4	
5	8	5	
6	9	12	
7	10	13	
8	11	14	
9	15	21	
10	16	22	
11	17	24	
12	18	25	
13	19	26	
14	20	28	
15	23	32	
16	27	33	
17	29	39	

Figure 3.7 Partial list of women who will receive each intervention

the same group. This is precisely why humans cannot carry out random selections. We are put off by a sequence of six in a row. But random numbers don't care. And in this case, the sequence of six from 6 to 11 was the result of random selection.

Other Random Sampling Mechanisms: =RANDBETWEEN() and the Data Analysis Add-In

Excel provides a number of different ways to draw random samples. The simplest is the =RAND() method, discussed earlier. A similar way is to use the =RANDBETWEEN (first, second) function, which returns a random integer between the two numbers specified as first and second. If the =RANDBETWEEN() function is to be used, it should be realized that the random numbers selected may be repeated if the range between the two numbers selected as first and second is small. This function recalculates just as =RAND() does, so it is necessary to use the Edit ≻ Copy and Edit ≻ Paste Special ≻ Values sequence prior to sorting if the satisfaction of seeing a sorted list is important.

The Data Analysis Add-In: Random Numbers from Different Distributions

Several other methods of selecting random samples can be found in Excel's Data Analysis add-in. For Excel, look in the Analysis group on the Data Ribbon and choose the Data Analysis option and then the Random Number Generation option in the Data Analysis dialog box.

Figure 3.8 Random Number Generation dialog box

If the Random Number Generation option is invoked in Excel 2013, the Random Number Generation dialog box (shown in Figure 3.8) appears. The Number of Variables field indicates the number of sets of random numbers that are to be generated. In the case shown in Figure 3.8, there will be five sets. The Number of Random Number field indicates the number of random numbers each set will contain. In this case, there will be 10 numbers in each set. The Distribution drop-down list indicates the type of distribution that will be generated. Seven different distributions of random numbers can be generated using this add-in. They are Uniform, Normal, Bernoulli, Binomial, Poisson, Patterned, and Discrete. More will be said of these later.

For each different type of distribution, corresponding parameters must be specified. For the *Uniform distribution*, selected in Figure 3.8, the parameters are the two numbers between which the random number will be generated. In the case shown, the numbers will be between 0 and 1, just as generated by the =RAND() function. Any real numbers can be used as the numbers between which random numbers will be generated, but the numbers generated will not be integer values, even if integers such as 5 and 25 are the numbers chosen for the range. Every distribution that can be generated has a separate set of parameters, which will be pointed out as each distribution type is discussed.

Random Numbers Generation: The Random Seed

Each Random Number Generation dialog box allows for the inclusion of a random seed. To understand the random seed, it is necessary to realize that no computer-driven random generating scheme can actually produce true random numbers. Computers can produce what are generally termed pseudorandom numbers. Any pseudorandom number–generating scheme takes some part of the last random number generated and uses that as a seed to begin the generation of the next random number. But in order for this to work, the computer has to have some number to work with as the first seed. Typically, the seed is taken from some source that is constantly changing in no predictable way. In the case of the =RAND() function, the seed is taken from the last several digits of the computer's time clock. These change so rapidly that it is impossible to predict what value they will have when the =RAND() function is invoked.

But the random number–generating schemes in the add-in all begin with a fixed seed by default. This means that every time Excel is started anew, these random number-generating schemes will produce exactly the same string of numbers. This is true for every one of the seven different random number–generating schemes—Uniform, Normal, Bernoulli, Binomial, Poisson, Patterned, and Discrete.

If the random number–generating schemes produced the same set of random numbers every time Excel was started anew, they would not seem to be producing very random numbers. But this problem has a relatively simple solution. Each of the seven random number–generating schemes allows for the specification of a random seed. Before using any of these random number generators, it would be best to use the =RAND() function to generate at least one random number. The first four digits of the result of =RAND() can then be used as an integer (i.e., without the decimal point) and as a random seed in whatever random number generation add-in is being used. Only the first four digits should be used, because the random seed value cannot exceed 9999. This strategy will produce a distinct and different set of random numbers each time the random number–generating schemes are invoked.

Random Numbers from the Uniform Distribution

The Random Number Generation dialog box (see Figure 3.8) will produce a set of random numbers, as shown in Figure 3.9. The 5 in the Number

	A	B	C	D	E
1	0.673757	0.557695	0.681936	0.914029	0.103977
2	0.273385	0.853511	0.429579	0.507523	0.089206
3	0.695853	0.92584	0.27131	0.073336	0.817316
4	0.638661	0.004639	0.947264	0.905637	0.448714
5	0.734123	0.125706	0.732475	0.492782	0.19425
6	0.470077	0.019074	0.191382	0.870235	0.785211
7	0.070009	0.973388	0.948454	0.592303	0.580065
8	0.479324	0.832057	0.207923	0.521836	0.52443
9	0.376659	0.661275	0.519242	0.602527	0.503525
10	0.48027	0.61388	0.212531	0.345408	0.878414

Figure 3.9 Five sets of 10 random numbers

of Variables box has produced 5 columns of numbers, and the 10 in the Number of Random Numbers box has produced 10 rows of numbers. It can be seen that all these numbers are between 0 and 1. It should be further noted that the Uniform distribution generates what are essentially random numbers. In other words, the numbers are generated to nine decimal places. The Uniform distribution was discussed earlier.

Random Numbers from the Normal Distribution

The Normal distribution dialog box looks exactly like that shown in Figure 3.8, except that in the Parameters field the user is asked to supply the mean and the standard deviation of the distribution. These terms will be discussed in detail in Chapter 6. For the present, it is sufficient to note that the Normal distribution option generates numbers that have no limit. The values generated most likely will be close to the mean value and will vary from the mean value as a function of the value of the standard deviation. The Normal distribution also generates continuous random numbers up to nine decimal places.

Within a spreadsheet, continuous random numbers are generated to nine decimal places.

Random Numbers from the Bernoulli Distribution

The *Bernoulli distribution* dialog box also resembles Figure 3.8, except for the Parameters field. For the Bernoulli distribution, only one parameter, p, is requested. The p stands for probability and must be between 0 and 1. The Bernoulli distribution option will generate a random sequence of ones and zeros, with the average number of ones being equal to p. So, if you were to generate 10 random ones and zeros using the Bernoulli option with a p of 0.5, it would be like flipping a coin 10 times. You would expect to get five heads (ones) and five tails (zeros), but you would not be surprised if you got four ones and six zeros, or three zeros and seven ones. Because the Bernoulli option generates only 0 or 1, it can be considered as generating discrete random numbers.

Discrete random numbers can take on only integer values (e.g., 0 or 1).

Random Numbers from the Binomial Distribution

The Binomial distribution dialog box requests two parameters—the p value and the number of trials. Again, as with the Bernoulli distribution, the p value refers to the probability of an occurrence. "Number of trials" refers to the number of times the probability will be applied. In the coin-flipping example of the Bernoulli distribution mentioned previously, the number of trials was 10. Rather than generate a series of ones and zeros, the binomial distribution generates a single number between 0 and the number of trials (e.g., 10). That number represents the number of ones that would result from applying p for the number of trial times. In the case of flipping a coin 10 times, the binomial distribution result would be a number between 0 and 10. Because the probability of one's getting a head or a tail is equal, the random numbers generated by the binomial distribution will be predominantly fours, fives, and sixes. The binomial distribution option generates only integer values, so it generates discrete random numbers.

Random Numbers from the Poisson Distribution

The Poisson distribution dialog box requests a single parameter: lambda. "Lambda" refers to the mean value of the distribution, or the average number that will be generated by the distribution over a large number of trials. In a Poisson distribution, the value of lambda is also the variance of the distribution. The Poisson distribution will be discussed further in Chapter 5. The Poisson distribution also generates only integer values, so it, too, generates discrete random numbers.

The patterned distribution is not actually a random number generator at all; rather, it generates a list of numbers that repeat as many times as desired in a pattern that is set by the Parameters field. In terms of the materials in this book, the patterned distribution is not relevant.

Random Numbers from the Discrete Distribution

The *discrete distribution* requests two parameters: the value and the probability input range. The discrete distribution generates random numbers from a prespecified set of numbers (the value range), according to the probabilities assigned to these numbers (the probability range). So, for example, if the value range was that shown in cells A1 to A10 of Figure 3.10, and the probability range was that shown in cells B1 to B10, the discrete random number generator would generate values of 1 to 10 according to the probabilities shown in column B. It should also be pointed out that the probability range must sum to 1. So if you wanted to generate a random series of, for example, 20 numbers from the list in cells A1 to A10, you would expect, on average, that the random number generation would result in six ones, four twos, two each of three and four, and one each of five through 10. Of course, because this is a random number generation process, it is likely that the result will not be exactly as indicated in the previous sentence. But, in general, the result will be similar to this.

One point must be made about the random seed in the discrete distribution generator. For some reason, the space following the random seed will be grayed out so that it cannot be used in many instances. The solution is to change to another type of distribution, put in the desired random seed, and then go back to the discrete distribution. The random number generator will pick up the random seed as specified.

It is useful to know of these random number generation capabilities of Excel, in general. However, the material in this book will rely either on the =RAND() method of selecting random samples or, in some examples with regard to the consequences of selection of random samples, on the discrete sampling capability of the random number add-in. In order to provide some familiarity with sampling in general, and these options in particular, the following exercises are offered.

	A	B
1	1	0.30
2	2	0.20
3	3	0.10
4	4	0.10
5	5	0.05
6	6	0.05
7	7	0.05
8	8	0.05
9	9	0.05
10	10	0.05
11		

Figure 3.10   Value and probability input range (example)

EXERCISES FOR SECTION 3.2

1. Use the data set from Figure 3.2 (Chpt 3-1.xls) and do the following:

    a. Use the =RAND() function to draw a random sample of 5 patients from the 20 patients given in the file.

    b. Use the uniform distribution option in the Data Analysis add-in to generate random numbers between 0 and 1, and use these numbers to select a simple random sample of 7 patients from the 20 in the file. Specify a random seed of 1325.

    c. Use the normal distribution option in the Data Analysis add-in to generate random numbers with a mean of 0 and a standard deviation of 1, and use these numbers to select a simple random sample of 10 patients from the 20 in the file. Specify a random seed of 7936.

2. The file Chpt 3-2.xls contains data from the State and Metropolitan Area Data book for 1998 on nurses and health insurance coverage by state, plus the District of Columbia. Use the data from this file and do the following:

    a. Use the =RAND() function to draw a random sample of 10 states from among all the states, including the District of Columbia.

    b. Use the uniform distribution option in the Data Analysis add-in to generate random numbers between 1 and 100, and use these to select a random sample of 15 states from among all the states, including the District of Columbia. Specify a random seed of 1359.

    c. Use the normal distribution option in the Data Analysis add-in to generate random numbers with a mean of 20 and a standard deviation of 4, and use these numbers to select a simple random sample of 10 states from among all the states, including the District of Columbia. Specify a random seed of 8109.

3. Staff members at a prenatal clinic see many women who smoke. Staff have decided to assess the effectiveness of a video on the dangers of smoking during pregnancy. They have decided to divide the women smokers who come to the clinic into two groups: one that receives the normal warnings about the dangers of smoking and one that is asked to view the video. Over the next six months, the clinic expects to see about 40 women who are smokers. Use =RAND() to select a sample of 20 women who will view the film and 20 who will not out of the next 40 women to arrive at the clinic.

4. Use the Bernoulli distribution in the Data Analysis add-in to simulate the flip of a coin 50 times. Generate a random seed using =RAND(). If you consider a value of one to be a head, use the =SUM() function to determine the number of heads and tails flipped.

5. Use the binomial distribution in the Data Analysis add-in to simulate the distribution of men and women among the next 10 arrivals at an emergency room, assuming that, on average,

6 people out of 10 who arrive are men. Generate a random seed using =RAND(). Simulate the arrival of 50 sets of 10 people. Use the =COUNTIF() function to determine how many of the 50 sets of 10 people will be all men and how many will be 9 men and 1 woman.

6. Use the discrete distribution in the Data Analysis add-in to simulate the roll of a six-sided die 50 times. Generate a random seed using =RAND(). Use the =COUNTIF() function to determine how many of the 50 rolls will produce a six.

3.3   Data Access and Preparation

Data access can be the subject, just as sampling can, of an entire book. This section provides only a basic introduction to the issues involved. Essentially, data can be accessed and acquired in only two ways; they can be collected directly by the investigator (e.g., the user of this statistics text) or they can be obtained as secondary data. If they are to be collected by the investigator, the options available for collection include questionnaires that are filled out by respondents themselves (e.g., patients or hospital CEOs) or interview schedules to which answers are given by respondents. Direct data collection can also include observation in which the researcher observes and records these specific details on a predetermined schedule.

Secondary Data

Secondary data are data that have been collected for some purpose other than the study of interest to the researcher but can be accessed by the investigator for study purposes. Secondary data could include such information as patients' records (when appropriate clearances for use and informed consent have been obtained), operating data from a hospital or other health care organization, or data in the public domain, such as county-by-county statistics on median income, percentage below poverty, or low birth weight rates.

A major advantage of the use of directly collected data is that data can be collected in a way that is specific to the needs of the investigator. To take a relatively simple example, if the interest is in a patient's age, the investigator can ask the patient for his age. However, if secondary data are used to get a patient's age, the data actually available may not be age but, rather, date of birth. This leads to the general issue of turning those data into data that can be used in the application of other statistical analysis. Happily, Excel is a very useful tool in this process.

An Examination of Data Preparation Using Secondary Data

This section describes an example of the use of Excel in the preparation of some secondary data for analysis. The secondary data to be examined are actual data, but they are data from which all identifying information has been deleted. The data file represents information for 100 hospital discharges for Medicare-eligible persons randomly selected from a much larger file of discharges. There are nine different pieces of information included in the file. These are sex, date of birth, date of hospital admission, date of discharge, MS-DRG code, total hospital charges, actual Medicare payment, number of diagnoses for the hospital stay, and admitting ICD-9 code. (The ICD-9 code is one digit. Normally, ICD-9 codes are three digits or more, but this is the way the data were actually coded and made available, because the institution from which the data came was having trouble coding the ICD-9. Problems such as this are not uncommon in the use of secondary data.)

Importing Data with the Text Import Wizard

The data file is initially in a simple text format, and it must be put into spreadsheet format to be used by Excel. It is not uncommon to find data in a format other than the Excel format. Excel provides a *Text Import Wizard* with three steps to import text data into Excel. The Text Import Wizard will automatically come up in the Excel screen whenever Excel recognizes that the user is trying to open a text file. The first step of the Text Import Wizard is shown in Figure 3.11.

The Text Import Wizard will assume that the text file to be imported is a data file, as opposed to a conventional text file. It will also assume that each line of the text file represents a separate observation and that individual data elements (the variables) for any observation are all contained on the same line. It will first attempt to determine the way in which each data element is distinguished from every other data element. There are two ways in which data elements may be separated: by using a delimiter or by using a fixed-width field. A delimiter is a character (e.g., a tab or an ampersand) that generally will not be used to represent data but will simply be included in the text file to separate one variable from another. Data may also be stored in a text file in fixed width. Fixed width means that every variable will take up exactly the same number of spaces—for example, 10—in the text file. *Delimited* data is the most common format. A fixed-width file requires a certain number of spaces for each variable, even though there may be no

Figure 3.11   Text Import Wizard, Step 1

data in a particular field, or the actual data may be much shorter than the number of spaces allocated. The delimited data file takes up only as much space as is required for each data element.

Step 1

As you can see by the selected radio button in Figure 3.11, the Text Import Wizard has correctly determined, in the case of the data in the text file referenced here, that the data are delimited. The wizard further indicates that the importing of data to the spreadsheet will begin in row 1 and that the text file is actually contained in a Windows (ANSI) format. The other formats that can appear in the file origin window are Macintosh and MS-DOS. The preview area of the dialog box shows the data that will be imported by Excel with the delimiter (in this case, actually a tab character). Line 2 of the preview screen shows F as the first code (representing Female for sex); 1/5/15 representing the date of birth; 4/14/02 and 4/22/02 representing the date of admission and date of discharge, respectively; and 139 representing the MS-DRG code. The remaining information on the first line includes 6815.6 representing the total dollar charges for the stay, 1072.17 representing what Medicare actually paid, 4 indicating four separate diagnoses for the stay, and 4 indicating an admitting ICD-9 code.

Steps 2 and 3

Figure 3.12 shows the second step of the Text Import Wizard. This step allows the user to select the character that is actually used to delimit the data and see the result of the selection of this delimiter in the Data preview area. The check mark before Comma indicates that Excel has correctly determined on its own that the text file was delimited with commas.

The final step in the Text Import Wizard is shown in Figure 3.13. This dialog box provides an opportunity to do several things. These include setting the format of each imported column and indicating whether a column should not be imported. The highlighted first column will be acted upon by anything checked in the Column data format area. Each successive column in the data can be highlighted in turn, and its format can be set to General, Text, or Date. General is the most versatile format, as it treats numeric values as numbers, treats text values as text, and treats data in date format (i.e., 11/28/55) as dates.

In general, if Excel correctly recognizes that the data file is delimited (or is of fixed width) and there is no desire to change or delete the actual data elements, it is usually not necessary to go beyond the Step 1 dialog box. In fact, the first dialog box is all that is necessary to convert the file under discussion here to spreadsheet format. If you click the Finish button in the

Figure 3.12 Text Import Wizard, Step 2

Figure 3.13 Text Import Wizard, Step 3

Step 1 dialog box of the Text Import Wizard, the text file will automatically appear as an Excel spreadsheet.

Inspecting, Formatting, and Modifying Imported Data

The data as imported into Excel are shown, in their initial form, in Figure 3.14. Only the first 10 records in the file are shown, although the data file actually contains 100 records. On looking at the file as shown in Figure 3.14, you will immediately notice several things. First, columns B, C, and D contain several cells with number signs (#######) instead of recognizable data. This means that the formatting currently applied to the cell, including its width, is preventing Excel from displaying the data

	A	B	C	D	E	F	G	H	I
1	F	#######	9/11/2002	9/15/2002	294	2426.48	2003.62	2	0
2	F	1/5/2015	4/14/2002	4/22/2002	139	6815.61	1072.17	4	4
3	F	3/16/1932	5/1/2002	5/11/2002	34	7596.68	4096.98	6	0
4	M	5/15/2029	2/5/2002	2/10/2002	140	6450.77	1710.79	5	0
5	F	#######	4/9/2002	4/12/2002	141	3542.79	1914.9	3	7
6	F	#######	1/13/2002	1/15/2002	15	2590.86	2601.14	5	4
7	F	6/23/2028	2/9/2002	2/14/2002	294	5082.83	2035.31	7	2
8	M	#######	9/11/2002	9/17/2002	241	3580.55	2320.42	6	0
9	M	8/7/2029	#######	11/6/2002	335	11045.79	4184.26	1	0
10	F	1/3/2008	#######	#######	148	19708.11	12158.49	4	0
11	F	7/2/2007	6/1/2002	6/12/2002	89	8953.38	4345.84	4	0

Figure 3.14 Data as initially imported from a text file

properly. You can correct this situation easily by widening the column (put the cursor between the letters heading any two columns and drag it to the right or double-click). You will also notice as you look at column B that several of the dates (e.g., 5/15/2029, in row 4) have not even occurred yet. But this is the date-of-birth column. Excel has misinterpreted the date 5/15/29 (which obviously meant May 15, 1929) and has made it a complete century later. This problem is one that should be anticipated when using date data that are for a date prior to 1930. Any date prior to that time that is not given as the entire date (i.e., is given only as the last two digits of the year) is treated by Excel on being imported as a date in 20xx rather than a date in 19xx. But because we know that this is a date of birth, it is obvious that we will have to change any dates shown in the imported file as 20xx to dates in the form 19xx.

Adjusting Dates in Excel

The solution to this problem is a little tricky, but it depends on the fact that Excel stores dates as a number beginning with 1/1/1900 as 1. The number that corresponds to 1/1/2000 is 36526. In order to convert the dates in column B in Figure 3.14 that are given as 20xx to numbers in the form 19xx, it will be necessary to subtract 36525 from each of the dates that are in the form 20xx. Figure 3.15 shows the data from Figure 3.14. The columns containing dates have been widened to show all the dates (no #######). In addition, a column has been inserted between B and C (with column C in Figure 3.14 becoming column D in Figure 3.15) in which the corrected date of birth has been calculated. (In order to insert a column or a row between two other columns or rows, left-click the letter [column] or number [row] where you wish to make the insert. Then right-click the cursor while it is still on the letter or number and select Insert from the pop-up menu. A column will be moved to the left and a new one inserted, or a row will be moved down and a new one inserted.)

	C1		=IF(B1<36526,B1,B1-36525)							
	A	B	C	D	E	F	G	H	I	J
1	F	11/28/1955	11/28/1955	9/11/2002	9/15/2002	294	2426.48	2003.62	2	0
2	F	1/5/2015	1/5/1915	4/14/2002	4/22/2002	139	6815.61	1072.17	4	4
3	F	3/16/1932	3/16/1932	5/1/2002	5/11/2002	34	7596.68	4096.98	6	0
4	M	5/15/2029	5/15/1929	2/5/2002	2/10/2002	140	6450.77	1710.79	5	0
5	F	11/27/2019	11/27/1919	4/9/2002	4/12/2002	141	3542.79	1914.9	3	7
6	F	11/22/2016	11/22/1916	1/13/2002	1/15/2002	15	2590.86	2601.14	5	4
7	F	6/23/2028	6/23/1928	2/9/2002	2/14/2002	294	5082.83	2035.31	7	2
8	M	12/27/1936	12/27/1936	9/11/2002	9/17/2002	241	3580.55	2320.42	6	0
9	M	8/7/2029	8/7/1929	10/31/2002	11/6/2002	335	11045.79	4184.26	1	0
10	F	1/3/2008	1/3/1908	11/11/2002	11/25/2002	148	19708.11	12158.49	4	0
11	F	7/2/2007	7/2/1907	6/1/2002	6/12/2002	89	8953.38	4345.84	4	0

Figure 3.15 Making imported dates century-correct

The =IF() statement that was used to produce the correct date is shown in the formula line of Figure 3.15, and is =IF(B1<36526, B1,B1-36525). The =IF() statement says that if the date given in column B is less than (<) 36526 (i.e., if it is a date prior to 1/1/2000), it should remain as in column B. But if it is not, it should be changed to whatever is in column B minus 36525 (a century of days). There is one small drawback to this strategy. In the unlikely event that a person was actually born in the 1800s rather than in the 1900s, this would change his or her date of birth to a date near the end of the 1900s. This can possibly be checked for in these data, however, because anyone who had a birthdate in the late 1900s would not likely be eligible for Medicare yet. With other types of data, it might be more difficult to determine if a date of birth should be prior to 1900.

Values versus Formulas, Deleting Extra Columns, $ Formatting

Having corrected the date of birth in column C, we should now make several additional modifications to the imported data set. First, the current column C, which gives the corrected date of birth, should be changed from a formula dependent on column B to the value shown in column C. This can be done by right-clicking column C and selecting Copy, then right-clicking column C again and selecting Paste Special ➤Values for the data in column C (and it can be done while the data are still highlighted, as shown in Figure 3.15). Once this has been done, it is a good idea to eliminate column B by left-clicking the B at the top of the column and then right-clicking and selecting Delete from the pop-up menu. This will put the corrected date of birth in column B. A new first row (row 1) should be added as a place to put an identifier for each variable. A new first column (column A) should be added as a place to put a unique identifier for each hospital stay (an ID number).

Finally, the formatting for the hospital charges and actual Medicare payments can be changed from general to dollar format to clearly appear as dollar amounts. To do this, first highlight the cells that should be in dollar format, in the Home ribbon select the $ pull-down menu from the Number menu, and select the appropriate currency, in this case "$ English (United States)" from the menu. The completed transformation of the data is shown (again, for the first 10 observations only) in Figure 3.16. At this point the data should be saved as an Excel file.

Finally, the formatting for the hospital charges and actual Medicare payments can be changed from general to dollar format to clearly appear

	A	B	C	D	E	F	G	H	I	J
1	ID	Sex	DOB	DOA	DOD	DRG	Charges	Medicare	Diag	ICD-9
2	1	F	11/28/1955	9/11/2002	9/15/2002	294	$ 2,426.48	$ 2,003.62	2	0
3	2	F	1/5/1915	4/14/2002	4/22/2002	139	$ 6,815.61	$ 1,072.17	4	4
4	3	F	3/16/1932	5/1/2002	5/11/2002	34	$ 7,596.68	$ 4,096.98	6	0
5	4	M	5/15/1929	2/5/2002	2/10/2002	140	$ 6,450.77	$ 1,710.79	5	0
6	5	F	11/27/1919	4/9/2002	4/12/2002	141	$ 3,542.79	$ 1,914.90	3	7
7	6	F	11/22/1916	1/13/2002	1/15/2002	15	$ 2,590.86	$ 2,601.14	5	4
8	7	F	6/23/1928	2/9/2002	2/14/2002	294	$ 5,082.83	$ 2,035.31	7	2
9	8	M	12/27/1936	9/11/2002	9/17/2002	241	$ 3,580.55	$ 2,320.42	6	0
10	9	M	8/7/1929	10/31/2002	11/6/2002	335	$11,045.79	$ 4,184.26	1	0
11	10	F	1/3/1908	11/11/2002	11/25/2002	148	$19,708.11	$12,158.49	4	0

Figure 3.16 Text file imported to Excel with ID and Variable labels

as dollar amounts. To do this, first highlight the cells that should be in dollar format and then select Format ➤ Cells ➤ Currency. The completed transformation of the data is shown (again, for the first 10 observations only) in Figure 3.16. At this point the data should be saved as an Excel file.

The ID number given in Figure 3.16 (column A) may not seem important, because each record is in a different row and it is not likely that one row will be confused with another. But the ID number can be used to return the data set to the original order if it is sorted on some variable, such as hospital charges or Medicare payments. It can be used to ensure that data stay with the right observation if a subset of observations and variables is moved to another spreadsheet. In general, it is good practice to include an ID number. It takes up little space in a file, and if you do not include it, you will wish that you had.

Performing Data Checks

Usually, importing any data set to Excel and getting it into a format that looks like an Excel spreadsheet (and ensuring that such things as date of birth reflect reality) are not the last step in getting data ready for analysis. In certain cases (e.g., with date of birth), it might be desirable to perform some data checks to see if the data are all within a reasonable range (e.g., not a date that represents one in the future or a date signifying someone was born 100 years from now). We mentioned earlier that in the unlikely event that someone represented in the data file was born before 1900, the method used here to give the correct date of birth would give a date incorrectly recorded as 19xx rather than as 18xx. But this would show up in the data file as a date in the 1990s (assuming that no one is over 112 years of age). So one way to ensure that no one has been incorrectly shown as having been born in the 1990s, when he or she was actually born in the 1890s, is to check the date-of-birth column (DOB) for a date in the 1990s.

Checking Date of Birth with an =IF() Statement

A date in the 1990s in the date-of-birth column can be found simply by looking at each individual entry in column C. But even with only 100 records, this is unnecessarily time-consuming. A better choice is to use the =IF() statement as shown in Equation 3.1.

$$= IF(C2 < 32874, 1, 0) \tag{3.1}$$

where C2 references the first data cell in column C (date of birth) and 32874 is the number corresponding to the date 1/1/1990.

This =IF() statement will record a 1 for dates of birth prior to 1990 and a zero for any dates of birth shown as after 1990. The =IF() statement should be put into an unused column in the spreadsheet (e.g., column K). It should then be copied to the end of the data file (in this case, the first 101 rows in the spreadsheet). An easy way to determine if any of the dates are in the 1990s is to sum the column containing the =IF() statement. If the sum is 100, then it is likely that no dates of birth should have been recorded as in the 1800s. If the sum is less than 100, it is easy to find the records for which date of birth should probably have been recorded as 18xx by sorting the entire data set on the column containing the =IF() statement.

In the case of the hospital data being discussed here, none of the dates of birth are recorded as being in the 1990s, so it is probably unlikely that there are any records in the data file with a true date of birth prior to 1900. Once the =IF() statement has done its job of determining if the data in the date-of-birth column are correct, the column containing the =IF() statement can be deleted.

Checking M or F with an =IF() Statement and an =OR() Statement

Other logical checks might be made on the initially imported data. For example, it might be useful to be certain that every entry in the column representing sex is coded either M or F. This can be done by using either the =IF() statement (in this case, a nested =IF() statement) or an =OR() statement. The two statements that can check for either an M or an F in column B are as those shown in Equation 3.2.

$$= IF(B2 = \text{``F''}, 1, IF(B2 = \text{``M''}, 1, 0))$$

or

$$= OR(B2 = \text{``F''}, B2 = \text{``M''}) \tag{3.2}$$

where B2 references the first data cell in column B.

In the case of the =IF() statement in Equation 3.2, Excel first checks to see if the entry in B2 (or whatever cell is being referenced) is an "F." The quotation marks are necessary if Excel is to recognize a text character. If Excel finds an "F," it will put a 1 in the cell in which the =IF() statement appears. If the entry in the referenced cell is not an "F," Excel then checks to see if it is an "M." If it finds an "M," it will record a 1. If Excel finds neither an "F" nor an "M," it will record a 0. The entries in the column in which =IF() is invoked can then be summed to determine if the sum is equal to the number of observations. If not, the entire data file can be sorted on the =IF() column to find the anomalous data entries in column B. It should be pointed out that "F" and "f" are the same character to Excel, as they are in general to you and to us. So the statement in Equation 3.2 will also find an "f."

The =OR() statement operates much the same way as =IF(). But it checks both "F" and "M" and if it finds either, it records a TRUE in the column in which it is invoked. If it finds neither "F" nor "M," it records FALSE. If there are any entries that are not "F" or "M" in the column, recording sex can be determined by counting the number of TRUE entries in the column in which the =OR() statement was invoked. If this is equal to the number of observations, then sex is recorded as "F" or "M" (or "f" or "m") for each observation. Counting the number of TRUE entries is easier than looking at each entry in the column in which =OR() is invoked. It can be done with the =COUNTIF() function, as shown in Equation 3.3.

$$= COUNTIF(K2:K101, TRUE) \qquad (3.3)$$

where K2:K101 references the data cells in which the =OR() function has been invoked.

Again, once the data checks indicated here have been made, the column in which the check has been carried out can be deleted. This helps keep the data set from becoming cluttered with unneeded information.

Other Possible Data Checks for Medical Data

A number of other data checks might be warranted. These would depend entirely on whether it is possible to specify what codes should appear in given cells. For example, it could be possible to see if date of discharge (in column E) is always later than date of admission (column D). It might be possible to determine if the code given for MS-DRG was, in fact, a legitimate MS-DRG code. But that could require a large number of nested =IF() statements, and it still might not work. Incidentally, it is possible to nest up to 16 =IF() statements.

After you've checked for data errors, it is time to think about the kind of analysis that will be done with the data. As an initial step, it is likely that at some point in any analysis involving this data set, length of hospital stay will be important information. Similarly, it is quite possible that the age of the patient at the time of hospitalization will be of interest. So, at a minimum, these two pieces of information should be developed from what is already in the data.

Calculating Length of Stay (LOS)

Length of hospital stay (LOS) can be determined simply by subtracting the date of discharge (DOD) from the date of admission (DOA). Just as Excel can deal with addition or subtraction in regard to a date and a number, it can also deal with addition and subtraction in regard to two dates. Figure 3.17 shows the calculation of the length of stay in days by subtracting the date in column D from the date in column E (see =E2-D2 in the equation line in the figure). A new column was first inserted between DOD and DRG, and then the subtraction was carried out in the new column F, labeled LOS. When the calculation was made, the initial result was not 4 (for cell F2) but rather 1/4/1900. It was necessary to reformat the data in column F from date to general in order for it to appear as days of stay.

Calculating Age at Admission: Using the =YEARFRAC() Function

Calculation of age at admission by subtracting the date of birth from the date of admission would work, in general, but it would be a little more complicated. First, it would be necessary to make the subtraction, and then convert the resulting age in days from a date format to general format. Finally, it would be necessary to divide the resulting age in days by 365 (or 365.25, allowing for leap years). This would still not give exactly the right

	F2		▼	=	=E2-D2		
	B	C	D	E	F	G	
1	Sex	DOB	DOA	DOD	LOS	DRG	Cha
2	F	11/28/1955	9/11/2002	9/15/2002	4	294	$ ₂
3	F	1/5/1915	4/14/2002	4/22/2002	8	139	$ 6
4	F	3/16/1932	5/1/2002	5/11/2002	10	34	$ 7
5	M	5/15/1929	2/5/2002	2/10/2002	5	140	$ 6
6	F	11/27/1919	4/9/2002	4/12/2002	3	141	$ ₃
7	F	11/22/1916	1/13/2002	1/15/2002	2	15	$ ₂
8	F	6/23/1928	2/9/2002	2/14/2002	5	294	$ 5
9	M	12/27/1936	9/11/2002	9/17/2002	6	241	$ ₃
10	M	8/7/1929	10/31/2002	11/6/2002	6	335	$11
11	F	1/3/1908	11/11/2002	11/25/2002	14	148	$1C

Figure 3.17 Calculation of length of stay

age in years and fractions of years, because the number of leap years one has lived through will not always be exactly one-fourth of the years lived. An easier way to find the age is to use the Excel function =YEARFRAC(), which will give the number of years and fractions of years between two dates.

The use of =YEARFRAC() is shown in Figure 3.18. A new column has been inserted between DOB and DOA and labeled Age. Age has been calculated as is shown in the formula line of the spreadsheet. It does not matter in what order the two columns are referenced in the =YEARFRAC() function—the function calculates the number of years between the two dates in either order. An additional function is included in the calculation of age and shows how function statements in Excel can be used together to accomplish a desired data goal. The function =TRUNC() truncates (i.e., cuts off) a number at a specified number of decimal digits. If no number of decimal digits is specified (as in this case), the number is assumed to be zero. Unless the person we are referring to is a child, we cease to refer to people as being a certain number of years old and fractions of years; we refer to them only as the number of years they have attained. So even though the second person on the list (who was born on January 5, 1915, and entered the hospital on April 14, 2002) was actually 87.332 years old at the time of admission, we would refer to her as being 87 years old.

Table 3.1, Table 3.2, and Table 3.3 illustrate the Excel formulas associated with the aforementioned operations.

	D2		▼		= =TRUNC(YEARFRAC(E2,C2))		
	A	B	C	D	E	F	
1	ID	Sex	DOB	Age	DOA	DOD	LO
2	1	F	11/28/1955	46	9/11/2002	9/15/2002	
3	2	F	1/5/1915	87	4/14/2002	4/22/2002	
4	3	F	3/16/1932	70	5/1/2002	5/11/2002	
5	4	M	5/16/1929	72	2/5/2002	2/10/2002	
6	5	F	11/27/1919	82	4/9/2002	4/12/2002	
7	6	F	11/22/1916	85	1/13/2002	1/15/2002	
8	7	F	6/23/1928	73	2/9/2002	2/14/2002	
9	8	M	12/27/1936	65	9/11/2002	9/17/2002	
10	9	M	8/7/1929	73	10/31/2002	11/6/2002	
11	10	F	1/3/1908	94	11/11/2002	11/25/2002	

Figure 3.18 Calculation of age

Table 3.1   Formula for Figure 3.17

Cell	Formula	Action
F2	=E2-D2	Copy cell down to F101

Table 3.2   Formula for Figure 3.18

Cell	Formula	Action
D2	=TRUNC(YEARFRAC(E2,C2))	Copy cell down to D101

Table 3.3   Formula for Figure 3.19

Cell	Formula	Action
C2	=IF(B25"F",1,0)	Copy cell down to C101

Inserting a New Worksheet in a Current Workbook

Now that the age at admission and length of stay have been calculated, it is reasonable to assume that we will not need DOB, DOA, or DOD (date of birth, date of admission, and date of discharge, respectively) any further in our data analysis. So we can now create a spreadsheet that does not include these variables. To do this, we insert a new spreadsheet in the existing Excel workbook by using the Insert ➤ Sheet option from the Cells menu in the Home ribbon. We then highlight the entire original worksheet (containing the data as originally imported to Excel). This is accomplished by right-clicking the box in the extreme upper left-hand corner of the spreadsheet (the intersection of the letters designating the columns and the numbers designating the rows) and right-click ➤ Copy. We then move to the new spreadsheet (which is probably labeled "Sheet1") and left-click in cell A1. Finally, we right-click ➤ Paste. The entire data set will now be copied to the new spreadsheet.

Having copied the data set to the new spreadsheet, we can now delete the columns DOB, DOA, and DOD. But before we do that, it is necessary to convert the two variables—Age and LOS—from formulas dependent on DOB, DOA, and DOD to actual numbers. To do this, first highlight the entire Age column, and while the column is highlighted right-click and select Copy, then right-click the column again and select Paste Special ➤Values. This will change the entries in the Age column from a formula dependent on DOB and DOA to actual numbers. Repeat the process for LOS. Now, finally, you can delete DOB, DOA, and DOD by clicking the appropriate column letter (C for DOB in Figure 3.18) and selecting Edit ➤ Delete.

Transforming Categorical Variables into Numerical Variables

One last data modification should be discussed before we leave the topic of importing data and making them ready for analysis. This is the transformation of categorical variables to numeric variables. Certain data analysis techniques to be discussed later in the book—such as cross-tabulations and chi-square statistics, t tests, and analysis of variance—can accept categorical variables—in the form, for example, of sex as "F" or "M." Other techniques,

	A	B	C	D	E	F	G	H	I	J
			C2			=IF(B2="F",1,0)				
1	ID	Sex	Sex1	Age	LOS	DRG	Charges	Medicare	Diag	ICD-9
2	1	F	1	46	4	294	$ 2,426.48	$ 2,003.62	2	0
3	2	F	1	87	8	139	$ 6,815.61	$ 1,072.17	4	4
4	3	F	1	70	10	34	$ 7,596.68	$ 4,096.98	6	0
5	4	M	0	72	5	140	$ 6,450.77	$ 1,710.79	5	0
6	5	F	1	82	3	141	$ 3,542.79	$ 1,914.90	3	7
7	6	F	1	85	2	15	$ 2,590.86	$ 2,601.14	5	4
8	7	F	1	73	5	294	$ 5,082.83	$ 2,035.31	7	2
9	8	M	0	65	6	241	$ 3,580.55	$ 2,320.42	6	0
10	9	M	0	73	6	335	$11,045.79	$ 4,184.26	1	0
11	10	F	1	94	11	148	$10,708.11	$12,158.49	4	0

Figure 3.19 Imported file ready for analysis

particularly regression, cannot accept categorical variables. But a variable such as sex can be included as an independent variable in regression if it is recoded as what is called a *dummy variable*. A dummy variable is one that takes on two values (as does sex) but is coded 1 for one of the values and 0 for the other.

The result of the import process with the data modified for analysis might be as shown in Figure 3.19. The figure shows Sex1 as modified to a 1/0 variable (with the =IF() statement that produces that change shown in the formula bar). It also shows the ID number and the other variables—Sex, Age, LOS, MS-DRG, Charges, Medicare (payments), Diag (diagnosis), and ICD-9. This working file no longer contains any dates. But if the dates become important at some time during the analysis, it will always be possible to recover them from the original imported worksheet by matching the ID numbers on both worksheets.

EXERCISES FOR SECTION 3.3

1. Using the data in Chpt 3-3.txt (this is the data set discussed in Section 3.3), do the following:

   a. Import the data to a spreadsheet by using the Text Import Wizard.

   b. Make the data century-correct as discussed in relation to Figure 3.15.

   c. Provide a label line above the data (it will become row 1) and label the data, as shown in Figure 3.16.

   d. Insert a column after DOD, as shown in Figure 3.17, and calculate the LOS for each observation.

   e. Insert a column after DOB and calculate Age for each person, as shown in Figure 3.18.

   f. Insert a column after Sex and create a variable Sex1, as shown in Figure 3.19.

   g. Save the result as an Excel file.

2. Chpt 3-4.txt is a data file for 50 people from which the first 20 were selected, as shown in Figure 3.2. Use the Text Import Wizard to bring the data into Excel and do the following:

    a. Insert a column at A and give every observation an ID number.

    b. Insert a column at B and, using Date of Birth and Date of Visit, calculate an Age for each person.

    c. Insert a column at D and, using Opinion 1, convert the words to numbers, with All of the time being 5, Most of the time being 4, and so on. Name this variable Opinion 1a.

    d. Insert a column at E and, using Opinion 2, convert the words to numbers, with Strongly agree being 5, Agree being 4, and so on. Name this variable Opinion 2a.

    e. Insert a column at F, name it Charges, and accumulate the costs for Procedure 1 through Procedure 4 in that column.

    f. Insert a column at G, name it Visit Time, and, using Arrival time and Departure time, calculate the number of minutes for each visit. (Hint: Format Visit time using the second format option under Time.)

    g. Use Edit ➤ Copy, Edit ➤ Paste Special ➤ Values to fix all the calculations, and save the result as an .xls file.

3.4 Missing Data

One thing we have not yet discussed in regard to the use of data—either collected by the investigator or taken from an existing source—is missing data. The term "missing data" refers to the situation in which some of the observations have no data at all for some or all of the variables under study. In the example given in Section 3.3, the missing data issue was not considered because it was known at the outset that no data were missing. But in most real applications, it is likely that some of the observations will be missing some data. The question then is what to do about this.

First, it is important to recognize that virtually all statistical techniques assume complete data. If one wished to use a statistic to determine, for example, if males had greater or lesser hospital charges than females, based on the data discussed in the previous section, it would be assumed that complete data were available for sex and hospital charges for all 100 observations. But let us now assume that complete data were not available for all 100 observations. Let us assume that some of the data for charges are missing—specifically, that there are no charge data for 9 of the 100 observations. How might we deal with that situation?

Remedy for Missing Data: Case Deletion

The simplest way to deal with the missing charges in this case would be to delete those observations from the data set and base the analysis on 91 rather than 100 observations. There are difficulties with this strategy, however. The first and, in this case, the least important is that dropping the observations with no charge data from the data set reduces the number of observations under consideration. Consequently, the likelihood of finding a statistically significant difference between males and females, if one exists, is also reduced. In general, the more observations one has made, the more likely it is that statistical significance could be found. But going from 100 to 91 cases is likely to have little effect on statistical outcomes. The decrease is a proportionally small one in an already relatively large number for statistical purposes. However, going from 100 cases to 30 or from 30 cases to 20 would have a substantial effect on the ability to find statistically significant results.

Dropping observations can become even more of a problem if there are missing values in more than one of the variables that are to be considered in the statistical analysis. Perhaps there might be nine missing values for charges and five for sex. Unless all the missing values for sex are also missing for charges, there will be more than nine total cases with missing values. All hypothesis testing requires at least two variables, so the number of nonoverlapping missing values in the two variables will determine the number of cases without data. In regression analysis a number of variables may be involved. The total number of missing values will be the total of nonoverlapping missing values for all variables. In some cases, this will act to reduce the total data set to unacceptable levels. In such a case, there are two strategies. The first is to try to go back to the original source to obtain data for the missing values. But this is often impossible.

Remedy for Missing Data: Imputation

The second strategy is to impute—or "fill in"—missing values. There are a number of ways that this may be done, none of which gets high marks from statisticians but which are nevertheless used. The simplest and least time-consuming is to use the mean of the available data to fill in the missing values. So if there are 9 missing values for charges and the mean value for charge for the 91 other observations is $5,676.24, then that value could be assigned to the observations with missing values. There are a number of other strategies, such as using the median or a regression model, that can be used to assign values to missing data. All of these techniques provide somewhat more sophisticated ways of assigning values than does using the simple mean but do require increasingly complex steps. In general, this text will not cover these techniques in any detail.

There is a significant problem with assigning any type of imputed value to data that are missing. Regardless of how it is done, assigning a value to a missing data element will inevitably reduce the variance in that variable. In addition, imputation will be more likely to produce statistically significant results than if the missing values were simply deleted from the data. With this fact in mind, some investigators have used what is known as a *Monte Carlo technique* to randomly assign values within reasonable ranges to the missing elements. They then observe how these assigned values affect the statistical results over a large number of trials. While this is probably the ideal method for assigning missing values, it is both time-consuming and costly in terms of data analysis.

The bottom line with regard to missing data, then, is that it is probably best to drop cases with missing values. However, this rule of thumb applies only if fewer than 10 percent of cases will be dropped and the overall sample size remains relatively large—for example, over 30. If these circumstances do not prevail, randomly assigning reasonable values to the missing elements is probably the best strategy.

KEY TERMS

=OR ( )

=TRUNC ( )

=YEARFRAC ( )

Bernoulli distribution

binomial distribution

delimited

discrete distribution

dummy variable

Monte Carlo technique

patterned distribution

Poisson distribution

Text Import Wizard

uniform distribution

CHAPTER 4

DATA DISPLAY: DESCRIPTIVE PRESENTATION, EXCEL GRAPHING CAPABILITY

Statistics are to baseball what a flaky crust is to Mom's apple pie.

—Harry Reasoner

One of the most important aspects of statistical analysis is to be able to present your results in a way that is easily accessible to your audience. Microsoft Excel provides several useful tools to create accessible presentations. These include, in particular, the Excel frequency function, the Excel pivot table report capabilities, and the Excel graphing capability.

4.1 Creating, Displaying, and Understanding Frequency Distributions

One recurring need in statistical analysis is the need to be able to summarize quickly and efficiently the data that are under analysis. Later sections of the book, particularly Chapter 6, discuss measures of central tendency and dispersion (the mean and the standard deviation). Mean and standard deviation are useful devices for summarizing numerical data. This section discusses the Excel =FREQUENCY() function that was introduced in Chapter 2.

Recall the data file that was imported to Excel in Chapter 3. When the import process was finished, that file contained an ID number for each record and nine variables. The variables were *Sex* (as indicated by "F" and "M"), *Sex* (the *Sex* variable recoded to 1 and 0), *Age*,

LEARNING OBJECTIVES

- Understand how to create and display frequency distributions
- Understand how to create and display cumulative frequency distributions
- Be able to identify skewed, normal, and uniform distributions
- Understand how to create a pivot table
- Understand how to create a Pareto diagram

LOS (length of hospital stay), *MS-DRG*, *Charges*, *Medicare* (payments), *Diag* (number of diagnoses), and *ICD-9* (the admitting ICD-9 code). Although the file consisted of only 100 records selected from a much larger set, it was still impossible in the original presentation of the data import discussion to show more than a few of the records in the figures that were presented. Those figures gave some indication of what the data were like. For example, Age tended to be above the average age of the general population; this is not surprising, given that this is a Medicare-eligible population. Charges—for the records that were visible in the tables—were in the thousands of dollars. Length of stay ranged from 2 days to more than 10 days. But viewing the small portion of the records shown in the tables does not provide a very good idea of what the data actually look like.

Of course, if one has access to the Excel data file, it is possible to view all 100 observations to get a better idea of the nature of the data. But an alternative to viewing all the data as 100 separate observations is to use the =FREQUENCY() function to summarize the data. To see the use of the =FREQUENCY() function for summarizing data, consider the variable Age, for which we are going to generate a frequency distribution. The frequency distribution groups the ages into a small number of categories that include all the ages in the 100 observations. The first step in creating the frequency distribution is to determine the minimum and maximum ages represented in the data. To do this, we use the Excel =MIN() and =MAX() functions. For example, Figure 4.1 displays the minimum and maximum of the data set while actually showing the =MIN() function.

The =MIN() and =MAX() Functions

The =MIN() and =MAX() functions are a way of determining the minimum and maximum values in any set of data. In Figure 4.1, it can be seen that the minimum age is 39 (cell C2) and the maximum age is 96 (cell C3). The way in which the =MIN() and =MAX() functions are written is shown for

Figure 4.1 =MIN() and =MAX() functions

=MIN() in the formula line. Basically, the =MIN() and =MAX() functions each take a single argument, but this argument represents a *data range*. In Excel, data ranges are indicated by the two cell references that define the range separated by a colon (e.g., cell C2 is =MIN(B2:B101)).

In developing a frequency distribution, it is important to have the proper amount of categories. You wish to ensure that there will be enough categories but not too many. In general, having five to eight categories is probably useful in developing a frequency distribution. Fewer than five will not give enough categories to show a meaningful picture of the data, and many more than eight is difficult to conceptualize at a single glance. Having determined that the minimum age in the 100 records is 39 and the maximum age is 96, it is necessary to decide how many categories the frequency distribution will contain. In this case, we will develop a frequency distribution with six categories—in general, one category for each 10-year age group (e.g., 40, 50, 60, 70, 80, and 90).

Defining Bins for the Frequency Distribution

Figure 4.2 shows the completed frequency distribution with six categories. The individual cells contain the following information. Cell C4 contains the difference between 96 and 39. This age separation (57 years) will be divided into six categories for the frequency distribution. Cell C5 is 57 divided by 6. Each category for the frequency distribution will include 9.5 years of age. Column D represents what Excel refers to as *Bins*. Bins are the categories that define the frequency distributions. The first Bin value is the minimum age (cell C2) plus the size of the first frequency category (9.5 years in cell C5) or =C2+C5. Each observation with an age of 48.5 years or less (actually, 48 years, because the years are given in whole numbers only) will be recorded in cell E2 to represent that it is in that age category.

Cell D2 is simply cell C2 plus cell C5. The additional Bin values make use of the F4 function key and the dollar sign ($) convention. This convention

E2			= {=FREQUENCY(B2:B101,D2:D7)}		
	A	B	C	D	E	F
1	ID	Age		Bins	Freq	
2	1	46	39	48.5	2	
3	2	87	96	58.0	4	
4	3	70	57	67.5	5	
5	4	72	9.5	77.0	36	
6	5	82		86.5	33	
7	6	85		96.0	20	
8	7	73				
9	8	65				
10	9	73				
11	10	94				

Figure 4.2 Frequency distribution of age

	A	B	C	D	E
1	ID	Age		Bins	Freq
2	1	46	=MIN(B2:B101)	=C2+C5	=FREQUENCY(B2:B101,D2:D7)
3	2	87	=MAX(B2:B101)	=D2+$C$5	=FREQUENCY(B2:B101,D2:D7)
4	3	70	=C3-C2	=D3+$C$5	=FREQUENCY(B2:B101,D2:D7)
5	4	72	=C4/6	=D4+$C$5	=FREQUENCY(B2:B101,D2:D7)
6	5	82		=D5+$C$5	=FREQUENCY(B2:B101,D2:D7)
7	6	85		=D6+$C$5	=FREQUENCY(B2:B101,D2:D7)
8	7	73			
9	8	65			
10	9	73			
11	10	94			

Figure 4.3 Formulas for frequency distribution of age

is employed so that the formula for these Bins need be written only once (in cell D3). The formula can then be copied into the remaining four cells by dragging or double-clicking the lower right corner of cell D3. Figure 4.3 shows the formulas that have been used to create the frequency distribution shown in Figure 4.2. Essentially, the BIN range (9.5 years) has been added successively to each of the previous Bin values.

The Structure and Use of the =FREQUENCY() Function

When the =FREQUENCY() function is invoked, Excel looks at each data value and compares it with each Bin value. If the data value is equal to or less than any Bin value but larger than any other Bin value, Excel adds 1 to the total for that Bin. It is important to remember that the value of a Bin that appears on the spreadsheet is the largest value that will be recorded in any specific Bin. The =FREQUENCY() function is shown in the formula line of Figure 4.2 and in cells E2 to E7 of Figure 4.3. The format of the =FREQUENCY() function can be seen in either view. The function takes two arguments, the first being the DATA range (in this case, B2:B101, representing the Age data) and the second being the BIN range (in this case, D2:D7). In the formula line of Figure 4.2, the two curly braces that surround the =FREQUENCY() function indicate that it is an Excel function you invoke by pressing Ctrl+Shift and then Enter.

The formulas view of the spreadsheet is available in Excel at any time by clicking the Formula ribbon ➤ Formula Auditing tab ➤ Show Formulas menu (icon in top right). The same process can be accomplished by clicking the File tab and then clicking the Excel Options button ➤ Advanced option ➤ Display options for this worksheet ➤ Show formulas in the cells instead of their calculated results.

Using the Histogram Tool to Graph a Frequency Distribution

Given the spreadsheet in Figure 4.2, use the following steps to create a frequency distribution with Excel's Histogram tool.

1. On the Data ribbon select the Data Analysis menu from the Analysis tab to display the Data Analysis dialog box (see Figure 4.4). In this dialog box, select Histogram and click OK. The Histogram dialog box will appear, and you now need to input your data (see Figure 4.5).

2. Click in the text box to the right of the Input Range label, and enter the range for the data, including the label, by typing B1:B101 or by clicking on cell B1 and dragging to cell B101.

3. Click in the text box to the right of the Bin Range label, and enter the range for the Bin Ranges, including the label, by typing D1:D7 or by clicking cell D1 and dragging to cell D7.

4. Click the Labels checkbox to select it. This informs the Histogram tool that you have included labels with your data entries.

5. In the Output Options area, click the radio button corresponding to the appropriate output option. Generally, the best option is to select New Worksheet Ply. This option cuts down on the clutter of your main data sheet.

6. In the area at the bottom of the dialog box, click the checkboxes to select Cumulative Percentage and Chart Output.

7. Click OK to dismiss the dialog box, and Excel will compute and display output resembling that in Figure 4.6.

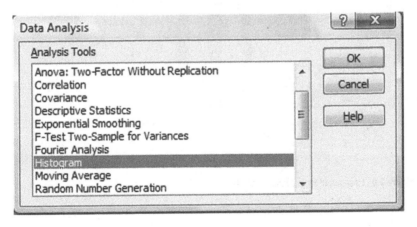

Figure 4.4 Data Analysis dialog box

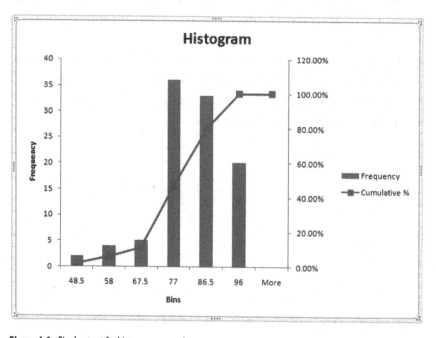

Figure 4.5   Histogram dialog box

Figure 4.6   Final output for histogram example

Figure 4.6 shows a *histogram* overlaid with a cumulative percentage diagram. The scale on the left depicts the frequency, and the scale on the right depicts the cumulative percentile. The data table in the upper left of the spreadsheet displays the Bin and frequency data (refer to Figure 4.6). This type of graph can also be created using the Charts function in Excel and is presented next.

Using the Chart Function to Graph a Frequency Distribution

The frequency distribution shown in cells E2:E7 of Figure 4.2 displays a distribution that has only a few observations in the lower ages and many more in the upper ages. This type of distribution is said to be skewed to the left because it seems to tail off to the left. This tailing off can be seen in Figure 4.7 as the bars on the left of the chart are smaller in height than the bars on the right of the chart. The fact that most people in the data set are in the older ages is not surprising because, as noted earlier, this is a Medicare-eligible population. But seeing the actual numbers in a frequency distribution is only one way of picturing (and hence understanding) the data. An additional valuable tool for viewing a frequency distribution is the Charts function or graphing capability of Excel, which was also discussed in Chapter 2. Click the Insert tab to construct a column chart of the data in cells E2:E7, as shown in Figure 4.7.

Creating a Column Chart

The y-axis in the chart—labeled Observations—was supplied automatically by Excel from the number of observations in each age group. The two labels Age Categories and Observations were entered in the Excel sheet in cells D1 and E1. The numbers on the x-axis represent the Bin values in cells D2:D7. We included these in the chart by selecting cells D1 through E7 and clicking the Column icon on the Insert ribbon. A two-dimensional column chart is then chosen, and an initial column chart is created. However, the

Figure 4.7 Chart of the age frequency distribution

initial column chart needs to be formatted to look like the one in Figure 4.7. Right-click the column chart and choose the Select Data option, and the Select Data Source dialog box will appear (see Figure 2.18). Within this dialog box select Age Categories in the Legend Entries area and click the Remove button. Also, in the Horizontal (Category) Axis Labels area click Edit; when the Axis labels range box appears, highlight cells D2 through D7 and click OK. This deletes the Age Categories as data to be graphed and adds the proper x-axis scale. The titles Graph of Age, Observations, and Age Categories can be modified by using any of the style buttons on the Design ribbon (e.g., adding a title for the y-axis).

In any chart, such as the one shown in Figure 4.4, the y-axis is always considered to be the vertical axis on the left and the x-axis is always considered to be the horizontal axis on the bottom.

The view of the data in Figure 4.7 clearly shows the tail to the left that makes these data skewed to the left. It also shows that the largest single category is the age group with the x-axis value of 77.0. It should be remembered that the x-axis designation 77.0 actually refers to all observations with ages between 67.5 years and 77.0 years. This characteristic of Excel, to use the largest value in a frequency as the Bin value, can be confusing when displayed in a chart such as that shown in Figure 4.7. Because the x-axis values are supplied by the creator of the chart, the x-axis labels can be made more descriptive.

Figure 4.8 shows part of the spreadsheet for the Age frequency distribution. The figure includes the graph of the frequency distribution with new x-axis designations. You put these into the chart by first entering them as a set of categories in cells E9: E14. Change the x-axis in the chart by right-clicking the column chart and choosing the Select Data option. The Select Data Source dialog box will appear (see Figure 2.18). Within this dialog box select the Horizontal (Category) Axis Labels area and click Edit; when the Axis labels range box appears, highlight cells E9 through E14 and click OK. This makes the x-axis labels much more descriptive of what is actually in those categories and what the bars in the graph actually represent. It is worth mentioning that the chart shown in Figure 4.8 is the same chart (in the original spreadsheet) as that shown in Figure 4.7. This demonstrates an extremely useful and important characteristic of the Charts function: When you change the data or labels that make up the chart, the corresponding changes appear in the Excel chart. This applies

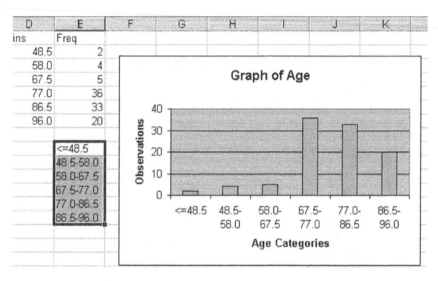

Figure 4.8 Chart of age showing BIN ranges

whether different data or labels are selected or when changes to the actual data or labels are made.

It is important to mention that the categories shown in Figure 4.8 are still not exactly right. The range 48.5 to 58.0, for example, is actually any age greater than 48.5 to 58.0, because if there were an age recorded as 48.5, it would be in the <=48.5 category. This is true in every other Age category as well.

Various Charting Types within Excel

Data can be displayed in a number of other ways using the Charts function. In fact, Excel offers 14 standard types of graphs and 20 of what Excel calls custom types. All of the standard types have a number of subtypes. For most of the work in this book, the simple column chart (frequently called a histogram) is all that will be used. However, it is also useful to look at four other of the charts that Excel can produce.

Creating a Line Chart The first alternative chart type is the line chart, a column chart in which the presentation is made with a single line rather than with a number of columns. The data charted in Figure 4.9 are the same as those charted in Figures 4.7 and 4.8, but the columns have been changed to a single line. This is done by selecting the chart in Figure 4.8, selecting the Change Chart Type icon in the Type group on the Design ribbon, and then choosing the Line chart option. It is not uncommon to make the addition to the line chart by dropping the line to the *x*-axis at each end. This was

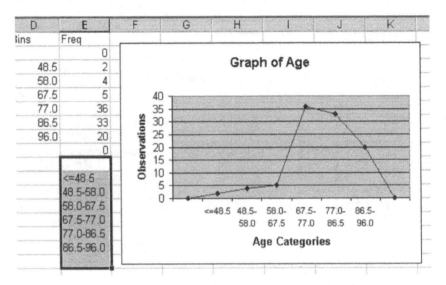

Figure 4.9 Line chart depiction of age frequencies

done by inserting a zero cell at both ends of the frequency distribution and a blank cell at each end of the Age categories that form the x-axis values. Then, both the zero values and the blank cells were included as part of the chart. The result is the data depiction in Figure 4.9.

Creating a Bar Chart   A second chart of interest is the bar chart, as shown in Figure 4.10. The bar chart shows exactly the same information as that shown in the column chart, but it shows it in a different orientation. To put the data into this chart, it was necessary only to select the chart in Figure 4.8, choose the Change Chart Type icon in the Type group on the Design ribbon, and then choose the Bar chart option. Notice that with the bar chart the smallest charted value is always at the lower end of the vertical column.

Figure 4.10 Bar chart depiction of age frequencies

Creating a Pie Chart   A third chart that is useful to consider is the pie chart. The pie chart presents data as the pieces of a pie, each piece representing its proportional part of the whole. The notion that each piece represents its proportional part of the whole is a significant factor in the use of a pie chart. The pie chart assumes that the material depicted represents the entire set of information and, furthermore, that all the pieces accumulate to the total. This is true with the Age data. Each frequency category represents a part of the entire frequency distribution, and all taken together add to all 100 observations. The pie chart can be created from the original chart shown in Figure 4.8 by selecting the chart again, choosing the Change Chart Type icon in the Type group on the Design ribbon, and then choosing the Pie chart option. The result, after some manipulation of labels and axes, is shown in Figure 4.11.

It is important to reiterate that the pie chart, by its very nature, implies that 100 percent of observations of any type are being included in the graph. This is further depicted by the percentages that are shown in the chart in Figure 4.11, which add to 100 percent. A pie chart should never be used to depict a total amount and its subcomponents together, or part of a total amount.

Creating an XY(Scatter) Chart   To this point, the discussion has focused on looking at the frequency distribution of a single variable at a time. Excel offers an entirely different type of chart that can be very useful in examining the relationship between two separate variables at the same time. This is what Excel calls the XY(Scatter) chart. The XY chart requires two separate variables. The XY chart of Age and LOS (length of stay) is shown in Figure 4.12. Several points about this chart should be mentioned. First, this chart is not based on frequencies in categories, as the other charts discussed here have been, but on the actual values of the two variables. The horizontal

Figure 4.11   Pie chart depiction of age frequencies

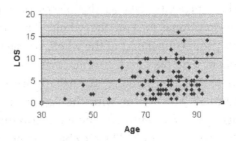

Figure 4.12 XY(Scatter) chart of age and LOS

axis, or x-axis, represents the values of the variable Age. The lowest value of Age in the data set is 39 and the highest value of Age is 99. The vertical axis, or y-axis, represents the values of the variable LOS (length of stay). LOS ranges from the shortest length of stay of 1 day to the longest stay of 16 days.

Excel always treats the left-most variable in the spreadsheet as the x-axis variable when constructing an XY chart and the right-most variable as the y-axis variable. The variables do not have to be in contiguous columns to construct the XY chart, but the data must begin in the same row in order to successfully construct an XY chart. Each diamond in the XY chart represents one observation. For example, the left-most diamond in the chart represents the single person who was 39 years of age and had a hospital stay of one day. The only diamond above the line marked 15 on the vertical axis is the single person who had a 16-day hospital stay. The person staying 16 days appears to have been 83 years old. The person's age is read from the horizontal axis. Each of the other points in the chart is interpreted in the same way, although one would not count on the chart to know the actual values. The chart works more to provide a general view of what the entire data distribution looks like. This information is valuable, particularly in deciding whether regression analysis (discussed in Chapters 11 to 13) will be appropriate to the data.

Cumulative Frequencies and Percentage Distributions

Obtaining a frequency distribution of a numerical variable is one way to understand the nature of the data. It is often useful to look also at the *cumulative frequency* distribution, the percentage distributions, and cumulative percentage distributions. This section considers these three distributions.

Creating a Cumulative Frequency Distribution

A cumulative frequency distribution begins with the smallest Bin value. It then accumulates observations so that the first category contains only the

	D	E	F	G	H
1	Bins	Freq	Cum Freq	Perc	Cum Perc
2	48.5	2	2	2%	2%
3	58.0	4	6	4%	6%
4	67.5	5	11	5%	11%
5	77.0	36	47	36%	47%
6	86.5	33	80	33%	80%
7	96.0	20	100	20%	100%

Figure 4.13 Cumulative frequency and percentage distributions

	D	E	F	G	H
1	Bins	Freq	Cum Freq	Perc	Cum Perc
2	=C2+C5	=FREQUENCY(B2:B101,D2:D7)	=E2	=E2/$F$7	=G2
3	=D2+$C$5	=FREQUENCY(B2:B101,D2:D7)	=F2+E3	=E3/$F$7	=H2+G3
4	=D3+$C$5	=FREQUENCY(B2:B101,D2:D7)	=F3+E4	=E4/$F$7	=H3+G4
5	=D4+$C$5	=FREQUENCY(B2:B101,D2:D7)	=F4+E5	=E5/$F$7	=H4+G5
6	=D5+$C$5	=FREQUENCY(B2:B101,D2:D7)	=F5+E6	=E6/$F$7	=H5+G6
7	=D6+$C$5	=FREQUENCY(B2:B101,D2:D7)	=F6+E7	=E7/$F$7	=H6+G7

Figure 4.14 Formula view of Figure 4.13

observations in that Bin, the second category contains observations in both the first and second Bins, the third contains observations in the first three Bins, and so on. Figure 4.13 shows a cumulative frequency distribution for the variable Age in cells F2:F7. The cumulative frequency was calculated by making cell F2 equal to cell E2 and then adding each successive cell in column E to the current total in column F. For example, cell F3 is =F2+E3 and cell F4 is =F3+E4.

The formulas used to construct the cumulative frequency are shown in the formula view of Figure 4.13, which is given in Figure 4.14. Cell F2 in this view shows that it is simply equal to E2. Cell F3 shows that the number in that cell was developed with the formula =F2+E3. Once =F2+E3 has been entered into cell F3, the remainder of the cells in column F can be entered by copying cell F3 down. This can be accomplished by placing the cursor in the lower right corner of cell F3 and either dragging the cell references down to cell F7 or double-clicking the lower right corner of cell F3. As the formula moves down each cell, it becomes the correct formula for that cell by virtue of relative cell referencing. It is extremely important to remember that, in general, you need enter any formula into Excel only once. You are doing way too much work if you enter the formulas for cells F3:F7 separately in each cell.

Creating a Percentage and Cumulative Percentage Distribution

Cells G2:G7 and H2:H7 in Figures 4.13 and 4.14 show the percentage distribution and the cumulative percentage distribution for the *Age*

frequency data. Because the original data involved exactly 100 observations, the percentage values are the same as the actual frequencies. In
general, this will not be the case. In any event, the formulas for the percentage distribution are clearly different from the formulas for the actual
frequencies (cells E2:E7), which rely on the =FREQUENCY() function. The
formulas for the percentage distribution (column G) rely on the dollar sign
($) convention (cycle through with function key F4) to fix cell F7 as the
cell by which each value in column E is divided. Again, it is necessary only
to enter the formula =E2/$F$7 (F7 is the cumulative total value) into
cell G2. Then the formula can be copied into each of the other five cells
in column G. The relative reference to each cell in E in the numerator
changes as the formula is copied down column G, but because of the dollar
signs before the F and before the 7 in the denominator, that reference does
not change.

The formulas for the cumulative percentage distribution (H2:H7) are
the same as the formulas for the cumulative frequency distribution. Because
of this, it is necessary only to copy the range F2:F7 and then paste the copy
into cell H2. That will enter all the values for the cumulative percentage
distribution in H2:H7. It should be mentioned that the actual values that
will appear in both G2:G7 and H2:H7 will be decimal values until they are
reformatted to percentages. This can be done by highlighting G2:H7 and
from the Home ribbon choosing the Cells tab ➤ Format menu ➤ Format
Cells menu and choosing Percentage on the Number tab, or by highlighting
G2:H7 and clicking the % icon on the Number tab in the Home ribbon.

It may be useful to look at a graph that includes both the actual
frequency and the cumulative frequency. Figure 4.15 shows such a graph.
The actual frequency is in light gray, and the cumulative frequency is shown
in dark gray. It should be mentioned that a number of things were done

Figure 4.15 Graph of age showing actual and cumulative values

to this graph to make it look as it does (and almost all graphs need some modifications to make them look good when they are first created).

Modifying a Chart

When a graph is first generated, it frequently is too narrow vertically to provide a very good view of the comparative length of the columns, so this graph was stretched out both vertically and horizontally. (After clicking on the chart, grab one of the black squares on the chart border to resize it.) The data labels, Freq and Cum Freq, were initially given as Series 1 and Series 2. These were modified by changing and/or including the cell references for the names in the data series. This is accomplished using the Select Data Source dialog box. Once the name has been changed, the new name will appear in the Series window. Series 2 was renamed Cum Freq in the same way.

The Age categories shown in Figure 4.15 were originally given in too large a font to be displayed entirely in the graph. They were also displayed at an angle because of their larger size. To put them into the form in which they now appear, it was first necessary to right-click anywhere in the set of numbers that appeared as the Age categories (the horizontal scale) to invoke a pop-up menu that allows you to access areas such as Font or the Format Axis dialog box. After that Font option was selected, the font size was changed to 9 from 12. Then the Format Axis dialog box was chosen, the Alignment tab was selected, and the cursor was used to move the diamond on that tab from the horizontal and back again. That produced the Age category format, as shown in the figure.

The initial graph, before reformatting, also had a vertical scale that went to 120. As there are only 100 total observations, and in order to indicate that the last dark gray column represented all of the observations, the vertical scale was changed so that it would go only to 100. This was done by right-clicking anywhere in the numbers on the vertical scale to invoke the Format Axis dialog box for the vertical axis. After left-clicking that menu, select the Axis Options tab and change the maximum to 100. The graph as it appears in Figure 4.15 is the result of all these operations.

The total number of changes and modifications that can be made to a graph to serve the purposes desired is extremely large—far beyond what can be described in this text. The plot area itself can be reformatted in a number of ways, the colors of the columns can be changed, and many other modifications can be made. The only way to get a good notion of the modifications that can be made in an Excel graph is to create a graph and experiment with the various options. Sooner or later, you will hit on a series of style changes that will best serve your purposes.

Types of Distributions

Frequency distributions can take on many different shapes, but four different distribution configurations deserve mention. These are *skewed left, skewed right, normal,* and *uniform distributions,* examples of which are shown in Figure 4.16. The distribution that is skewed left appears to have a tail that moves off to the left side of the distribution while the bulk of the observations are to the right. The distribution that is skewed right appears to have a tail to the right while the bulk of the observations are to the left. The distribution that is generally referred to as normal will be discussed in detail in Chapters 5 and 6, but it essentially has tails of equal length, and the bulk of the observations are in the center of the distribution. The uniform distribution (sometimes called a flat distribution) has equal numbers of observations at each point in the distribution.

Skewed Distributions

The graph of Age shown in Figure 4.7, as well as subsequent graphs, is skewed to the left because the distribution shows the characteristic tail on the left side of the distribution. Data distributions may also be skewed to the right. In the data file under discussion thus far in this chapter, *LOS*

Figure 4.16   Four distribution types

Graph of Medicare Payments

Figure 4.17　Graph of Medicare payments

(length of stay), *Charges* (total hospital charges), and *Medicare* (Medicare payments) are all skewed to the right.

Figure 4.17 shows the distribution of Medicare payments in six categories. It is clear that this distribution has a tail that moves off to the right, thus making it right-skewed. In general, it is more common to encounter distributions that are right-skewed than distributions that are left-skewed. Costs of health services (office visits, hospital stays, emergency room visits, or any other categories of cost) are likely to be skewed to the right. This is because most costs will be more or less similar, but there will be a few encounters with very high costs. This produces a distribution that is skewed to the right. Disease or morbidity patterns are similar.

The State of the World's Children 2001 (2000) provides one example of a distribution that is skewed to the right. UNICEF reports data on infant mortality for countries of the world at https://www.unicef.org/media/84781/file/SOWC-2001.pdf. According to UNICEF, infant mortality for 149 countries of the world with more than 1 million inhabitants ranged in 1999 from a high of 182 deaths per 1,000 live births (Sierra Leone) to a low of 3 deaths per 1,000 live births (Sweden and Switzerland). But the distribution of infant mortality by countries of the world is skewed to the right, as demonstrated in Figure 4.18.

As Figure 4.18 shows, more than 70 countries of the world have infant mortality rates of 33 or less. The number of countries with infant mortality rates in each of the higher categories decreases monotonically to the 153-to-183 deaths category. There are exactly five countries in this category. This distribution is decidedly skewed to the right.

Normal Distributions

The *normal distribution* is one that is skewed neither to the right nor to the left but, rather, has tails of approximately equal length. Exact characteristics of normal distributions will be discussed in Chapters 5 and 6. But for the

Figure 4.18   Infant mortality for 149 countries of the world

current presentation, the notion that the normal distribution is skewed in neither direction is sufficient. Approximately normal distributions are found in many health care–related types of data. The body temperature of healthy human beings, for example, is probably normally distributed around 98.6 degrees. Not every person's body temperature is exactly 98.6 degrees; body temperature varies from that normal temperature by a fraction of a degree or more. This variance is probably as likely to be below 98.6 as it is likely to be above 98.6. Average height of adults is another example of data that are generally normally distributed with a more or less equal number of persons on each side of the distribution.

Data on infant mortality for the world are skewed to the right. But data on infant mortality for the United States by state more closely approximate a normal distribution. Infant mortality in the United States ranged in 1998 from a low of 4.4 deaths per 1,000 live births (New Hampshire) to 10.2 deaths per 1,000 live births (Alabama) (U.S. Census Bureau, 2001, p. 89).

The graph of infant mortality by state in the United States is shown in Figure 4.19. This graph clearly shows that the bulk of states have infant mortality rates in the center of the distribution rather than at the left side. The number of states that have infant mortality rates at each end of the continuum is, while not exactly equal, certainly in the same order of magnitude. The infant mortality rate by state in the United States is much closer to normal than that for the same measure by countries of the world.

Uniform Distributions

Although uniform distributions are not often found in health statistics, it is still useful for comparative purposes to show an example of one. A uniform distribution is one that has approximately equal numbers at each interval. To give an example of a uniform distribution, the random number generation selection in the Data Analysis add-in was used and

Figure 4.19 Infant mortality for states of the United States

Figure 4.20 Simulation of the roll of a fair die 100 times

the Uniform distribution option was selected. This option allows one to generate a random number between any upper and lower limits. One hundred random numbers were generated in the range zero to six. The random number generation add-in produces numbers to nine decimal places. Then the =FREQUENCY() function is used to put these numbers into the six categories—1, 2, 3, 4, 5, and 6. This is a reasonable simulation of the roll of a fair die 100 times. The result is shown in Figure 4.20. An actual uniform distribution (or a simulated one as in Figure 4.20) will not look exactly like the example in the lower right quadrant of Figure 4.16, but it will look approximately like that example.

EXERCISES FOR SECTION 4.1

Use the data file created in Exercise 1 of Section 3.3 or use the Hospital Charges sheet in the file Chpt 4-1.xls. This data set corresponds to the data set discussed in Section 4.1.

1. Select the variable Age, and do the following:

    a. Using the =MIN(), =MAX(), and =FREQUENCY() functions, replicate Figure 4.2.

b. Using the results just obtained, generate the chart shown in Figure 4.8 and put in the relevant labels as shown in that chart. Show this chart on the spreadsheet.

c. Modifying the data as shown in Figure 4.9, generate a line chart as shown in that figure, and show this chart on the spreadsheet.

d. Create a bar chart as shown in Figure 4.10, and show it on the spreadsheet.

e. Create a pie chart as shown in Figure 4.11, and modify it to look as much like that figure as possible; show this chart on the spreadsheet.

f. Replicate the chart of Age and LOS as shown in Figure 4.12. Show this chart on the spreadsheet.

g. Generate a cumulative frequency for the variable Age as well as percentage and cumulative percentage distributions as shown in Figure 4.13.

h. Create a chart showing the actual and cumulative values of Age as given in Figure 4.15, and show this chart on the spreadsheet.

2. Select the variable Charges and do the following:

a. Using the `=MIN()`, `=MAX()`, and `=FREQUENCY()` functions, create a frequency distribution with seven categories.

b. Using the results just obtained, generate a column chart for the data and put in relevant labels; show this chart on the spreadsheet.

c. Transform the chart into a line chart, and include the necessary additions to make the line drop to the horizontal axis at each end; show this chart on the spreadsheet.

d. Create a bar chart from the data, and show this chart on the spreadsheet.

e. Create a pie chart from the data, put in appropriate labels, and then show this chart on the spreadsheet.

f. Create an XY(Scatter) chart for LOS and Charges, and show this chart on the spreadsheet.

g. Generate a cumulative frequency for the variable Charges as well as percentage and cumulative percentage distributions.

h. Create a chart showing the actual and cumulative values of Charges, and show this chart on the spreadsheet.

3. Use the SWC worksheet in the file Chpt 4-1.xls, and do the following:

a. Generate the appropriate frequency distribution for infant mortality (IMR), and with it replicate Figure 4.18.

b. Generate a frequency distribution of five Bins for under-five mortality (U5MR), and produce a column graph for that variable. Is it normal, flat, or skewed, and if it is skewed, in which direction?

    c. Generate a frequency distribution of eight Bins for life expectancy at birth (LEB), and produce a column graph for that variable. Is it normal, flat, or skewed, and if it is skewed, in which direction?

4. Use the US IMR sheet in the file Chpt 4-1.xls, and do the following:

    a. Generate the appropriate frequency distribution to replicate Figure 4.19, and replicate the figure.

    b. Generate a frequency distribution with 12 Bin categories, and use the column chart option to graph that frequency distribution.

    c. Which of (a) or (b) seems to you to provide the most useful information about the distribution?

5. Use the data from the Hospital Charges worksheet in Chpt 4-1.xls and do the following:

    a. Generate an XY chart for Age and LOS, and show this chart on the spreadsheet.

    b. What conclusions might you draw from this chart about any possible relationship between Age and LOS?

    c. Generate an XY chart for LOS and Charges, and show this chart on the spreadsheet.

    d. What conclusions might you draw from this chart about any possible relationship between LOS and Charges?

6. Use the data from the SWC worksheet in Chpt 4-1.xls, and do the following:

    a. Generate an XY chart for IMR and LEB, and show this chart on the spreadsheet.

    b. What conclusions might you draw from this chart about any possible relationship between IMR and LEB?

4.2   Using the Pivot Table to Generate Frequencies of Categorical Variables

Thus far, the data discussed in this chapter have been numerical data. We are going to turn now to the discussion of frequency distributions for categorical data. There are actually three categorical variables in the data on hospital charges that have been discussed thus far in this chapter. These are Sex, MS-DRG, and ICD-9. In the original data, Sex was given as F or M and was later converted to 1 and 0. But MS-DRG and the ICD-9 code were given as numbers. But despite the fact that they are given as numbers, MS-DRG and ICD-9 remain categorical variables. The numbers simply represent a category rather than having meaning as a number.

Using the categorical variable Sex1 in the data set to create a frequency distribution is fairly easy with the =FREQUENCY() function. Because that variable is coded 0 and 1, it is necessary only to create two Bin values—0 and 1—and use the =FREQUENCY() function to accumulate all 100 observations into these two Bins. But categorical data are not always that easy to work with. If the data were left with the sex variable coded only "F" and "M," the =FREQUENCY() function could not be used.

Access and Setup of the Pivot Table

The alternative, for most categorical data, would be to use what Excel calls the *pivot table*. The interface for pivot tables in Excel has changed since the introduction of Microsoft Office. The following sections will detail only pivot tables using Excel.

Using Excel to Generate Pivot Tables with One Variable

The pivot table function in Excel produces the same output as the pivot table function in earlier versions of Excel. However, the steps and the look of the screens in getting to that output differ. The following are the steps to generate one-variable pivot tables. Another example is given that corresponds to two-variable pivot tables.

Figure 4.21   Create PivotTable dialog box

1. Highlight your data range.
2. On the Insert ribbon, click the PivotTable icon on the far left side in the Tables group.
3. The Create PivotTable dialog box (Figure 4.21) appears. Because your data were highlighted, the Select a table or range radio button is selected and the Table/Range field is filled in. Also, the New Worksheet radio button is selected, signifying where the pivot table will be placed. Click OK.
4. A display resembling Figure 4.22 will appear. This is the pivot table layout screen.
5. In the new worksheet created, you will see that the fields from our source spreadsheet were carried over to the PivotTable Field List on the right.
6. Drag an item, such as Sex, from the PivotTable Field List down to the Rows quadrant. The left side of your Excel spreadsheet should show a row for each Sex value. You should also see a check mark appear next to Sex.
7. To see the count for each Sex, drag the same field to the Values quadrant (see Figure 4.23).
8. In this case, Excel has determined that we wanted a Count of Sex. However, if you click the entry Count of Sex, and then the Value Field Settings option, the Value Field Settings dialog box (Figure 4.24) will appear. Here you can choose another value field from the Summarize value field by scroll menu.

Figure 4.22 Pivot table layout screen

Figure 4.23 Finished pivot table for Sex category

Figure 4.24 Value Field Settings dialog box

EXERCISES FOR SECTION 4.2

1. Use the variable Sex on the Hospital Charges sheet in Chpt 4-1.xls, and do the following.

    a. Create a frequency distribution using the pivot table that replicates the one in Figure 4.23, using Count of Sex in the DATA field.

    b. Create a frequency distribution using the pivot table that replicates the one in Figure 4.23, using Count of Age in the DATA field.

    c. Is there any difference between the two tables you just created? Why or why not?

2. Use the variable LOS on the Hospital Charges sheet in Chpt 4-1.xls, and do the following:

    a. Using a nested =IF() function, create a new variable, LOS1, which will take on the value "Short" when LOS is less than 4 days, "Medium" when LOS is 4 days to 9 days, and "Long" when LOS is 10 days or more.

    b. Create a frequency distribution of LOS1 using the pivot table.

3. Use the MS-DRG worksheet in Chpt 4-2.xls, and do the following:

    a. Create a pivot table for MS-DRG categories.

    b. Sort the data in the pivot table by the frequency of each MS-DRG category.

    c. Generate a cumulative distribution for the MS-DRG data from (a) and a Pareto chart.

4. Use the Late Delivery worksheet in Chpt 4-2.xls. This worksheet is adapted from Figure 4.8 on page 84 of Veney and Kaluzny's *Evaluation and Decision Making for Health Services* (1998). The data in the worksheet show the reason for late delivery of the noon meal for 474 patients on three hospital wards.

    a. Use the pivot table to develop a frequency distribution for reasons for late delivery of the meal.

    b. Sort the frequency distribution so that the reason with the most instances is first, the second next, and so on, and create a chart showing the reasons from most to least.

    c. Generate a cumulative frequency for the data in (a), and construct a Pareto chart of the result.

4.3 A Logical Extension of the Pivot Table: Two Variables

The last topic to consider in this chapter is the logical extension of the pivot table to two variables. A frequency distribution of Sex categories is interesting, but it might also be interesting to know how males and females compare on MS-DRG categories. Of course, certain categories, such as Female reproductive and Male reproductive, will be limited to one sex only.

But how are the admissions in the other categories distributed? The pivot table can provide this information.

When the pivot table is created, the variable Sex will produce a table with two columns instead of the one column that was created in Figure 4.23. A pivot table with two variables when referred to in statistical parlance is more likely to be called a contingency table or a cross-tab (short for *cross-tabulation*).

An important point should be made about the two-variable pivot table that is to be created. There is a reason that Sex is the column heading rather than the row heading, and it goes beyond the fact that MS-DRG was the row heading in the original frequency distribution. This reason has to do with the notion of causality. In general, if one variable may be the cause of the level of another variable, the variable that may be a cause is typically used to define the columns. The other variable is typically used to define the rows.

What is meant by the idea that one variable may be the cause of the level of another variable? In the case of the MS-DRG category and Sex, there is every reason to expect that Sex has some causal relation to who is characterized in which MS-DRG category. Female reproductive disorders, for example, can be relevant only to women. But the pivot table will also show that there are many more women than men with heart and circulatory disorders (there are also twice as many women as men in the sample). On the other hand, there are more men in the respiratory disorder category. These differences can be attributed to Sex. However, it would be unreasonable to imagine the contrary. Only in rare instances would the MS-DRG category a person falls into somehow determine the person's sex. The next section details the steps to create a two-variable pivot table in Excel.

Using Excel to Generate Pivot Tables with Two Variables

The following example is the logical extension of the pivot table example in Section 4.2. The two-variable pivot table considering MS-DRG category and Sex from Section 4.2 is illustrated here using Excel. These are the steps for obtaining the pivot table output.

1. Highlight your data range after you open the Excel spreadsheet.

2. On the Insert ribbon, click the PivotTable icon on the far left side in the Tables group.

3. The Create PivotTable dialog box appears (refer to Figure 4.21). Because your data were highlighted, the Select a table or range radio button is selected and the Table/Range field is filled in. Also, the New Worksheet

button has been selected, signifying where the pivot table will be placed. Click OK.

4. A display resembling Figure 4.25 will appear. This is the pivot table layout screen.

5. In the new worksheet created, you will see that the fields from our source spreadsheet were carried over to the PivotTable Field List on the right.

6. Drag the item DRG Categ from the PivotTable Field List down to the Rows quadrant. In addition, drag the item Sex from the PivotTable Field List down to the Columns quadrant. The left side of your Excel spreadsheet should show a row for each DRG category and a column for each Sex value. You should also see check marks appear next to DRG Categ and Sex.

7. To see the count for each DRG and Sex combination, drag the DRG Categ field to the Values quadrant. Figure 4.26 illustrates what the finished two-variable pivot table looks like.

Working with Pivot Tables: Creating a Pareto Chart

Although pivot tables provide an important means to organize and subsequently analyze data, one other chart that may be interesting to look at

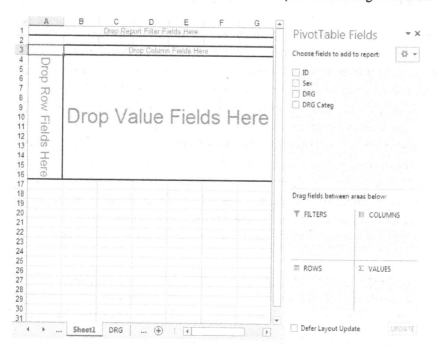

Figure 4.25 Pivot table layout screen

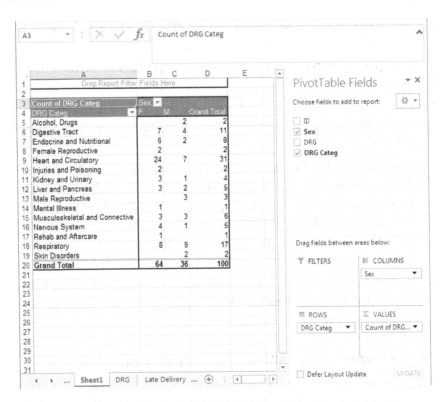

Figure 4.26 Two-variable pivot table for DRG category and Sex

is what is known as a *Pareto chart*. A Pareto chart is a way of looking at both the individual frequencies and the cumulative frequencies at the same time, and it is typically confined to categorical data. The Pareto chart is often used in quality assurance efforts to see where the major problems in some process may lie. However, it can also be used to look at major classes of hospital admission, for example. A Pareto chart combines the actual frequency distribution with the cumulative frequency distribution, as was the case in Figure 4.15. But with a Pareto chart, the categorical data are always arranged in order, from the most frequent to the least frequent, and the cumulative frequency is always shown as a line graph (refer to Figure 4.27 as an example of a Pareto chart for DRG categories).

The easiest way to construct a Pareto chart from a pivot table is as follows:

1. Copy the pivot table, and paste it somewhere else on the spreadsheet, using Edit ➤ Paste Special ➤ Values. This eliminates the interactive nature of the pivot table and allows the inclusion of the cumulative line.

2. Calculate a set of cumulative frequency values, as was done in Figures 4.13 and 4.14.

Note: Use only the Grand Total column from the pivot table (refer to Figure 4.26) to calculate the cumulative frequencies. The female (F) and male (M) columns can be ignored in the creation of the cumulative frequencies.

---

3. Select both the actual and the cumulative frequencies, and click the Column chart icon on the Insert tab of the Excel ribbon to create a new chart. This new chart will be created in the same spreadsheet as the data.

4. Right-click the cumulative frequency data, and select the Change Series Chart Type option.

5. From the Change Chart Type menu, which appears when the data is right-clicked, select the type of chart you wish the cumulative frequency data to resemble. In this case, choose the Line option.

6. Format the x- and y-axes to produce the chart shown in Figure 4.27.

A Pareto chart is typically used in situations where it is useful to be able to see the major problems easily and quickly at the left side of the chart. Of course, with hospital admissions, it is not surprising to see that the major problems are heart/circulatory and respiratory disorders. In other cases, the major problems may not be so obvious until the chart is constructed.

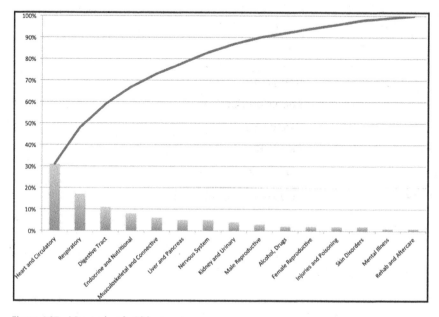

Figure 4.27 A Pareto chart for DRG categories

The cumulative line indicates that all observations are included in the chart, and, as there are 100 observations, the cumulative line ends at 100.

EXERCISES FOR SECTION 4.3

1. Use the data on the MS-DRG worksheet in Chpt 4-2.xls, and use the pivot table capability to replicate Figure 4.26.

2. Use the data on the Late Delivery worksheet in Chpt 4-2.xls, and do the following.

   a. Generate a cross-tabulation using the pivot table capability with Ward as the column heading and Reason as the row heading.

   b. Add a new variable, Reason1, to the Late Delivery worksheet, assigning Other as the label for all but the two most common reasons for late delivery, and generate a cross-tabulation with Ward as the column headings and the reasons in Reason1.

3. Use the data on the SWC worksheet in Chpt 4-1.xls. Create a new variable IMR1, where IMR1 is 0 if IMR is less than 25, 1 if IMR is 25 to 74, and 2 if IMR is greater than 74.

   a. Create a new variable LEB1, where LEB1 is 0 if LEB is less than 50, 1 if LEB is 50 to 69, and 2 if LEB is greater than 69.

   b. Use the pivot table capability to produce a cross-tabulation for IMR1 and LEB1, with IMR1 as the column variable and LEB1 as the row variable. (Be sure to count the data field rather than sum it.)

KEY TERMS

=FREQUENCY ()	histogram
=MAX ()	normal distribution
=MIN ()	Pareto chart
Bins	pivot table
cross-tabulation	skewed left distribution
cumulative frequency	skewed right distribution
data range	

CHAPTER 5

BASIC CONCEPTS OF PROBABILITY

If your experiment needs statistics, you ought to have done a better experiment.

—Ernest Rutherford

LEARNING OBJECTIVES

- Understand initial concepts and definitions associated with the basic concepts of probability

- Understand and apply the principles associated with marginal probabilities, joint probabilities, and conditional probabilities

- Understand the definition of and concepts associated with binomial probability

- Understand the definition of the Poisson distribution and how it is different from a binomial distribution

- Understand the definition of the normal distribution and how it differs from the Poisson and binomial distributions

Probability is just a formal way of referring to chance. If, for example, we were to flip a coin, we would know that there is some chance that it will come up heads and, by implication, some chance that it will come up tails. We know, in general, that this chance is fifty-fifty for either heads or tails occurring. But we also know that there is no certainty at all to the way the coin will come up. If the coin is flipped in what any of us would think of as the normally appropriate way, we are pretty sure that the resulting head or tail will have come up totally by chance or, in statistical terms, randomly. This random occurrence of heads or tails makes the result of a coin flip conform to what statisticians call a *stochastic process*. Simply put, a stochastic process is one for which any result has a certain probability of occurrence. In this case, the probability of any result of the flip of a single coin (either heads or tails) is 0.5.

5.1 Some Initial Concepts and Definitions

Any discussion of probability requires agreement on some initial concepts and definitions. The following sections provide working definitions for probability concepts.

All statistics are based on probability. Probability is a formal way of talking about chance. Therefore, we need probability to help us link chance and statistics.

Events, Independent Events, Outcomes, and Sample Space

An observation to which a probability can be assigned is often referred to as an *outcome*. If we flip a coin, we might reasonably think of that as an outcome (i.e., the flip). But in this chapter we will actually think of the outcome as the viewing of the results of the flip. To understand how we will consider this, think of the story of the three umpires—the traditionalist, the pragmatist, and the existentialist. The traditionalist umpire, in calling balls and strikes, says, "I call 'em as they are." The pragmatist says, "I call 'em as I see 'em." The existentialist says, "They ain't nothin' until I call 'em." We will take the existentialist view. The result of a coin flip is nothing until we view it and "call" the result.

An outcome is defined as an observation to which a probability can be assigned.

Independent Events

If we flip a coin twice, it is generally assumed that the *outcome* of the first flip will have no bearing on the outcome of the second flip. The first event does not influence the second event in any way. In statistical terms, it is said that the two events (flip one and flip two) are independent of each other. When we flip the coin the first time, the probability of our getting either a head or a tail is 0.5. When we flip the coin the second time, the probability of either a head or a tail is again 0.5. There are four possible outcomes of the flip of two coins: HH, HT, TH, or TT. The probability of any one of these four outcomes is 0.25, because each is equally likely and one divided by four is 0.25. But we can also arrive at the probability of any one of these four outcomes by the rule that says the probability of any outcome of two independent events is the multiplication of the probability of each separate event. Thus, the probability of the outcome HH is 0.5 times 0.5, which is 0.25, which is also the probability of the outcome TH, HT, or TT. This rule is referred to as the simple multiplication rule.

In general we will talk of individual observations as outcomes and the accumulation of those observations as events. However, a single event—the flip of a coin that results in a tail—may also be considered an event if there is only one coin flip. In general we will talk of individual observations as outcomes and the accumulation of those observations as events. However, a single event—the flip of a coin that results in a tail—may also be considered an event if there is only one coin flip.

Just in passing, it might be interesting to think about what the multiplication of probabilities of independent events may mean for long sequences of coin flips. If we were told that a person had flipped a coin five times and gotten the sequence HTTHT, we would not be particularly surprised. But if we were told that the person had gotten the sequence HHHHH, we would perhaps question the accuracy of the reporting or the honesty of the reporter. But the probability of either of these two outcomes as the result of five flips of a coin is exactly the same: $0.5 \times 0.5 \times 0.5 \times 0.5 \times 0.5$, or 0.5^5, or 0.03125.

Why, then, are we not surprised by the first outcome but are surprised by the second? The answer lies in the fact that we would expect the result of five flips of a coin to include some heads and some tails, even though we would not necessarily expect any particular order of heads and tails. When we see a specific ordering that includes both heads and tails, our expectation is confirmed without our recognizing that the specific ordering we see is no more likely than five heads in a row.

Sample Space

The two possible outcomes from the flip of a coin—heads or tails—are frequently called the *sample space* for this process. The sample space refers to all the possible outcomes of a particular process. The sample space for two flips of a coin includes the outcomes HH, HT, TH, and TT. For five flips of a coin, the sample space includes 2^5, or 32, separate outcomes. As we have seen, each of these individual outcomes has the same probability (0.03125) of occurring. But it is often less the specific outcome than the mix of heads and tails that will interest us in the flip of five coins.

"Sample space" refers to all the possible outcomes of a particular process.

From the perspective of the mix of heads and tails, the outcomes of five flips of a coin include five heads, four heads and one tail, three heads and two tails, two heads and three tails, one head and four tails, and five tails. There is only one way that an outcome of five heads can occur—if each flip is a head. The outcome of four heads and one tail can occur five ways. For example, the first four flips could come up heads and the last a tail; or there could be three heads, a tail, and then a head, or two heads, then a tail, and then two heads, and so on. There are actually 10 ways that the results could be three heads and two tails, 10 ways to get two heads and three tails, 5 ways to get one head, and 1 way to get no heads (all tails).

Mutually Exclusive Outcomes

Figure 5.1 shows the 32 ways that the five flips of a coin can come out in terms of the number of heads realized. As the table shows, there is one way to obtain five heads, five ways to obtain four heads, and so on. In five flips of a coin, each of the 32 outcomes is *mutually exclusive* of all others. Being mutually exclusive means, for example, that the result HHHHH and the result HTTHT cannot both occur. One can occur or the other can occur, but the occurrence of one precludes the occurrence of the other (and, similarly, all other outcomes).

Mutual exclusivity means that only one event in a sample space can occur at a time.

A Venn diagram uses circles to represent sets, with the position and overlap (if any) of the circles indicating the relationships between the sets. Figure 5.2 displays a Venn diagram for two events that are mutually exclusive. For our coin example, there are two circles. One circle represents heads, H, and one circle represents tails, T. Notice in Figure 5.2 that the two circles do not overlap. In the context of a Venn diagram, this illustrates that the two events, heads and tails, are mutually exclusive.

When outcomes are mutually exclusive, their probabilities can be summed. For example, there are five ways in which four heads can occur,

	A	B	C
C8		=	=SUM(C2:C7)
1	Outcome	Ways	Probability
2	Five Heads	1	0.03125
3	Four Heads	5	0.15625
4	Three Heads	10	0.3125
5	Two Heads	10	0.3125
6	One Head	5	0.15625
7	No Heads	1	0.03125
8		32	1

Figure 5.1 Possible combinations of five coin flips

Figure 5.2 Venn diagram for two mutually exclusive events

each of the ways having a probability of 0.03125. The sum of these five ways is the total probability of getting four heads in any one of the five ways, which is shown in Figure 5.1 as 0.15625. The probability of getting three heads or two heads is given in Figure 5.1 as 0.3125, which is the sum of the probability of getting any combination of either three or two heads. The probabilities of all mutually exclusive outcomes in the sample space must add to 1. This is considered one of the rules of probability.

The discussion of Figure 5.1 allows us to better understand why we would probably not be surprised by a sequence of HTTHT from the flip of five coins, whereas we would be surprised by the sequence HHHHH. The probability of seeing two heads and three tails from five flips of a coin is 0.3125, almost one-third. In looking at the sequence HTTHT, we ignore the specific pattern and think only of the combination of heads and tails. The probability of seeing five heads, however, is only 0.03125, or about 3 chances out of 100. Consequently, we would be much more surprised to see that result. Be careful not to confuse the concept of independence and the concept of mutual exclusivity. Think of *independence* when you have successive events (e.g., two flips of a coin) and think of mutual exclusivity when you think of events in the event space (e.g., in any one flip I can obtain a head or a tail, but not both at the same time).

A Priori Probability and Empirical Probability

There are two types of probability to consider. The first of these is the probability associated with the flip of a coin or, for example, with the roll of a die or the draw of a card from a deck. The nature of the object or objects upon which the random process is based determines the probability of the outcome. The probability of the outcome of a head after the flip of a coin is 0.5 given the nature of the coin (it has only two sides). The probability that a two will come up on the roll of a fair six-sided die is approximately 0.1667 (1/6) given the nature of the die. The probability of drawing an ace from the top of a well-shuffled deck is approximately 0.0769 (4/52) given the nature of the deck of cards (there are four aces in a 52-card deck). This type of probability is called *a priori* probability. Virtually all games of chance are based on a priori probabilities.

A priori probabilities are objective and are known "a priori" or before the event has occurred.

The second type of probability is probability associated with a set of objects about which we do not have the necessary knowledge to specify a probability a priori. These probabilities are referred to as subjective probabilities or probabilities that are random in nature. For example, if we were to consider people arriving for treatment at a hospital emergency room, they could be divided into two types: those who are coming for true emergencies, however defined, and those coming for nonemergency conditions. If we are interested in the probability that the next person arriving at the emergency room will have a true emergency, we cannot generally call upon some a priori knowledge of the people arriving and the propensity for their conditions to be emergencies or nonemergencies in determining that probability.

Subjective probabilities are random in nature and thus not known before the occurrence of an event.

Frequency of Occurrence and Empirical Probability

What we can rely on to gauge this probability of occurrence is some historical record of persons arriving at the emergency room. Suppose we have a record of all the arrivals at the emergency room for the past six months, during which time there were 7,320 total emergency room visits (about 40 per day). We also have information about whether the visit was for a true emergency as assessed by the attending physician, physician's assistant, or nurse. Suppose the record indicates that 4,729 of the visits were true emergencies. Now we can say that for the past six months, the probability that a person coming to the emergency room came for a true emergency was 0.646 (4,729/7,320). Based on this, and assuming that the future is like the past, we could predict that when the next person arrives at the clinic, that person has about a 0.65 probability of having a true emergency and about a 0.35 probability of having a nonemergency problem. This type of probability is known as *empirical probability*.

An empirical probability is one based on actual observations or event occurrences.

To consider another example of empirical probability, suppose we have records on 2,556 married women, and for each of these women we have recorded the number of children born to that woman. Thinking back to the definition of event that was given in the first subsection of Section 5.1, the recording of the number of children born to each woman is the event. The distribution of women by number of children born might look something like Figure 5.3. This table shows that 256 of the women have had no children born, 682 have had one child, 796 have had two children, and so on. Among these 2,556 women, no woman has had more than seven children born.

Figure 5.3 also shows the proportion of women with no children, one child, two children, and so on. This proportion also represents an empirical probability. In this case, it is the empirical probability that any woman drawn at random from our group of 2,556 will have no children, or one child, and so on. For example, the empirical probability that a woman drawn at random from among the 2,556 would have four children is 0.0865. The probability that a woman drawn at random would have no children is 0.1001. The other probabilities follow similarly.

If our 2,556 women had been a random sample from some larger population, we would be able to ascribe the probabilities associated with numbers of children to that larger population as well. In particular, if we were to select another woman from that larger population, we would be

	A	B	C
1	Children Born	3 Women	Proportion
2	0	256	0.1002
3	1	682	0.2668
4	2	796	0.3114
5	3	531	0.2077
6	4	221	0.0865
7	5	59	0.0231
8	6	10	0.0039
9	7	1	0.0004
10		2556	

Figure 5.3 Children ever born to 2,556 women

able to anticipate that the probability was about 0.0004 that the woman selected would have seven children, based on the empirical probabilities for our 2,556 women. Similarly, we would be able to say that the probability was about 0.2076 that she would have three children, again based on the empirical probabilities.

Sequential Events and Empirical Probabilities

Empirical probabilities work just like a priori probabilities in regard to sequential events. For example, if we looked at the record of the sequential arrival of any two people at the emergency room, we would see four possible events. If we classify true emergencies as E and nonemergency conditions as O (other), then the results of the arrival of two sequential people could be EE, EO, OE, and OO. Now, however, despite the fact that there are four possible outcomes, the probability of each outcome is not 0.25. If we do assume for the moment that the outcome of the arrival of the first person (i.e., E or O) does not influence the outcome of the arrival of the second person, then we can say that the arrival outcomes are independent of one another. Under the assumption of independence, the probability that the outcome will be EE is 0.65×0.65, or 0.42. The probability of EO is 0.65×0.35, or 0.23. The probability of the outcome OE is the same as that of EO, and the probability of the outcome OO is 0.35×0.35, or 0.12. Because these four mutually exclusive outcomes represent the entire sample space, the reader can confirm that the probabilities for the four sum to 1. Figure 5.4 displays the probability tree associated with emergency and nonemergency situations. Per the probability tree, marginal probabilities are listed first, followed by conditional probabilities and finally joint probabilities.

Independence and Empirical Probabilities

With empirical probabilities, though, unlike the case with a priori probabilities, we may not always be justified in viewing many events as independent. It is likely that several persons arriving at an emergency room in a sequential manner may be dependent on one another in regard to their emergency or nonemergency status. If, for example, there occurred a large highway accident that sent a number of persons to emergency rooms, several persons arriving at the same time might all be related (and hence not independent) emergencies. In fact, one of the most important capabilities of statistics is the ability to assess whether events are independent of or dependent on one another. The concept of independence is one that we will return to over and over in the course of this book.

Marginal Probabilities	Conditional Probabilities	Joint Probabilities

Emergency given Emergency
P(E|E) = 0.65

Emergency and Emergency
P(E and E) = 0.65*0.65 ≈ 0.42

Emergency

P(E) = 0.65

Non-Emergency given Emergency
P(O|E) = 0.35

Emergency and Non-Emergency
P(E and O) = 0.65*0.35 ≈ 0.23

Emergency given Non-Emergency
P(E|O) = 0.65

Non-Emergency

P(O) = 0.35

Non-Emergency and Emergency
P(O and E) = 0.35*0.65 ≈ 0.23

Non-Emergency given Non-Emergency
P(O|O) = 0.35

Non-Emergency and Non-Emergency
P(O and O) = 0.35*0.35 ≈ 0.12

E=Emergency
O=Non-Emergency
Assumption: Emergency and Non-Emergency are independent events

Figure 5.4 Sequential events

Empirical Probability and Probability Distributions

In many instances, data of interest to health workers can be viewed only from the standpoint of empirical probability. Whether an arrival at an emergency room is an emergency can be understood only as an empirical probability. But, interestingly, once we know what the overall probability of being an emergency is, and if we assume that the arrival of an emergency is independent of whether the last person arriving was an emergency, we can apply a priori probability assumptions to the arrival of several people at a time. In other words, those arrivals could be modeled using a probability distribution, and the a priori assumption we apply is that those arrivals are from a *binomial distribution*. The binomial distribution is discussed in detail later in this chapter. In fact, numerous distributions can be used to model data depending on the specific character or shape of the data. Another very important distribution is the *normal distribution*. The normal distribution is important in that one of the most important assumptions for statistics is that both discrete numerical data and continuous numerical data will somehow follow, a priori, a normal distribution. Normal distributions are discussed further in this chapter, and also in Chapter 6.

EXERCISES FOR SECTION 5.1

1. Calculate the probability of the following:

   a. The sequential roll of the die faces 2, 4, and 3

   b. The sequence of coin flips HTHH

   c. Assuming a probability of any arrival at an emergency room being an emergency as 0.646, and assuming that arrivals are independent, the probability of the next four arrivals being all emergencies

   d. Assuming (c), the probability of the next five arrivals being all nonemergencies

   e. Assuming (c), the probability of the next four arrivals being two emergencies and two nonemergencies, in that order

   f. Assuming a probability of 0.5 that any child born will be a boy, the probability of any family of five children having no girls

2. Lay out on a Microsoft Excel spreadsheet the possible outcomes of two rolls of a fair die and calculate the following:

   a. The probability that the two faces of the dice will equal 7

   b. The probability that the two faces of the dice will equal 11

   c. The probability that the two faces of the dice will equal 8 or more

3. Lay out on an Excel spreadsheet the possible outcomes of a visit by three persons to an emergency room. Assuming that the visits are independent, with a probability of 0.646 of being an emergency, calculate the following:

   a. The probability of two emergencies out of three arrivals

   b. The probability of no emergencies out of three arrivals

   c. The probability of at least two emergencies out of three arrivals

5.2   Marginal Probabilities, Joint Probabilities, and Conditional Probabilities

To continue with the discussion of probability, it will be useful to distinguish three different types of probabilities: marginal probabilities, joint probabilities, and conditional probabilities. Marginal probabilities are those associated with a single event. "Joint probability" refers to the simultaneous occurrence of two or more types of events. "Joint probabilities" and "conditional probabilities" refer to the outcomes of two different types of events that may or may not be independent of each other.

Marginal probabilities are those associated with a single event. "Joint probability" refers to the simultaneous occurrence of two or more types of events. "Conditional probability" refers to the occurrence of one event given that another event has occurred.

Marginal Probability

The probability (proportion) shown in Figure 5.3 is often referred to as *marginal probability*. Marginal probability is the probability of the occurrence of a single outcome. The probability that any single woman selected at random from among the 2,556 women will have no children is the number of women with no children divided by the total number of women. "Marginal probability" refers to the probability of an occurrence of any single outcome. By the same token, whether the next person appearing at the emergency room arrives with a true emergency or a nonemergency condition is also a single outcome (or event if we are counting only that one person). The marginal probability for true emergencies, according to the discussion earlier in this chapter, is 0.65, and for nonemergency conditions it is 0.35.

"Marginal probabilities" refers to outcomes that are mutually exclusive of one another. For example, a woman cannot at the same time have no children and three children. These categories are mutually exclusive. Those arriving at an emergency room can be coming either for a true emergency or for a nonemergency condition. In this context, they could not be coming for both. As was noted earlier, the probabilities of mutually exclusive events can be added together. Furthermore, the sum of the probabilities of all possible mutually exclusive marginal probabilities will always be 1. To see the consequences of these two points, consider again Figure 5.3. If we wished to know the probability that a woman would have at least four children, we could add together the probability of any woman having four, five, six, and seven children. The resulting probability, 0.1138, is the probability that a woman will have at least four children. In regard to the second point, it is relatively easy to verify that the sum of all probabilities in Figure 5.3 is 1.

Joint Probability

"Marginal probability" refers to the outcome of a single event or type of event (the birth of children, the arrival at an emergency room). *Joint probability* refers to the simultaneous occurrence of two or more types of events. Return to the example of persons arriving at an emergency room. Figure 5.5 shows the first 20 observations in a file that contains records of 7,320 emergency room visits. Column C shows whether the visit was for an

	A	B	C
1	Visit	Shift	Emergency Status
2	1	3rd	Emergency
3	2	1st	Emergency
4	3	2nd	Emergency
5	4	2nd	Emergency
6	5	3rd	Emergency
7	6	1st	Other
8	7	1st	Emergency
9	8	1st	Other
10	9	1st	Other
11	10	2nd	Emergency
12	11	2nd	Emergency
13	12	1st	Other
14	13	1st	Emergency
15	14	1st	Emergency
16	15	2nd	Other
17	16	2nd	Emergency
18	17	2nd	Emergency
19	18	1st	Other
20	19	3rd	Emergency
21	20	2nd	Emergency
22	21	2nd	Emergency

Figure 5.5 First 20 observations in an emergency room visit file

emergency. Column B is labeled Shift. The first shift (labeled 1st) is from 7 A.M. to 3 P.M. The second shift (labeled 2nd) is from 3 P.M. to midnight, and the third shift (labeled 3rd) is from midnight to 7 A.M.

Building a Joint Probability Table Using a Spreadsheet

In this example, we might, in addition to determining whether the visit was for a true emergency or a nonemergency condition, determine when during the day the arrival took place. The pivot table option in Excel was used to produce Figure 5.6, which shows the joint occurrence of a true emergency or a nonemergency condition and the shift during which the visit took place. It should be easy to recognize that Figure 5.6 is an example of a *contingency table*. A contingency table is one that shows the simultaneous occurrence of two or more events. In this case, the events are whether the

	A	B	C	D	E
1					
2					
3	Count of Shift	Shift			
4	Emergency Status	1st	2nd	3rd	Grand Total
5	Emergency	1504	1852	1373	4729
6	Other	1148	980	463	2591
7	Grand Total	2652	2832	1836	7320
8					

Figure 5.6 Contingency table of shift and emergency status

arrival at the emergency room is or is not an emergency and the shift during which the arrival occurred.

Figure 5.6 shows that of the 4,729 visits that were true emergencies, 1,504 occurred during the first shift, 1,852 occurred during the second shift, and 1,373 occurred during the third shift. Similarly, for visits to the emergency room that were not for true emergencies (the Other category), 1,148 occurred during the first shift, 980 occurred during the second shift, and 463 occurred during the third shift. The probability that, for example, a visit took place during the first shift and was for a true emergency is a joint probability. The joint probability for the simultaneous occurrence of a visit during the first shift and for a true emergency is 1,504/7,320, or 0.205.

Figure 5.7 shows the contingency table for all the joint probability combinations as well as the marginal probabilities for both reason for visit (true emergency or other) and time of day. The calculation of the joint probability is shown in the formula line at the top of the figure. Notice that the dollar sign ($) convention is used to fix the divisor as cell E7 for every internal cell.

The probabilities shown in Figure 5.7 can also be obtained directly from the pivot table capability. In the PivotTable Field dialog box, you can click an Options button (see Figure 4.25). If you click this button, you can then select a "Show Data as" dialog box that allows you to select any one of nine ways to display the data in the pivot table cells. One of these is the normal view, which is given in Figure 5.6. Another is "as percent of the total," which displays the data as shown in cells A11:E13 of Figure 5.7.

Mutual Exclusivity and the Simple Addition Rule

It can be confirmed from the table that the marginal probability (p) that the visit was for a true emergency is equal to the sum of the joint probabilities for the first, second, and third shifts. This can be seen in Equation 5.1. Equation 5.1 is referred to as the simple addition rule. The simple addition

	A	B	C	D	E
B11		=B5/$E$7			
1					
2					
3	Count of Shift	Shift			
4	Emergency Status	1st	2nd	3rd	Grand Total
5	Emergency	1504	1852	1373	4729
6	Other	1148	980	463	2591
7	Grand Total	2652	2832	1836	7320
8					
9	Count of Shift	Shift			
10	Emergency Status	1st	2nd	3rd	Grand Total
11	Emergency	0.205	0.253	0.188	0.646
12	Other	0.157	0.134	0.063	0.354
13	Grand Total	0.362	0.387	0.251	1.000

Figure 5.7   Joint probabilities for shift and emergency status

rule can be applied here since the first, second, and third shifts are mutually exclusive (i.e., they cannot occur at the same time).

$$p(\text{True}) = p(\text{True and First}) + p(\text{True and Second}) + p(\text{True and Third})$$

$$p(\text{True}) = 0.205 + 0.253 + 0.188 = 0.646 \tag{5.1}$$

In general, it is always possible to find the marginal probability of occurrence of an event from the joint probabilities of its occurrence when viewed in a contingency table, such as that shown in Figure 5.7. The reader can confirm that the marginal probabilities for the other categories are the sum of the relevant joint probabilities.

Mutual Exclusivity and the Addition Rule

Thus far, the discussion has concerned a joint probability that is represented by the conjunction "and." It is also possible to discuss a joint probability that is represented by the conjunction "or." The joint probability "or" would be stated in regard to true emergencies and time of day. For example, a visit was for a true emergency or it occurred during the first shift. The joint probability "or" is the sum of the appropriate marginal probabilities minus the appropriate joint probability. At times this is referred to as "avoiding the double count." We must subtract the joint probability of the two events if those two events are not mutually exclusive. In our example, a visit for a true emergency is not mutually exclusive of time of day. Figure 5.8 is a Venn diagram representing the events from our example, true emergency (TE) and first shift (FS). Notice that the two circles overlap. The overlap represents the intersection of the two events or the joint probability. The overlap indicates that these two events are not mutually exclusive.

Therefore, the probability that a visit was for a true emergency or that it took place during the first shift can be calculated by the formula shown in Equation 5.2.

$$p(\text{True or First}) = p(\text{True}) + p(\text{First}) - p(\text{True and First})$$

$$p(\text{True or First}) = 0.646 + 0.362 - 0.205 = 0.803 \tag{5.2}$$

Notice that if we did not subtract the $p(\text{True and First})$, the probability of True or First would be well over 1.0, violating the rules of probability.

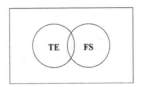

Figure 5.8 Venn diagram of two events that are not mutually exclusive

B17	▼	=	=B$13+$E11-B11	
	A	B	C	D	E
9	Count of Shift	Shift			
10	Emergency Status	1st	2nd	3rd	Grand Total
11	Emergency	0.205	0.253	0.188	0.646
12	Other	0.157	0.134	0.063	0.354
13	Grand Total	0.362	0.387	0.251	1.000
14					
15	Count of Shift	Shift			
16	Emergency Status	1st	2nd	3rd	Grand Total
17	Emergency	0.803	0.780	0.709	2.292
18	Other	0.559	0.607	0.542	1.708
19	Grand Total	1.362	1.387	1.251	4.000

Figure 5.9 Joint probability "or" for shift and emergency status

Calculating Joint Probability "or" Values in a Spreadsheet

Figure 5.9 shows all the joint probability "or" values for arriving during one of three shifts or for coming for an emergency or for a condition that is not an emergency. The formula line shows the calculation of the joint probability p(True or First) as B$13+$E11-B11. This formulation lets us drag the formula in cell B17 to the other five cells and generates the joint probability "or" for each of the cells in the table. The joint probabilities "or" for each row and column have been summed in cells B19:D19 and in cells E17 and E18. At first glance, these numbers mean nothing, because all probability values must be equal to or less than 1 to have meaning. However, the sum of the row probabilities or the sum of the column probabilities can be summed to the total of the joint probabilities "or" in cell E19. For a two-by-three table, such as the one shown in Figure 5.9, the sum of the joint probabilities "or" will always be 4. Four turns out to be the number of rows in the figure plus the number of columns minus 1. In fact, for any contingency table of any size, the sum of all joint probabilities "or" is always equal to the number of rows plus the number of columns minus 1.

It is possible to determine if the calculation of joint probabilities "and" is correct by determining if the probabilities sum to 1. It is equally possible to ensure that the calculation of joint probabilities "or" is correct by determining whether the probabilities sum to the number of rows plus the number of columns minus 1. For example, in a three-by-four table (three rows and four columns), the sum of all joint probabilities "or" would be $3 + 4 - 1$, or 6.

Conditional Probability

The discussion of probabilities given thus far has involved the development of probabilities with essentially no prior knowledge of events. The discussion has focused, for example, on the probability that a visit to the emergency room would be for a true emergency and would occur during the first shift.

Now the discussion turns to another point of probability—the probability of one event occurring if it is known that another event has occurred. For example, suppose we know that an emergency room visit has taken place during the third shift. The task then might be to determine the probability that the visit would be a true emergency, given that it is already known that it took place during the third shift. We might also ask, what is the probability that the visit was an emergency conditional on its having taken place during the third shift? This is known as *conditional probability*.

Bayes's Theorem and Conditional Probability

The calculation of conditional probabilities can be taken directly from our discussion of marginal and joint probabilities and may be shown as given in Equation 5.3. In Equation 5.3, $p(A|B)$ is read as "the probability of A given B," which means the probability of A is conditional on B having occurred, or having been known. This is also known as Bayes's theorem.

$$p(A \mid B) = p(A \text{ and } B)/(B) \tag{5.3}$$

In regard to our example of emergency room visits, the conditional probability that a visit was for a true emergency, given that it occurred during the third shift, would be calculated as is shown in Equation 5.4.

$$p(\text{True}|\text{Third}) = p(\text{True and Third})/(\text{Third})$$

$$p(\text{True}|\text{Third}) = 0.188/0.251 \approx 0.748 \tag{5.4}$$

The calculation of all the conditional probabilities, given that the arrival took place either during the day or during the night, is shown in Figure 5.10. Cell B17, for example, shows the calculation of the conditional probability that the arrival was for an emergency, given that it took place during the first shift. The formula used for that calculation is =B11/B$13 and is shown in the formula line above the spreadsheet. The formula can be copied into all the cells in the table to calculate the associated conditional probabilities. It is important to note that the conditional probabilities in Figure 5.10 are calculated for the columns. This means that each conditional probability is the probability that the arrival is or is not an emergency, given that it took place during either the first, second, or third shift. Because these probabilities are calculated by column, the total of column conditional probabilities is 1 for each column. It is also possible to calculate row conditional probabilities. The row conditional probabilities would be interpreted as the probability of coming during a particular shift, given that the visit was for an emergency or not. If conditional probabilities were calculated

B17	▼	=	=B11/B$13		
	A	B	C	D	E
9	Count of Shift	Shift			
10	Emergency Status	1st	2nd	3rd	Grand Total
11	Emergency	0.205	0.253	0.188	0.646
12	Other	0.157	0.134	0.063	0.354
13	Grand Total	0.362	0.387	0.251	1.000
14					
15	Count of Shift	Shift			
16	Emergency Status	1st	2nd	3rd	Grand Total
17	Emergency	0.567	0.654	0.748	0.646
18	Other	0.433	0.346	0.252	0.354
19	Grand Total	1.000	1.000	1.000	1.000
20					

Figure 5.10 Conditional probabilities for arrival during any shift

this way, they would sum to 1 by rows rather than by columns. In general, however, conditional probabilities are usually calculated for columns.

Conditional Probabilities and Data Frequencies

Conditional probabilities can also be calculated directly from data frequencies. It should be noted that the conditional probability of the visit to the emergency room being for a true emergency, given that it took place during the first shift, is just the number of visits for true emergencies taking place during the first shift divided by all the visits taking place during the first shift. If we look at Figure 5.6, for example, we can see that there were 2,652 visits during the first shift, of which 1,504 were for true emergencies. If we divide 1,504 by 2,652, the result is 0.567, which is the same as what we found using the formula in Equation 5.4, or as calculated in Figure 5.10.

Conditional Probability and Independent Events

This introduction of the concept of conditional probability provides another opportunity to talk about the notion of independent events and independence. Earlier, independence was defined as being a situation in which the occurrence of one event had no relation to the occurrence of a second event. In particular, if a coin is flipped twice, the second flip is generally assumed to be independent of the first because the result of the first will not influence the result of the second. If the first is a head, we should not expect that a second flip will be any more likely a tail than a head.

The introduction of conditional probability provides another way to look at the independence of events. Two events are independent if all the conditional probabilities of the event are equal to the marginal probabilities of the event. This general relationship is expressed in Equation 5.5. Consider the conditional and marginal probabilities for emergency room visits, shown in Figure 5.10. The conditional probability of a true emergency, given that the visit took place during the first shift, is $p(\text{True}|\text{First}) = 0.567$.

The marginal probability of a true emergency is $p(\text{True}) = 0.646$. Because these are not equal, arrival for an emergency and arrival during a particular shift are not independent of each other.

$$p(A|B) = p(A) \qquad \text{(condition for independence)} \qquad (5.5)$$

The condition of independence, as shown in Equation 5.5, holds for the earlier discussion of the flip of two coins. A first coin, B, is flipped, and its outcome is observed (head or tail). For the first flip, the probability of flipping a head, $p(H_B) = 0.5$, or a tail, $p(T_B) = 0.5$. On the second toss, coin A is flipped and the probability of flipping a head, $p(H_A) = 0.5$, or a tail, $p(T_A) = 0.5$. In fact, there is no difference in the probability of flipping a head or tail on the second coin given the first flip had or had not been observed. Regardless of the results of flip B, the probability of flip A does not change, so $p(H_A|H_B) = p(H_A)$. The previous equation reads: Given that coin B flipped a head, then the probability of coin A flipping a head is simply equal to the marginal probability of coin A flipping a head. This statement illustrates that the events are independent.

This is contrary to our previous example. Considering visits to emergency rooms, the probability that a visit was for a true emergency, given that it took place during the first shift, is $p(\text{True}|\text{First}) = 0.567$, but the probability that a visit is a true emergency is $p(\text{True}) = 0.646$. In this case, $p(\text{True}|\text{First}) \neq p(\text{True})$ and therefore emergency status and shift are dependent upon each other.

Conditional Probability Tables via Spreadsheet to Test Independence

If we had been dealing with a table of two rows and two columns, any conditional probability that did not equal the marginal probability would have forced all conditional probabilities to be different from the marginal probabilities. The nature of a two-by-two table is such that if $p(A|B) \neq p(B)$ for any individual conditional probability in the table, the principle of independence will hold for all other conditional probabilities in the table. In a table with more than four internal cells, we cannot make that claim.

Consider, again, children ever born to 2,556 women. Suppose these women were divided into low and high income and the number of children ever born was categorized as 0, 1, 2, 3, and 4+, as shown in Figure 5.11. The number of women in the high- and low-income groups, with their respective numbers of children, is shown in cells H2:I5. The column conditional probabilities (the conditional probability, e.g., of having 0 children, given that the woman is high income) are given in cells H10:I14. It is possible to

H10	▾	=	=H2/H$7	
	G	H	I	J
1	Children Born	High	Low	Total
2	0	102	154	256
3	1	380	302	682
4	2	317	479	796
5	3	189	342	531
6	4+	32	259	291
7		1020	1536	2556
8				
9	Children Born	High	Low	Total
10	0	0.100	0.100	0.100
11	1	0.373	0.197	0.267
12	2	0.311	0.312	0.311
13	3	0.185	0.223	0.208
14	4+	0.031	0.169	0.114
15		1.000	1.000	1.000

Figure 5.11 Conditional probabilities for high- and low-income women and number of children

see that the conditional probability of having 0 children, given high income (cell H10), is essentially the same as the marginal probability of having no children within three decimal points (cell J10).

Similarly, the conditional probability of having two children, given high income (cell H12), is the same as the marginal probability of having two children (cell J12).

But in other cells, the conditional and marginal probabilities are not equal. For example, the conditional probability of having one child, given high income (cell H11), is not the same as the marginal probability for one child (cell J11). Therefore, it can be concluded that income and number of children born are dependent. It is necessary to show only one occurrence that a conditional probability does not equal a marginal probability to prove dependence.

Mathematical versus Statistical Independence

It is important to point out, however, that the concept of independence discussed thus far is mathematical independence. If Equation 5.5 does not hold, then two events are not mathematically independent. By this definition, the two events, arrival for an emergency and arrival during a particular shift, are not independent. But the conditional probabilities for arrival for an emergency or for a nonemergency condition, given a shift during the day, are not much different from the marginal probabilities. As Figure 5.10 shows, the conditional probability of arriving for an emergency during any particular shift is in every case no more than 0.1 different from the marginal probability. Mathematically speaking they are different; however, viewed another way, are they statistically different? Could we think of those probabilities in terms of statistical independence? The answer to this question is yes. Chapter 8 discusses statistical tests for categorical data. These tests allow us to determine whether the differences between conditional and marginal probabilities can be considered statistically independent.

EXERCISES FOR SECTION 5.2

1. Use the data in file Chpt 5-2.xls. This is the data file from which the discussion in Section 5.2 was developed. Do the following:

   a. Generate a contingency table such as that shown in Figure 5.6, using the pivot table capability of Excel.

   b. Calculate the marginal probabilities for both Shift and Emergency Status, as is shown in Figure 5.7.

   c. Calculate the joint probabilities "and" for each of the cells in the table, as is shown in Figure 5.7. Confirm that the sum of the cells is 1.

   d. Calculate the joint probabilities "or" for each of the cells in the table, as is shown in Figure 5.9. Confirm that the sum of the joint probabilities "or" is equal to rows + columns − 1.

   e. Calculate the conditional probabilities of reason for arrival, given that the patient arrives in the first, second, or third shift (replicate Figure 5.10) and confirm that reason for arrival and time of arrival are not independent.

2. Use the file created in Exercise 2 of Section 3.3 of Chapter 3 (or use Chpt 5-3.xls), and do the following:

   a. Generate a contingency table with Sex as the column variable and Insurance as the row variable, and calculate the marginal probabilities of each variable.

   b. Calculate joint probabilities "and" for the two variables, and show them in a separate table. Confirm that the joint probabilities "and" sum to 1.

   c. Calculate joint probabilities "or" for the two variables, and show them in a separate table. Confirm that the joint probabilities "or" sum to rows + columns − 1.

   d. Calculate conditional probabilities of having a particular type of insurance, given Sex, and determine if the two variables are independent.

3. Use the file in Exercise 2 (preceding), and do the following:

   a. Generate a new variable, Charges 2, where Charges 2 is 1 if Charges is greater than the average and 0 if less.

b. Generate a contingency table with Insurance as the column variable and Charges 2 as the row variable, and calculate marginal probabilities for each variable.

c. Calculate joint probabilities "and" for the two variables, and show them in a separate table. Confirm that the joint probabilities "and" sum to 1.

d. Calculate joint probabilities "or" for the two variables, and show them in a separate table. Confirm that the joint probabilities "or" sum to rows + columns − 1.

e. Calculate conditional probabilities for charges, given insurance, and show these in a separate table. Determine if the two variables are independent.

5.3   Binomial Probability

As has been discussed thus far, a person comes to the emergency room for one of two reasons: either for an emergency or for a nonemergency reason. Because arrival can be for one of two reasons, this can be considered a binary event. The occurrence of binary events generally follows a known distribution, called the binomial distribution. Consider, again, a most common binary event—the flipping of a coin. The result can be either a head or a tail, and either outcome is equally likely (i.e., either outcome has a 0.5 probability of occurrence). But suppose we are flipping the coin five times. Figure 5.1 showed the number of different heads that could be obtained in five flips of a coin. That table indicates that the probability of getting all heads was 0.03125, the probability of getting four heads was 0.15625, the probability of getting three heads was 0.3125, and the probability of getting two, one, or no heads was exactly the same probabilities in reverse. These probabilities for five flips of a coin follow the binomial distribution.

Figure 5.12 shows all the possible outcomes of the flip of a coin five times. Column B shows the result of the first flip, column C shows the result of the second flip, and so on. By examining the figure, it can be seen that there is only 1 way that the result can be five heads, 5 ways that the result can be four heads, 10 ways that the result can be three heads, and so on, to 1 way to obtain no heads. The probability of any 1 of the 32 outcomes is given in column H. Each of these outcomes has exactly the same probability: 0.03125. But because there are five ways to get four heads, each of these 0.03125 probabilities can be added together to get the probability of getting four heads. The same can be done for three heads, and so on. The results will be exactly those shown in Figure 5.1.

	A	First	Second	Third	Fourth	Fifth	# Heads	Prob
2	1	H	H	H	H	H	5	0.03125
3	2	H	H	H	H	T	4	0.03125
4	3	H	H	H	T	H	4	0.03125
5	4	H	H	H	T	T	3	0.03125
6	5	H	H	T	H	H	4	0.03125
7	6	H	H	T	H	T	3	0.03125
8	7	H	H	T	T	H	3	0.03125
9	8	H	H	T	T	T	2	0.03125
10	9	H	T	H	H	H	4	0.03125
11	10	H	T	H	H	T	3	0.03125
12	11	H	T	H	T	H	3	0.03125
13	12	H	T	H	T	T	2	0.03125
14	13	H	T	T	H	H	3	0.03125
15	14	H	T	T	H	T	2	0.03125
16	15	H	T	T	T	H	2	0.03125
17	16	H	T	T	T	T	1	0.03125
18	17	T	H	H	H	H	4	0.03125
19	18	T	H	H	H	T	3	0.03125
20	19	T	H	H	T	H	3	0.03125
21	20	T	H	H	T	T	2	0.03125
22	21	T	H	T	H	H	3	0.03125
23	22	T	H	T	H	T	2	0.03125
24	23	T	H	T	T	H	2	0.03125
25	24	T	H	T	T	T	1	0.03125
26	25	T	T	H	H	H	3	0.03125
27	26	T	T	H	H	T	2	0.03125
28	27	T	T	H	T	H	2	0.03125
29	28	T	T	H	T	T	1	0.03125
30	29	T	T	T	H	H	2	0.03125
31	30	T	T	T	H	T	1	0.03125
32	31	T	T	T	T	H	1	0.03125
33	32	T	T	T	T	T	0	0.03125

Figure 5.12 All possible outcomes of the flip of a coin five times

Applying Binary Logic to Flips of a Coin

But is it possible to generalize the information found in Figure 5.12 to any number of coin flips or, for that matter, to any binary events, such as the arrival for an emergency or nonemergency condition? The answer is yes. To do so, let us first consider the probability of getting any number of heads in five flips of the coin. Let us say that we flip a coin five times and we get the outcome HHTHT. This is outcome number six in Figure 5.12. It can then be asked, "What is the probability of getting that outcome?"

The solution is as follows: the probability of a head on the first flip (0.5) times the probability of a head on the second flip (0.5) times the probability of a tail on the third flip (0.5) times the probability of a head on the fourth flip (0.5) times the probability of a tail on the fifth flip (0.5). Because the probabilities of heads or tails are both 0.5, the probability of the outcome HHTHT is $0.5 \times 0.5 \times 0.5 \times 0.5 \times 0.5$, or 0.5^5. But it is also the probability of heads raised to the third power times the probability of tails raised to the second power, or $0.5^3 \times 0.5^2$. Think of the number of flips of a coin as being designated by n; think of the occurrence of a head—the outcome we wish to track—as the index value (I) and the number of heads that come up as being designated by x. Then, the probability of any single outcome (i.e., of any number of heads in a specific order) in n flips of a coin is given in Equation 5.6.

$$p \binom{n}{I^*}{}_{x} = p(I)^x (1 - p(I))^{(n-x)} \qquad (5.6)$$

where $p(I)$ is the probability of the event I (e.g., the probability of a head in one flip of a coin) and $p \binom{n}{I^*}{}_x$ is the probability of any single outcome of x events in n tries (e.g., the outcome HHTHT in five flips of a coin).

For example, the probability of the specific pattern of heads and tails HHTHT is

$$p \binom{5}{H^*}{}_{3} = 0.5^3 \times 0.5^{(5-3)} = 0.03125$$

Applying Binary Logic to Emergency and Nonemergency Visits

For the flip of a coin where the probability of heads and one minus the probability of heads are the same (0.5), the result of Equation 5.6 is exactly the same for any single value of x (i.e., for any single number of heads, such as one head, two heads, and so on). If we consider again the visit of people to an emergency room and use the empirical probabilities shown in Figure 5.6, $p(I)$ and $1 - p(I)$ are not equal (e.g., $p(E) = 0.646$ and $p(O) = 1 - 0.646 = 0.354$). Consequently, the result of the application of Equation 5.6 will not be the same for every different number of true emergencies (x) and nonemergency conditions. Figure 5.13 shows all the possible outcomes of the visit to an emergency room of five people and their emergency or nonemergency status. We assume that each visit is independent of all other visits. The probability of five emergencies is given as 0.113. You can confirm that this is 0.646^5 or $p(I)^5 \times (1 - p(I))^{(5-5)}$. The equation in cell H2 would resemble this: $= (0.646^{\wedge}(G2))^*((1-0.646)^{\wedge}(5-G2))$. The probability of four emergencies out of five (e.g., outcome number 2 or outcome number 3) is 0.062. It is possible to confirm that this is $0.646^4 \times 0.354^1$ or $p(I)^4 \times (1 - p(I))^{(5-4)}$, as expressed in Equation 5.6.

Now that we have calculated the probabilities of occurrence of each of the 32 different ways in which five persons can present emergencies

	A	B	C	D	E	F	G	H
1		First	Second	Third	Fourth	Fifth	# Emerg	Prob
2	1	E	E	E	E	E	5	0.113
3	2	E	E	E	E	NE	4	0.062
4	3	E	E	E	NE	E	4	0.062
5	4	E	E	E	NE	NE	3	0.034
6	5	E	E	NE	E	E	4	0.062
7	6	E	E	NE	E	NE	3	0.034
8	7	E	E	NE	NE	E	3	0.034
9	8	E	E	NE	NE	NE	2	0.019
10	9	E	NE	E	E	E	4	0.062
11	10	E	NE	E	E	NE	3	0.034
12	11	E	NE	E	NE	E	3	0.034
13	12	E	NE	E	NE	NE	2	0.019
14	13	E	NE	NE	E	E	3	0.034
15	14	E	NE	NE	E	NE	2	0.019
16	15	E	NE	NE	NE	E	2	0.019
17	16	E	NE	NE	NE	NE	1	0.010
18	17	NE	E	E	E	E	4	0.062
19	18	NE	E	E	E	NE	3	0.034
20	19	NE	E	E	NE	E	3	0.034
21	20	NE	E	E	NE	NE	2	0.019
22	21	NE	E	NE	E	E	3	0.034
23	22	NE	E	NE	E	NE	2	0.019
24	23	NE	E	NE	NE	E	2	0.019
25	24	NE	E	NE	NE	NE	1	0.010
26	25	NE	NE	E	E	E	3	0.034
27	26	NE	NE	E	E	NE	2	0.019
28	27	NE	NE	E	NE	E	2	0.019
29	28	NE	NE	E	NE	NE	1	0.010
30	29	NE	NE	NE	E	E	2	0.019
31	30	NE	NE	NE	E	NE	1	0.010
32	31	NE	NE	NE	NE	E	1	0.010
33	32	NE	NE	NE	NE	NE	0	0.006

Figure 5.13   All possible outcomes of five emergency room visits

	T	U	V
1	Emergencies	Ways	Prob
2	5	1	0.113
3	4	5	0.308
4	3	10	0.338
5	2	10	0.185
6	1	5	0.051
7	0	1	0.006
8		32	1.000

Figure 5.14   Probabilities of number of visits that are actual emergencies

or nonemergency conditions in an emergency room, it is possible to add all of the ways that each number of emergencies may be generated to produce the result shown in Figure 5.14. The formula to calculate cell V2 in the column labeled Prob in Figure 5.14 is as follows: $=(0.646^{\wedge}(T2))$ $*((1-0.646)^{\wedge}(5-T2))*U2$. This formula can then be copied down through cell V7.

Equations for the Binomial Distribution

But there is a less tedious way of getting the result in Figure 5.14 than by enumerating every possible combination. As both Figures 5.13 and 5.14 show, the probability of getting any single number of emergencies is exactly the same for each one of the ways in which that number of emergencies can be obtained. For example, the probability of seeing three emergencies out of five arrivals at the emergency room is 0.034. This is true for any of the 10 ways to see three emergencies. Consequently, if there is a way to determine the number of ways that one can find three emergencies out of five visits, it would be possible simply to multiply this number times the probability of finding three emergencies in any single way (Equation 5.6).

Combinatorial Formulas

It turns out that there is a formula for finding the number of ways that one can get three emergencies out of five visits. More generally we wish to find x emergencies (I or the Index event) out of n observations. Therefore, we divide n factorial by the quantity x factorial times $(n - x)$ factorial. Equation 5.7 says that the total number of combinations, (C), for finding n emergencies (I or the Index event) out of n observations is n factorial divided by the quantity x factorial times $(n - x)$ factorial.

$$C\begin{pmatrix} n \\ I \\ x \end{pmatrix} = \frac{n!}{x! \times (n - x)!} \tag{5.7}$$

where $C\begin{pmatrix} n \\ I \\ x \end{pmatrix}$ is the number of different ways to get x results of I out of n observations (e.g., three emergencies out of five persons coming to the emergency room).

Factorials in Excel: The =FACT () Function

The term "factorial" means to multiply the number to which the factorial refers by every number less than it in the number sequence. So, for example, 5! is $5 \times 4 \times 3 \times 2 \times 1$, or 120. The Excel =FACT () function will provide the value of factorials up to 170! (about 7.257E+306 or 7,257 followed by 303 zeros). Now if we wish to know the probability of seeing, for example, x emergencies in the next n persons who come to the clinic, the complete formula is as given in Equation 5.8.

$$p\begin{pmatrix} n \\ I \\ x \end{pmatrix} = C\begin{pmatrix} n \\ I \\ x \end{pmatrix} p\begin{pmatrix} n \\ I^* \\ x \end{pmatrix} \tag{5.8}$$

	A	B	C	D	E	F
1	Emergencies	n!	x!*(n-x)!	Ways	p(I*) (1 way)	prob
2	5	120	120	1	0.113	0.113
3	4	120	24	5	0.062	0.308
4	3	120	12	10	0.034	0.338
5	2	120	12	10	0.019	0.185
6	1	120	24	5	0.010	0.051
7	0	120	120	1	0.006	0.006
8						1.000
9	p(I)		0.646			
10						

Figure 5.15 Probabilities of number of visits using formulas

where $p\begin{pmatrix} n \\ I \\ x \end{pmatrix}$ is the total probability of n results of I out of x observations (the binomial probability).

Figure 5.15 shows the same probabilities as Figure 5.14, except that those in Figure 5.15 were developed using the =FACT() function and the formulas in Equations 5.6, 5.7, and 5.8. Column D in the figure is the result of the application of Equation 5.7. Column E is the result of the application of Equation 5.6. Column F is the binomial probability, which is the result of the application of Equation 5.8. The actual setup of the formulas as implemented in Excel is shown in Figure 5.16. You will recall that the table shown in Figure 5.16 can be generated by going to the File menu and clicking in the Options menu, then clicking on the Advanced menu and looking for the "Display options for this worksheet" category; within this menu click "Show formulas in cells instead of their calculated results."

The formulas for Figure 5.16 were entered only into row 2 and copied to the other rows. It is useful to look closely at Figure 5.16 to see how the $ convention was used to generate the correct cell references in each row.

Binomial Probabilities in Excel: The =BINOMDIST() Function

Figure 5.15 was calculated using the formulas in Equations 5.6, 5.7, and 5.8. Excel actually provides a function that produces an easier way

	A	B	C	D	E	F
1	Emergencies	n!	x!*(n-x)!	Ways	p(I*) (1 way)	prob
2	5	=FACT($A$2)	=FACT(A2)*FACT($A$2-A2)	=B2/C2	=$B$9^A2*(1-$B$9)^($A$2-A2)	=D2*E2
3	4	=FACT($A$2)	=FACT(A3)*FACT($A$2-A3)	=B3/C3	=$B$9^A3*(1-$B$9)^($A$2-A3)	=D3*E3
4	3	=FACT($A$2)	=FACT(A4)*FACT($A$2-A4)	=B4/C4	=$B$9^A4*(1-$B$9)^($A$2-A4)	=D4*E4
5	2	=FACT($A$2)	=FACT(A5)*FACT($A$2-A5)	=B5/C5	=$B$9^A5*(1-$B$9)^($A$2-A5)	=D5*E5
6	1	=FACT($A$2)	=FACT(A6)*FACT($A$2-A6)	=B6/C6	=$B$9^A6*(1-$B$9)^($A$2-A6)	=D6*E6
7	0	=FACT($A$2)	=FACT(A7)*FACT($A$2-A7)	=B7/C7	=$B$9^A7*(1-$B$9)^($A$2-A7)	=D7*E7
8						=SUM(F2:F7)
9	p(I)	0.646				
10						

Figure 5.16 Formulas used for calculations of probabilities

to determine binomial probabilities. This is the =BINOMDIST() function. The =BINOMDIST() function takes four arguments. These are the number of emergency visits (5, 4, 3, 2, 1, or 0), the number of visits observed (five), the probability of an emergency (0.646), and a 0 or 1 to indicate whether the value to be determined is the actual probability or the cumulative probability. Figure 5.17 shows the result of using the =BINOMDIST() function to calculate binomial probabilities. The values in column B have been calculated by the formula shown in the formula bar. The values in column C have been calculated by dragging the equation from column B to column C and changing the 0 in the final argument to a 1.

Two additional things should be pointed out. First, the cumulative binomial function always accumulates from the lowest number of the index value (0 emergencies) to the highest. Consequently, column C accumulates from cell C7 to cell C2. Second, it is relatively easy to confirm that the cumulative probabilities are simply the accumulation of the probabilities at each of the number of emergencies. In other words, the cumulative value for two emergencies is the sum of the probabilities for zero emergencies, one emergency, and two emergencies. This seems logical, and it is true because the number of emergencies is a discrete numerical variable. There cannot be a half of an emergency or 3.2 emergencies. We will discuss distributions, particularly the normal distribution (see Section 5.5), where it is not possible to accumulate individual probabilities to get the cumulative probability.

A final note about Figure 5.17. It is instructive to examine how the $ references have been used to be able to copy the original formula from cell B2 to cells B2:C7 to get all the correct probabilities by changing only the 0 in cell B2 to a 1 in column C.

Binomial Applications to the Health Care Professional

To this point there has been ample time spent on the development of the binomial distribution. Therefore, it is appropriate to relate the binomial

B2		= =BINOMDIST($A2,$A$2,$B$9,0)		
A	B	C	D	E
1 Emergencies	Actual	Cummulative		
2	5	0.113	1.000	
3	4	0.308	0.887	
4	3	0.338	0.579	
5	2	0.185	0.241	
6	1	0.051	0.056	
7	0	0.006	0.006	
8				
9 P(E)	0.646			

Figure 5.17 The =BINOMDIST() function

distribution to the health care professional. The binomial distribution can give the probability for the occurrence of any event that can have two outcomes. Let's continue with the emergency room visits example. Suppose a hospital emergency room administrator has data over the past year showing that exactly 20,278 true emergencies were seen in the emergency room out of 31,390 people who sought care from the emergency room. Suppose further that the emergency room administrator is pretty certain that most visits to the emergency room are independent events (i.e., they are not related to one another, such as patients from a train wreck or a multiple-car pileup). Using the binomial event logic, the emergency room administrator can figure out how many emergencies she might expect during an eight-hour shift.

She knows from existing data that on any given night on average 29 people will show up at the emergency room. In turn, for staffing purposes she may be interested in the probability that no more than 15 real emergencies will appear in the emergency room. By using the =BINOMDIST(15,29,0.646,1) function, she will learn that there is a probability of only about 0.106 that 15 or fewer true emergencies will show up at the emergency room. The administrator would have good reason, then, to be prepared for more than 15 emergencies, and staff accordingly. Although this is interesting information, the administrator is most likely interested in times when the emergency room is busy.

So, for example, what would be the probability that more than 25 emergencies would show up during her shift out of the 29 people who come in? That would be found by subtracting =BINOMDIST(25,29,0.646,1) from 1, the result of which is about 0.002. Assuming an eight-hour shift, an occurrence of more than 25 emergencies is going to happen only about three times per year. So she would be justified in assuming that only very rarely would she have to be prepared for more than 25 true emergencies. Figure 5.18 shows the entire binomial distribution for any number of emergencies (from 0 to 29) occurring during an eight-hour shift. As the figure shows, the administrator can expect between 13 and 25 true emergencies during any eight-hour shift. On virtually no days will the emergency room see fewer than 13 emergencies and rarely more than 25. This same logic can be applied to any other occurrences that can take on only two values.

Answering the Question of Correctly Documented Medicare Claims

In Chapter 1 there is a brief discussion of the problem of incorrectly documented Medicare claims at the Pentad Home Health Agency. The agency drew a random sample of 80 records from its files, and during an audit

Figure 5.18 Binomial distribution for emergencies in an eight-hour shift

of the records it was determined that only 75 percent of them had been correctly documented. The agency believed that any fewer than 85 percent correctly documented would lead to real reimbursement difficulties with the Medicare administration. They were concerned that they should initiate a training activity for staff to ensure that at least 85 percent of claims would be correctly documented in the future. But they were not completely convinced that just because only 75 percent were correctly documented in the audit, fewer than 85 percent of all records had been incorrectly documented. The training activity was not going to be cheap, and it would be a real waste to undertake the training if it was not really needed. What information could they call on to make a decision as to whether to undertake training?

Because any record can be either correctly or incorrectly documented, the outcome is binary. Let's assume that the probability of one record being correctly documented is independent of whether any other is being correctly documented (not a completely obvious assumption). In turn, we can consider that the probability of appearance in our random sample of any number of correctly or incorrectly documented records will follow the binomial distribution. So if we want to know the probability that the true proportion of correctly documented records is 85 percent when we discovered 75 percent correctly documented in our sample, we could approach the question in either of two ways.

Calculating the Binomial Probability of Correctly Documented Claims

The first way would be to ask, if we have found 75 percent of our sample correctly documented, what is the probability that 85 percent of the population from which the sample came was correctly documented? Considering 80 records, 85 percent would be 68 records. So we can use the binomial distribution equations given in Equations 5.6, 5.7, and 5.8, or the =BINOMDIST(67,80,0.75,1) function, to determine that the cumulative binomial probability of obtaining a value of 67 or fewer correctly documented in any random sample of 80 records is 0.978. We can also determine that 1−(=BINOMDIST(67,80,0.75,1)) is 0.022. Therefore, there is about a 2.2 percent chance that the true proportion of correctly documented records is 85 percent or more when the sample proportion is 75 percent.

Alternatively we could ask, if the true proportion of correctly documented cases in the population is 85 percent, what is the probability that only 75 percent of a sample will be correctly documented? Again, considering 80 records, 75 percent of 80 would be 60. So we can apply the binomial distribution equations or the =BINOMDIST(60,80,0.85,1) function in Excel. The result is that the cumulative binomial probability of obtaining 60 or fewer correctly documented records in any random sample of 80 records is 0.013. In other words, there is about a 1.3 percent chance that the true proportion of correctly documented records is 75 percent or less when the sample proportion is 85 percent. In either way of looking at this issue, the odds that 85 percent of the population of records could be correctly documented, given a sample proportion of 75 percent, are very small. A statistical consultant to the home health agency would almost certainly recommend initiating a training event.

Visualizing the Binomial Distributions of Correctly Documented Claims

Another way of considering either of these alternatives might be by visualizing the actual binomial distributions for each. Figure 5.19 shows the binomial distribution for 75 percent correct out of 80 observations (the light gray distribution on the left) and the binomial distribution for 85 percent correct out of 80 observations (the black distribution on the right). These

Figure 5.19 Binomial distributions for 0.75 and 0.85 correct

were generated using the =BINOMDIST(x,80,p,0) function, where x was all values from 50 to 80 and p was either 0.75 or 0.85. If we look first at the light gray distribution ($p = 0.75$), we can see that only a small proportion of that distribution (actually 2.2 percent) is to the right of the vertical black line that marks the number 68 (85 percent of 80). But if we look at the black distribution ($p = 0.85$), we can see that only a small proportion of that distribution (actually, 1.3 percent) is to the left of the vertical black line that marks the number 60 (75 percent of 80). This is graphic evidence that it is very unlikely that the true proportion of correctly documented records is 85 percent when the sample finds 75 percent.

One question that may remain is, why are the probabilities found from these two views not exactly the same? The answer lies in the fact that the binomial distribution is not symmetrical. The closer the actual proportion gets to 0 or to 1, the more the binomial distribution becomes skewed in the direction away from the 0 or 1 limit. This means that, in most cases, the probabilities examined in the two ways given earlier will not be exactly equal. An example of a situation in which they would be equal could be given as the following: What is the probability that the true proportion of the population is 0.55 if a sample of 80 finds a proportion of 0.45? In this case, the two proportions are equidistant from the center of the probability distribution, which is 0.5. The proportion 0.55 of 80 is 44 and 0.45 of 80 is 36. Now if we use =BINOMDIST(36,80,0.55,1), we discover that the probability of finding 36 or fewer out of 80 when the probability is 0.45 is 0.046. If we use $1 -$ BINOMDIST(43,80,0.45,1), we discover that the probability of finding 44 or more out of 80 is 0.046. This happens because 0.45 and 0.55 are equidistant on opposite sides of 0.5, so their "skewnesses" are mirror images of one another.

The fact that the two different decision rules may not always produce the same probability should not be a source of great concern. In most cases, the probabilities will differ only slightly. Only infrequently would a different decision be reached from one view versus the other.

EXERCISES FOR SECTION 5.3

1. Use Equation 5.6 to determine the probability of any one outcome of the following:
   a. $n = 5, x = 2, p = 0.646$
   b. $n = 11, x = 9, p = 0.42$
   c. $n = 11, x = 7, p = 0.42$
   d. $n = 120, x = 35, p = 0.5$
   e. $n = 120, x = 60, p = 0.5$

2. Use Equation 5.7 to determine the number of separate outcomes for the following:

    a. $n = 5, x = 2$

    b. $n = 11, x = 9$

    c. $n = 11, x = 7$

    d. $n = 120, x = 35$

    e. $n = 120, x = 60$

3. Use Equation 5.8 to determine the binomial probability of the following:

    a. $n = 5, x = 2, p = 0.646$

    b. $n = 11, x = 9, p = 0.42$

    c. $n = 11, x = 7, p = 0.42$

    d. $n = 120, x = 35, p = 0.5$

    e. $n = 120, x = 60, p = 0.5$

4. Use the =BINOMDIST() function to determine the binomial probability of the following and determine if they are the same as what is given in Exercise 3.

    a. $n = 5, x = 2, p = 0.646$

    b. $n = 11, x = 9, p = 0.42$

    c. $n = 11, x = 7, p = 0.42$

    d. $n = 120, x = 35, p = 0.5$

    e. $n = 120, x = 60, p = 0.5$

5. Use the formulas in Equations 5.6, 5.7, and 5.8 to replicate Figure 5.15.

    a. Add the comparable values as generated by the =BINOMDIST() function as column D.

    b. Add the cumulative probabilities as column E by accumulating column D from $x = 0$.

    c. Add the cumulative probabilities as column F by using =BINOMDIST() with 1 as the final argument.

    d. Do columns C and D and columns E and F match?

6. A local health department counsels expectant mothers coming to a prenatal clinic on cigarette smoking only if they are smokers. History has shown that about 27 percent of expectant mothers are smokers when they first come to the clinic. Assume that the clinic will see 11 new expectant mothers today.

    a. Use the formulas in Equations 5.6, 5.7, and 5.8 to determine binomial probabilities that the health department will see no women who smoke today, 1 woman who smokes, 2 women who smoke, and so on, up to 11 women who smoke.

b. Use =BINOMDIST() to determine the same values.

c. Accumulate the values found in (a) (preceding) from 0 to 11.

d. Use =BINOMDIST() to determine the cumulative probabilities.

e. Make sure that the two sets of probabilities are equal to each other.

7. A dentist sees about 15 new patients per month (the rest of her patients are repeats). She knows that on average, over the past year, about half of her patients have needed at least one filling on their first visit.

a. What is the probability that she will see 10 patients or more out of 15 who need fillings?

b. What is the probability that she will see five or fewer patients who need fillings?

c. What is the probability that she will see between 7 and 10 new patients who need fillings?

8. An emergency room administrator wants to know the proportion of emergency room patients who spend more than one hour before being attended to. He knows that the time of arrival at the emergency room and the time of seeing the first medical staff member are both recorded. He draws a random sample of 50 records and discovers 14 indicate that the person spent more than one hour waiting.

a. What is the probability that the true proportion of persons spending more than one hour is 36 percent or more?

b. What is the probability that the true proportion of persons spending more than one hour is 20 percent or less?

c. What is the probability that the true proportion of persons spending more than one hour is from 24 to 32 percent?

5.4   The Poisson Distribution

The *Poisson distribution*, like the binomial distribution, is a discrete distribution. It takes on values for whole numbers only. But whereas the binomial distribution is concerned with the probability of two outcomes over a number of trials, the Poisson distribution is concerned with the number of observations that will occur in a small amount of time or over a region of space. We have been discussing the probability of seeing a certain number of emergencies out of a number of persons who arrive at an emergency room. The binomial distribution describes these probabilities. But if we consider the actual arrival at the emergency room of anyone, emergency or not, the Poisson distribution is more likely to describe these probabilities.

Arrivals at the Emergency Room: Application of the Poisson Distribution

Consider again the emergency room that deals with 29 people, on average, during an administrator's eight-hour shift. The administrator can figure out that this is an average of just about 0.9 persons—or just less than one person—every 15 minutes. She also knows that it takes about 15 minutes to go through all the administrative paperwork—checking insurance coverage, inquiring about previous visits, and so on—entailed in getting a person into the system. She knows that she will have to be prepared to deal with about one person every 15 minutes, but she also knows that on occasion several people arrive within the same 15-minute time interval, even when they arrive for different reasons. She would like to know, then, how often she will have to be prepared to deal with two people, or three or four, in any 15-minute interval. She can determine this with the Poisson distribution.

The =POISSON() Function in Excel

Figure 5.20 shows the Poisson-predicted probabilities for the number of arrivals in any 15-minute period. The probabilities are calculated using the =POISSON() function, which takes three arguments. These are the number of arrivals (A2 in the formula line), the average number of arrivals during the period of time under consideration ($B$11 in the formula line, and generally termed 1 in the context of the Poisson distribution), and a zero to indicate that the actual probability is desired.

It is important to point out that the probabilities shown in Figure 5.20 are based on three assumptions:

1. The arrival of an emergency in any 15-minute interval is independent of arrivals in any other 15-minute interval.

	B2	▼	=	=POISSON(A2,$B$11,0)	
	A	B	C	D	
1	Arrivals	Probability			
2	0	0.407			
3	1	0.366			
4	2	0.165			
5	3	0.049			
6	4	0.011			
7	5	0.002			
8	6	0.000			
9		1.000			
10					
11	Average	0.9			
12					

Figure 5.20   Poisson distribution of emergency room arrivals in 15-minute intervals

2. The number of arrivals in the time interval is proportional to the size of the interval.

3. The likelihood of more than one arrival in the time interval is very small.

If the administrator accepts these assumptions, she can see from Figure 5.20 that in only a small number of 15-minute intervals will she have to deal with more than two arrivals in the same 15-minute interval. The specific number of arrivals is calculated as follows: $0.063 \times 32 = 2.01$, or about two in any eight-hour shift.

Note: The 32 is four 15-minute intervals over eight hours, and the 0.063 is the sum of cells B5 through B8 in Figure 5.20.

Moreover, she will have to deal with more than three arrivals in a 15-minute period in only about one 15-minute interval in any two eight-hour shifts ($0.013 \times 32 = 0.416$). On this basis, she may be well justified in being prepared to deal with up to two arrivals in a 15-minute period but in letting the arrival of three or more persons be treated as an unlikely event that will be handled by the mobilization of extra resources.

Equations for the Poisson Distribution

In the section on the binomial distribution, we spent a good deal of time showing where the binomial distribution comes from. This was for two reasons:

1. The binomial distribution is a relatively easy distribution to understand.

2. The number of different combinations of any outcome (HHTHT, for example) is a general formula that applies to many different aspects of statistics.

The Poisson distribution, however, is more difficult to derive. So in the case of the Poisson distribution, we will look at the formula for the distribution directly. The formula for the Poisson distribution is shown in Equation 5.9.

$$p(x) = \frac{\lambda^x e^{-\lambda}}{x!}, \quad x = 0, 1, 2, \ldots$$

$$P(x) = 0, \text{ otherwise}$$

(5.9)

Equation 5.9 says that the probability of any value x is equal to the quantity λ to the power of x times e to the power of $-\lambda$, divided by $x!$ for 0 and integer values of x, but 0 for noninteger values of x. Like the binomial distribution, the Poisson distribution is defined only for 0 and integers. The term *e raised to the* $-\lambda$ is the value of e (approximately 2.718) raised to the negative power of the mean number of arrivals in any given interval of time.

Calculating the Poisson Distribution with a Spreadsheet

Figure 5.21 shows the calculated values of the Poisson distribution for emergency room arrivals in 15-minute intervals. Column B gives the value of λ^x, where x represents zero to six arrivals. Column C is simply the value of e (2.718) raised to the power of $-\lambda$. Column D is the factorial value for each number of arrivals, zero to six. Column E uses the formula in Equation 5.9 to replicate the values in column B in Figure 5.20.

Figure 5.22 shows the Excel formulas for the calculations in Figure 5.21. The calculations in column C use the Excel $=$EXP () function, which raises the value of e to the power of the value in the parentheses. The calculations in column D use the $=$FACT () function, which provides the factorial of the number in parentheses. Both of these functions take only one argument. The formulas shown in Figure 5.22 are revealed in Excel by the selection of the File menu and clicking in the Options menu, then clicking on the Advanced menu and looking for the "Display options for this worksheet" category; within this menu click "Show formulas in cells instead of their calculated results."

Poisson distributions apply not only to the distribution of occurrences in short periods of time but also to occurrences in regions. For example,

	A	B	C	D	E	F
1	Arrivals	Lambda^x	e^-Lambda	x!	Probability	
2	0	1	0.4065697	1	0.407	
3	1	0.9	0.4065697	1	0.366	
4	2	0.81	0.4065697	2	0.165	
5	3	0.729	0.4065697	6	0.049	
6	4	0.6561	0.4065697	24	0.011	
7	5	0.59049	0.4065697	120	0.002	
8	6	0.531441	0.4065697	720	0.000	
9					1.000	
10						
11	Lambda	0.9				
12						

Figure 5.21 Calculated Poisson distribution of emergency room arrivals in 15-minute intervals

	A	B	C	D	E
1	Arrivals	Lambda^x	e^-Lambda	x!	Probability
2	0	=$B$11^A2	=EXP(-$B$11)	=FACT(A2)	=B2*C2/D2
3	1	=$B$11^A3	=EXP(-$B$11)	=FACT(A3)	=B3*C3/D3
4	2	=$B$11^A4	=EXP(-$B$11)	=FACT(A4)	=B4*C4/D4
5	3	=$B$11^A5	=EXP(-$B$11)	=FACT(A5)	=B5*C5/D5
6	4	=$B$11^A6	=EXP(-$B$11)	=FACT(A6)	=B6*C6/D6
7	5	=$B$11^A7	=EXP(-$B$11)	=FACT(A7)	=B7*C7/D7
8	6	=$B$11^A8	=EXP(-$B$11)	=FACT(A8)	=B8*C8/D8
9					=SUM(E2:E8)
10					
11	Lambda	0.9			
12					

Figure 5.22 Calculated Poisson distribution of emergency room arrivals: Excel formulas

suppose a hospital supply room is responsible for maintaining a supply of rubber gloves. The gloves come in boxes of 100, and quality control is advertised to be very good concerning these gloves. However, the hospital supply room manager has found that he gets reports of an average of about 2 gloves in every box of 100 that are not usable for one reason or another. Given this information, what is the probability that in any given box of gloves, all will be usable? What is the probability that only one will not be usable, or that more than five will not be usable? This can also be found by using the Poisson distribution.

Figure 5.23 charts the distribution of probabilities for the number of gloves that will be unusable in a box of 100 if the average number unusable in a box is 2 (e.g., for a spreadsheet model use =POISSON(x,2,0)). The supply room manager can expect about 14 percent of the boxes to have all good gloves ($x = 0$); an equal number, about 27 percent, to have one or two unusable gloves ($x = 1$ or $x = 2$); and about 18 percent to have three unusable gloves ($x = 3$). A very small percentage of boxes will have as many as eight unusable gloves.

Figure 5.23 Poisson distribution for gloves that are not usable in a box of 100

EXERCISES FOR SECTION 5.4

1. Replicate the Poisson distribution for persons arriving at the emergency room, as is shown in Figure 5.20, using

   a. The =POISSON() function

   b. The Poisson formula shown in Equation 5.9

2. Calculate the Poisson probabilities for finding unusable gloves in a box of 100 if the average is 2 per box.

   a. Use the =POISSON() function.

   b. Use the Poisson formula shown in Equation 5.9.

   c. Replicate the chart in Figure 5.23.

5.5   The Normal Distribution

The last topic that will be taken up in this chapter is the normal distribution. Both the binomial distribution and the Poisson distribution describe discrete numerical variables. That is, they give the probability of a certain number of true emergencies among visitors to an emergency room. Discrete events are individually distinct and take on a finite or countable number of values.

Continuous Probability Distributions

The normal distribution, however, provides probabilities for continuous numerical variables. Height of adult males, for example, is a continuous variable. Body temperature is another continuous variable as is systolic blood pressure. The amount of time spent in a physician's waiting room or with the physician is a continuous variable. All of these variables can be determined not by counting, which can be done with a discrete variable, but by measurement. In general, it is reasonable to say that a continuous numerical variable is the result of some measurement—say, with a watch, a ruler, or a scale.

Discrete distributions contain a finite or countable number of values. Continuous distributions contain an infinite or noncountable number of values.

The normal distribution is just one of a number of distributions that describe the properties of continuous numerical data. However, in terms of elementary statistical applications, it is by far the most important and is the only continuous distribution treated in any detail in this text. The chi-square distribution and the F distribution, both continuous distributions, will be discussed, but only as these apply to hypothesis testing.

An Introduction to the Normal Distribution

To briefly introduce the normal distribution, consider the chart shown in Figure 5.24. This chart represents the normal distribution. The normal distribution is discussed in detail in Chapter 6, but several points about it are noteworthy here. First, the normal distribution has often been called a *bell-shaped curve* because it looks like the cross section of a bell. Second, because the normal distribution looks like a bell, both sides of the distribution have exactly equal probabilities. In other words, the normal distribution is symmetrical. For example, if the probability of being at the point −1 on the horizontal scale is 0.024, then the probability of being at 1 on the horizontal scale is also 0.024. Moreover, the probability of being between −3 and 0 is exactly the same as being between 0 and 3.

Standard Deviation and the Normal Distribution

In Figure 5.24, the horizontal axis is given as standard deviations. The meaning of the term "standard deviation" is discussed in detail in Chapter 6. So, for now we will use the term in the context of the normal distribution. It

Figure 5.24 A normal distribution

is sufficient to say that in any normal distribution, approximately 68 percent of all observations will be within ±1 *standard deviations* of the center of the distribution. Let's assume we have a normally distributed data set of average height of adult males. Consequently, it can be expected that in a large sample of adult males, 68 percent will have heights no less than 1 standard deviation below the average and no more than 1 standard deviation above the average. Furthermore, if the average height of adult males is normally distributed, 95 percent of all adult males will have heights between ±2 standard deviations of the average. Following this logic, 99 percent will have heights between ±3 standard deviations of the average.

Three Common Characteristics of the Normal Distribution: 68 Percent, 95 Percent, and 99 Percent

The average height of adult males in the United States is about 69 inches. Let us say that virtually all adult U.S. males are at least 60 inches tall and no more than 78 inches tall. Of course, there are some U.S. adult males—professional basketball players, for example—who are notably taller than 78 inches. In fact, this is also a characteristic of normal distributions. Normal distributions have no upper or lower limits. If the range of adult male height is 60 to 78 inches and if height is normally distributed, then we could say that the standard deviation of height is about 3 inches (78 − 60 = 18, 18/6 = 3). Consequently, we could say that 68 percent of all U.S. males are between 66 and 72 inches tall (e.g., 69 ± 1 * 3 = 66 and 72). Furthermore, we could say that 95 percent of all adult males are between 63 and 75 inches tall (e.g., 69 ± 2 * 3 = 63 and 75). Finally, 99 percent are between 60 and 78 inches tall (e.g., 69 ± 3 * 3 = 60 and 78).

The following can be said about a normal distribution:

- Approximately 68 percent of the values lie between ±1 standard deviation from the mean.

- Approximately 95 percent of the values lie between ±2 standard deviations from the mean.

- Approximately 99 percent of the values lie between ±3 standard deviations from the mean.

The use of height to discuss the normal distribution is not accidental. Height is a measure. On the measurement scale of height, a person may be at any point. He does not need to be exactly 69 inches tall (although we might measure him as such). The normal probability distribution is a distribution of measurement. This is in contrast to both the binomial probability distribution and the Poisson probability distribution, which are both distributions of events or counts. Because the normal distribution is a distribution of measures, it is a continuous numerical probability distribution. More is said about the consequence of this fact in Chapter 6.

KEY TERMS

=BINOMDIST()	independence
=EXP()	joint probability
=FACT()	marginal probability
=POISSON()	mutually exclusive
a priori	normal distribution
bell-shaped curve	outcome
binomial distribution	Poisson distribution
conditional probability	probability
contingency table	sample space
empirical probability	standard deviation
event	stochastic process

MEASURES OF CENTRAL TENDENCY AND DISPERSION: DATA DISTRIBUTIONS

Statistics do not convey emotion. They shock us for a minute or two, and then we click again.

—Madeleine M. Kunin

There are three related, but quite different, uses of statistics. The first of these uses is descriptive. In a descriptive context, statistics are used to characterize either a total *population* or a sample from that population, but they go no further than characterization. The second use of statistics is inferential. In an inferential context, statistics from a sample are used to make inferences about the populations from which the samples were drawn. The third use of statistics is in hypothesis testing. Here, statistics are used to assign a probability to the likelihood that a particular statistical value could have come from some specifiable population, that two (or more) sample (or population) groups are different from one another, or that a measure taken from a sample (or from a population) is of a particular value. This chapter deals with the first of these uses of statistics: description. Subsequent chapters cover in detail both inferential statistics and hypothesis testing.

6.1 Measures of Central Tendency and Dispersion

This chapter is about data distributions. Two ways of characterizing any data distribution are by the central values around which the data cluster, measures of central tendency, and by the extent to which the data are variable, measures of *dispersion*.

LEARNING OBJECTIVES

- Understand the definitions and concepts associated with central tendency

- Understand measures of dispersion

- Understand the ways in which data are distributed over their range of values (frequency distribution)

- Understand the sampling distribution of the mean

- Understand the mean and standard deviation of a discrete numerical variable

- Understand the concepts associated with the distribution of a proportion

- Understand the concepts associated with the t distribution

Central Tendency: Mean, Median, Mode

One of the most important ways of characterizing either populations or samples is to provide information about what is called the *central tendency* of the data. There are three commonly employed measures of central tendency: the *mean*, the *median*, and the *mode*. These three measures can be illustrated with the data shown in Figure 6.1. This figure shows the amount of time—in one-minute intervals—that a physician may spend with patients who come to his office for treatment. Patient 1 received two minutes of the physician's time, patient 2 received eight minutes, and so on.

Central tendency is the degree of clustering of values in a statistical distribution and is usually measured by arithmetic mean, median, or mode.

Mean or Average

In statistical applications, the average is almost always called the mean and is defined formally for a sample as:

$$\bar{x} = \frac{\sum_{i=1}^{n} x_i}{n} \tag{6.1}$$

where $\bar{x}$ (pronounced x bar) designates the sample mean and $\sum$ (pronounced sigma) indicates a summation of all values x_i from $i = 1$ to $i = n$, with n being the sample size.

For the data shown in Figure 6.1, Equation 6.1 would be executed as $(2 + 8 + 11 + \cdots + 14)/12$ (the three dots mean to continue adding the numbers), and the result would be the mean, which is approximately 8.92.

	A	B
1	Patient	Minutes with patient
2	1	2
3	2	8
4	3	11
5	4	12
6	5	6
7	6	10
8	7	7
9	8	8
10	9	14
11	10	8
12	11	7
13	12	14

Figure 6.1 Time spent by physician with patients

In this example, the median is 8 and the mean is 8.92. The mean and the median are frequently different. For example, a large number of people stay in the hospital for short periods of time and incur relatively small charges, whereas a small number of people have relatively long hospital stays and incur high charges. Therefore, for hospital days and cost per admission, the mean is higher than the median, and the distribution of both is skewed to the right. If the mean of a data set is lower than the median, the data are skewed to the left.

"Mean" is also referred to as simple average.

Median

"Median" refers to the middle value in an ordered set of values, or, if there is an even number of values, it refers to the average of the two middle values. If we look at the data from Figure 6.1, as reordered in Figure 6.2, we can see that the sixth and seventh observations (out of 12, an even number) are both 8. The average of two values of 8 is also 8, so that the median for this set of data is 8. Typically, it is more likely that the median will be used to describe a set of data than the mode will be used. It is not uncommon to see the median referenced as the measure of central tendency in such examples as median family income, median age, and median inpatient days. It can be said that half the values of a data set lie above the median and half of the values lie below the median.

"Median" refers to the middle of the data set.

	A	B
1	Patient	Minutes with patient
2	1	2
3	5	6
4	7	7
5	11	7
6	2	8
7	8	8
8	10	8
9	6	10
10	3	11
11	4	12
12	9	14
13	12	14

Figure 6.2 Ordered time spent by physician with patients

Mode

"Mode" refers to the most commonly appearing value in a set of data. In this case, eight minutes is the most commonly appearing value and is the mode, or modal value. The physician spent eight minutes with each of three patients. Data sets can be bi- or multimodal if more than one value is represented an equal number of times. If, for example, patient 5 had received seven minutes of the physician's time, both eight minutes and seven minutes would have been modal values. In general, although the mode is usually listed as one of the three measures of central tendency, it rarely figures into any further statistical applications.

Mode is the most commonly appearing value in a data set.

The mode provides a measure of central tendency that uses only the most commonly appearing value. The median essentially provides a measure of central tendency that uses only the middle value (for an odd number of observations) or the two middle values (for an even number of observations) in an ordered array. The mean uses all the information in the data set to provide a measure of central tendency. The mean should be a familiar concept to most readers. It is the average. Few people taking their first statistics course are unfamiliar with how to obtain an average for a set of numbers; you just add them and divide by the total number of numbers.

Excel Functions for Central Tendency

Microsoft Excel provides a function for each of the three measures of central tendency. These are =MODE(), =MEDIAN(), and =AVERAGE() (not =MEAN()). The =MEDIAN() and =AVERAGE() functions work just as one would expect, producing the correct value. The =MODE() function will produce the correct value if the data set has only one mode. If it has more than one mode, it will produce a result that indicates only one of the modal values—the value that appears earliest in the data set.

Most of the work we do in this book with measures of central tendency will be done with the mean. The presentation in Equation 6.1 refers specifically to the mean of a sample of observations from some larger population. In the case of the data shown in Figure 6.1 or Figure 6.2, the population would presumably be all patients who ever did or ever will come to the office of the particular physician in question. If we were to consider the mean as a measure of central tendency for the entire population of patients who ever did or ever will visit this physician, it would be designated by slightly different symbols. The mean for a population is defined as shown in Equation 6.2. In Equation 6.2, the sample designation $\bar{x}$ has been replaced by the population designation μ and the sample designation for all the observations in the sample, n, has been replaced by the population designation for all possible observations in the population, N.

$$\mu = \frac{\sum_{i=1}^{N} x_i}{N} \qquad (6.2)$$

where μ (the small Greek letter μ, pronounced mu) designates the population mean and N represents all patients who ever have or ever will visit the physician. The value of x_i is summed from $i = 1$ to N.

The point of using the formula in Equation 6.1 to calculate the mean of the sample is that it is what is known as an unbiased estimator of the true population mean defined in Equation 6.2. An unbiased estimator is a sample estimator of a population parameter for which the mean value from all possible samples will be exactly equal to the population value. Thus, since $\bar{x}$ is an unbiased estimator of μ, the mean of the values of $\bar{x}$ from all possible samples taken from the population will be exactly equal to μ. More is said of this in the next section.

Dispersion

A measure of central tendency, whether it be the mode, median, or mean, can be produced for virtually any data set. Similarly, a measure of dispersion or variation in the data can also be produced for any data set. Dispersion describes how far values in the data set are from the measure of central tendency. Larger values of dispersion characterize data sets that are spread out (i.e., the data contain higher highs and/or lower lows than the mean). Smaller values of dispersion characterize data sets that have more values clustered closely together (i.e., the values in the data set tend to be clustered close to the mean). *Range*, *variance*, and *standard deviation* are all measures of dispersion.

> Range, variance, and standard deviation are all measures of dispersion. Dispersion describes how far values in the data set are from the measure of central tendency.

Range

A simple measure of dispersion is the range. The range is the difference between the largest and smallest values in the data set. There are also a number of modifications on the range, such as the range within which are found the lowest 25 percent of cases, the highest 25 percent of cases, the middle 50 percent of cases, and so on. The range is a measure of dispersion that is similar in concept to the median as a measure of central tendency. It uses only a limited amount of the data. Except for some descriptive purposes, the range is rarely used in statistical analysis applications and is therefore not discussed further in this book.

Variance and Standard Deviation

The measure of dispersion that, like the mean, uses all the information in the data is the variance, or its square root, the standard deviation. Both the variance and standard deviation are used extensively in statistical applications and are, in fact, the basis upon which much of statistics is constructed. The variance for a sample is defined mathematically as shown in Equation 6.3.

$$s^2 = \frac{\sum_{i}^{n} (x - \bar{x})^2}{n - 1} \tag{6.3}$$

where s^2 designates the variance and $\sum$ indicates a summation of all values of $(x - \bar{x})^2$ from $i = 1$ to $i = n$.

The standard deviation for a sample is calculated as shown in Equation 6.4.

$$s = \sqrt{\frac{\sum_{i}^{n} (x - \bar{x})^2}{n - 1}} \tag{6.4}$$

Calculating Variance and Standard Deviation with =VAR() and =STDEV()

Basically, the variance is a measure of the extent to which each observation differs from the mean of all observations. For the data shown in Figure 6.1, the variance calculation is shown in Figure 6.3, a spreadsheet representation of the calculation. In Figure 6.3, the patient number is shown in cells A3 to A14, and the minutes spent with the physician are shown in cells B3 to B14. Cells C3 to C14 show the calculation of the numerator portion of Equation 6.3. The mean value for the data (shown in cell B15) is subtracted from each cell B3 to B14, and the result is then squared (the Excel formula for cell C3, for example, is $=(B3-\$B\$15)^2$). The title in cell C2 is a convenient way to show this operation in Excel, because it is difficult to put bars above letters or to create superscripts to show the square process.

Figure 6.3 Calculation of variance

The ^2 is the Excel convention for raising a value to a power. Cell C15 is the sum of the squared differences (=SUM(C3:C14)), and cell C16 is the actual variance as calculated by the formula in Equation 6.3 and Figure 6.3 (=C15/11). The number in cell C17, which is identical to cell C16, is the variance as calculated using the =VAR() function. This function can be seen in the formula bar above the spreadsheet, because cell C17 was the highlighted cell when this image was captured. It is relatively easy to confirm the results shown in Figure 6.3. All that is required is to enter the data in column B into a spreadsheet and follow the formula given in Equation 6.3. Table 6.1 shows the formulas for Figure 6.3.

The variance is a measure of dispersion calculated on the basis of squared differences between each observation and the mean of all observations. This produces a measure of dispersion that is not on the same scale as the measure of central tendency (the mean). The variance actually corresponds more closely to the square of the mean than to the mean itself.

Table 6.1 Formulas for Figure 6.3

Cell	Formula
B15	=AVERAGE(B3:B14)
C3	Cell C3 is copied down to cell C14
C15	=SUM(C3:C14)
C16	=C15/11
C17	=VAR(C3:C14)

To get the measure of dispersion back to the same scale as the mean, the measure of dispersion that is typically used is the standard deviation, shown in Equation 6.4.

The value of the standard deviation for the data shown in Figure 6.3 is approximately 3.48. You can confirm this by using the =STDEV() function, which Excel provides for calculating the standard deviation on the data shown in Figure 6.3. You can also confirm that the =STDEV() function actually produces the square root of the variance by using the =SQRT() function to calculate the square root of the variance given in the same figure. You should find that the results of the two methods are the same.

The formulas in Equations 6.3 and 6.4 provide the variance and standard deviation for samples from a larger population. If we wished to calculate the variance and standard deviation for the entire population of patients who ever had or ever would attend the clinic in question, we would use the formula shown in Equation 6.5. The equation for the standard deviation of the population, designated σ^2, is just the square root of the value in Equation 6.5.

$$\sigma^2 = \frac{\sum_{i}^{N} (x_i - \mu)^2}{N} \tag{6.5}$$

where σ^2 designates the variance and N indicates that the summation of $(x_i - \mu)^2$ is over all observations in the entire population.

Why Is the Sample Variance Divided by *n* − 1?

In the calculation of the most frequently used measure of central tendency—the mean—the formulas for the sample estimate of the population parameter (Equation 6.1) and the population parameter itself (Equation 6.2) are calculated essentially the same way. All the values are summed and divided by the number of separate values. For the variance, however, and similarly for the standard deviation, the population value and the sample values are not calculated in the same way. The population variance as shown in Equation 6.5 is, logically, the sum of all the squared differences between actual values and the overall mean divided by the total number of observations; but the sample variance (Equation 6.3) is divided, instead, by the total number of observations less one. On the face of it, this does not seem logical. Why should it be so?

Interestingly, the answer to this question has to do, again, with unbiased estimators. As was mentioned earlier, the sample formula for the mean shown in Equation 6.1 is an unbiased estimator of the population value of the mean shown in Equation 6.2. Similarly, under the sampling with replacement assumption, the sample formula for the variance shown in Equation 6.3 will be an unbiased estimator of the population value of the variance calculated, as shown in Equation 6.5. In other words, if we took all possible samples from a population using the technique of sampling with replacement, the average variance for all possible samples calculated, as given in Equation 6.3, would be exactly equal to the population variance calculated, as given in Equation 6.5. This relationship has been proved mathematically, and the proof is given, for example, in Freund and Walpole (1987). Such a proof is beyond the scope of this book. But what this book does do is use the capabilities of Excel to demonstrate that the sample variance calculated, as given in Equation 6.3, is an unbiased estimate of the population variance calculated, as given in Equation 6.5. This holds true for a very small population as well as for a very small sample. Such a demonstration does not guarantee that it will work for any population or for any sample, but it at least demonstrates that it is reasonable.

An Example of Sampling with Replacement: In Other Words, Why n − 1?

Let us imagine a very small population that consists of only four observations. These four observations take on the following four values: 2, 4, 5, and 7. If this is the entire population, it is relatively easy to confirm that the mean, μ, for this population is 4.50, using the formula in Equation 6.2, and the variance σ^2 is 3.25, using the formula in Equation 6.5. To examine the effect of taking all possible samples, we can limit ourselves to all the possible samples of a given size. Whatever the outcome for a sample of any size, the outcome for all samples of other sizes will be the same.

First, what is sampling with replacement? Suppose we want a sample of size two, and we randomly select one observation from our very small population, which turns out to be 5. Now we will draw a second observation from the population to complete the sample of two. In sampling with replacement, we return the observation 5 to the population so that it has an equal chance, along with all other observations, of being drawn in the second selection. If we were sampling without replacement and drew the observation with the value of 5 on the first draw, that observation would not be available for the second draw, which would be limited to the observations with values of 2, 4, and 7.

If we are taking samples with replacement, there are N^m different samples of size n that can be taken from a population of size N. If we are sampling without replacement, there are different samples of size n that can be taken from a population of size N. This is a substantially smaller number than N^m. This is discussed in more detail later, but you should recognize

	A	B	C	D	E	F	G	H
1		Population	Sample	First	Second	Mean	Variance	
2		2	1	2	2	2	0	
3		4	2	2	4	3	2	
4		5	3	2	5	3.5	4.5	
5		7	4	2	7	4.5	12.5	
6			5	4	2	3	2	
7			6	4	4	4	0	
8	Mean	4.50	7	4	5	4.5	0.5	
9	Variance	3.25	8	4	7	5.5	4.5	
10			9	5	2	3.5	4.5	
11			10	5	4	4.5	0.5	
12			11	5	5	5	0	
13			12	5	7	6	2	
14			13	7	2	4.5	12.5	
15			14	7	4	5.5	4.5	
16			15	7	5	6	2	
17			16	7	7	7	0	
18								
19					Overall average	4.5	3.25	
20								

Figure 6.4 All samples of two from a population of four

this as being part of the binomial distribution formula. In the case of our population of four observations, there are 4^2, or 16, different samples of size two that can be taken from the population with replacement. These samples are shown in Figure 6.4.

Using Excel to Demonstrate Why n − 1 Is Used

Cells B2:B5 in Figure 6.4 are the values taken on by each of the four members of the population. The value in cell B8 is the mean of the population calculated with the =AVERAGE(B2:B5) function. The value in cell B9 is the variance of the population calculated with the =VARP(B2:B5) function, which calculates the population variance as given in Equation 6.5. The cells C2:C17 just number the 16 different samples of size two that can be taken from the population of four with replacement. Cells D2:D17 show the first observation in each sample, and cells E2:E17 show the second. Cells F2:F17 represent the means of each sample calculated, using =AVERAGE() for each of the corresponding two cells in D and E. For example, cell F2 is calculated as =AVERAGE(D2:E2). Cell F19 is calculated as =AVERAGE(F2:F17). It can be seen that it matches the value in B8. Similarly, cells G2:G17 are calculated by the =VAR() function, with the appropriate references in columns D and E. Note that the =VAR() function divides by $n − 1$ rather than by n. The number in cell G19 is calculated as =AVERAGE(G2:G17) and is the average of all the sample variances. It is equal to the number in cell B9. If, instead of using =VAR() to calculate the sample variances in G2:G17, we had used =VARP(), the average of all sample variances (cell G19) would have been not 3.25 but, rather, 1.625—a value much smaller than the true population variance.

This is a demonstration of the appropriateness of using the formulation in Equation 6.3 as the sample variance. This ensures that we obtain a measure that will be an unbiased estimate of the population variance as calculated in Equation 6.5. But two things should be remembered. First, although it is a demonstration (and it works every time), it is not a proof. Also, this relationship between Equation 6.3 and Equation 6.5 holds only for samples taken with replacement. In most cases, samples are not taken with replacement. If you drew a sample of people for interviews, you would not want to interview the same person twice if it happened by chance that he got into the sample twice. When one is sampling without replacement, the formulation in Equation 6.3 is not an unbiased estimate of the population variance. But, in general, the size of a sample relative to the size of a population makes it highly unlikely that any single population item will be selected more than once, so that sampling with replacement might be assumed. Interestingly, when one is sampling without replacement, the average of all sample variances calculated by Equation 6.3 turns out to be numerically equal to the variance of the population calculated by replacing N in Equation 6.5 with $N - 1$.

One other point should be made in regard to unbiased estimates of dispersion. The typical measure of dispersion used is the standard deviation or the square root of the variance. The average value of the standard deviation of all possible samples from any population will not be equal to the standard deviation of the total population, calculated by any means. This is because, in general:

$$\sqrt{\sum x_i} \neq \sum \sqrt{x_i}$$

Why Is the Measure of Dispersion So Complicated?

Why is it necessary to use something so complicated? Could there not be a simpler measure of dispersion that did not involve the complicated problem of squaring and taking square roots? For example, could we simply use the difference between each value and the mean or the absolute value of the difference between each value and the mean?

Cumulative Differences

One such possibility might be the sum of the differences between each value and the mean of all values, which could be shown as given in Equation 6.6.

$$\sum_{i=1}^{n}(x_i - \bar{x}) \tag{6.6}$$

Unfortunately, this strategy does not work well. Because the mean is the numerical midpoint of the distribution, the sum of all the negative numbers will always equal the sum of all the positive numbers derived from the operation given in Equation 6.6. In turn, the result of this operation is always zero for every data set. Because of this, Equation 6.6 cannot serve as a useful measure of dispersion.

Absolute Differences

But what if a measure of dispersion were the absolute value of the difference between each observation and the mean of all observations? Such a possibility would be expressed as Equation 6.7.

$$\sum_{i=1}^{n} |x_i - \bar{x}| \qquad (6.7)$$

Unfortunately, this criterion also does not work well for a measure of dispersion if our measure of central tendency is the mean. One assumption we are making is that any measure of dispersion we ultimately choose should be centered on the mean. This assumption is true for both Equations 6.6 and 6.7.

Measures of Dispersion and Being Centered at the Mean

To understand the notion of centered in the context of Equation 6.7, consider Figure 6.5. This table shows a column (cells A16 : A22) of seven data points that take on the values 1 through 7, respectively. It is easy to confirm that the mean of these seven items is 4. Cells B15 : H15 contain seven possible constants that may be substituted for the mean in Equation 6.7, including the true mean of 4. The formula line in Figure 6.5 shows that the value in cell B16 is the absolute difference between those in cells A16 and B15. Cell B17 is the absolute difference between cells A17 and B15. The remaining values are calculated in the same way. The sums of the absolute

	B16		= =ABS($A16-B$15)					
	A	B	C	D	E	F	G	H
14		Constant						
15	Data	1	2	3	4	5	6	7
16	1	0	1	2	3	4	5	6
17	2	1	0	1	2	3	4	5
18	3	2	1	0	1	2	3	4
19	4	3	2	1	0	1	2	3
20	5	4	3	2	1	0	1	2
21	6	5	4	3	2	1	0	1
22	7	6	5	4	3	2	1	0
23		21	16	13	12	13	16	21

Figure 6.5 Sum of absolute differences

differences in each column are given in cells B23 : H23. The value 12 in cell E23, which corresponds to the mean, is the smallest of the sum of absolute differences. In this sense, the result of Equation 6.7 is centered on the mean in this data set. If any number other than the mean is used as the constant subtractor, the result of the sum of absolute differences will be greater than the value when the mean is employed. In general, a working assumption is that whatever measure of dispersion is chosen, it should be centered on the mean. By being centered at the mean, the measure of dispersion then produces a minimum sum of differences at, and only at, the mean.

But Equation 6.7 does not always produce the minimum value at the mean. In fact, it turns out that Equation 6.7 always produces a minimum value at the median. To see an illustration of this, consider the data shown in Figure 6.6. This table again shows seven observations (cells A30 : A36). In this case, it is not difficult to confirm that the mean of the data elements is 4, whereas the median is 2. Again, the values in cells B30 : H36 are the absolute differences between each data point and the constant values listed in cells B29 : H29. Now it can be seen that the minimum value of the absolute differences (16 in column C) is centered not on the mean of 4 but, rather, on the median of 2. This is the primary reason that the absolute differences between each value and the median are not generally used as a measure of dispersion when the mean is the measure of central tendency. (It can also be shown that for data sets that have even numbers of cases, the absolute difference is centered in the sense discussed here on both values that define the median and on all possible numerical values between them.)

Now what of the sum of squared differences (Equation 6.3) as a measure of dispersion? Does it provide a measure that is centered on the mean? Consider Figure 6.7, which shows the sum of squared differences for the data displayed in Figure 6.6. Now, the minimum value of the sum of differences (squared) is at the mean of 4, so the sum of squared differences is centered at the mean. The reader might wish to confirm that for the data in Figure 6.5, the sum of squared differences is a minimum at the mean.

B30			= =ABS($A30-B$15)					
	A	B	C	D	E	F	G	H
28		Constant						
29	Data	1	2	3	4	5	6	7
30	1	0	1	2	3	4	5	6
31	2	1	0	1	2	3	4	5
32	2	1	0	1	2	3	4	5
33	2	1	0	1	2	3	4	5
34	7	6	5	4	3	2	1	0
35	7	6	5	4	3	2	1	0
36	7	6	5	4	3	2	1	0
37		21	16	17	18	19	20	21

Figure 6.6 Sum of absolute differences, second example

B44	▼	■ =($A44-B$15)^2						
	A	B	C	D	E	F	G	H
42		Constant						
43	Data	1	2	3	4	5	6	7
44	1	0	1	4	9	16	25	36
45	2	1	0	1	4	9	16	25
46	2	1	0	1	4	9	16	25
47	2	1	0	1	4	9	16	25
48	7	36	25	16	9	4	1	0
49	7	36	25	16	9	4	1	0
50	7	36	25	16	9	4	1	0
51		111	76	55	48	55	76	111

Figure 6.7 Sum of squared differences

It will turn out that for any data set, the sum of squared differences has the desirable property that it is centered at the mean in the sense that the sum of squared differences between the data elements and any constant will be a minimum when the true mean is the constant.

EXERCISES FOR SECTION 6.1

1. Use the Hospital charges worksheet in the file Chpt 4-1.xls.

   a. Calculate the mean and median for Age, LOS, and Charges by using the =AVERAGE() and =MEDIAN() functions.

   b. Based on these, in what direction are these distributions skewed, if at all?

   c. Calculate the variance and standard deviation of Age, LOS, and Charges by using the formulas in Equations 6.3 and 6.4.

   d. Calculate the variance and standard deviation of Age, LOS, and Charges by using the =VAR() and =STDEV() functions. Make sure that the results in (c) match those in (d).

2. Use the SWC worksheet in the file Chpt 4-1.xls.

   a. Calculate the mean and median for U5MR, IMR, and LEB by using the =AVERAGE() and =MEDIAN() functions.

   b. Based on these, in what direction are these distributions skewed, if at all?

   c. Calculate the variance and standard deviation of U5MR, IMR, and LEB by using the formulas in Equations 6.3 and 6.4.

   d. Calculate the variance and standard deviation of U5MR, IMR, and LEB by using the =VAR() and =STDEV() functions. Make sure that the results in (c) match those in (d).

3. A complete population consists of the values 1, 2, 5, 6, and 9.

   a. Demonstrate that the mean of the means of all samples of size two, taken with replacement from the population, will equal the true population mean.

b. Demonstrate that the mean of the variances of all samples of size two, taken with replacement from the population, will equal the true population variance. (The sample variance in Excel is =VAR ( ) and the population variance is =VARP ( ) .)

c. Demonstrate that the mean of the variances of all samples of size two, taken without replacement from the population, will equal a value for the true population calculated using the sample variance formula.

4. Use the population given in Exercise 3.

a. Demonstrate that the mean of the means of all samples of size three, taken with replacement from the population, will equal the true population mean.

b. Demonstrate that the mean of the variances of all samples of size three, taken with replacement from the population, will equal the true population variance. (The sample variance in Excel is =VAR ( ) and the population variance is =VARP ( ) .)

c. Demonstrate that the mean of the variances of all samples of size three, taken without replacement from the population, will equal a value for the true population calculated using the sample variance formula.

5. Fourteen women delivering at a hospital on a single day had made the following number of prenatal visits prior to their delivery:

3	4	6	4	15
4	6	12	5	5
4	4	9	3	

a. Using the model given in Figures 6.5, 6.6, and 6.7, show that $\sum_{i=1}^{n} |x_i - \bar{x}|$ is centered at the median in the sense discussed previously.

b. Using the same model, show that $\sum_{i=1}^{n} (x_i - \bar{x})^2$ is centered at the mean.

6.2   The Distribution of Frequencies

The measures of central tendency and dispersion discussed in Section 6.1 represent one way to characterize a set of data. A second way to characterize a data set is by the manner in which it is distributed over its range of values, commonly known as a frequency distribution. The frequency distribution was discussed in some detail in Chapter 4. In that discussion, the frequencies generated with the =FREQUENCY ( ) function were based on BIN ranges. The BIN ranges are developed by dividing the range from highest to lowest data values by some arbitrary number, such as six, to create six frequency intervals. This section discusses the frequency distribution further, basing the BIN ranges on standard deviations of the data.

Frequency Distributions and Standard Deviations

A frequency distribution can be based on arbitrary BIN ranges (e.g., six equal-size ranges, from the smallest to the largest value in the data set). But they can also incorporate information about the mean and standard deviation of the data to help in the understanding of those data. The example considered here will use the Human Development Index (HDI) for the countries of the world, as given by the United Nations Development Program (UNDP) for 1999 (https://hdr.undp.org/content/human-development-report-1999). The HDI is developed from measures of life expectancy, literacy, and gross domestic product (GNP) per capita for each country. The entire data set used in developing the HDI and the HDI for each country for which UNDP gives an HDI value for 1999 are contained in the Excel file Chpt 6-1.xls.

The HDI is given in column J in the Excel file Chpt 6-1.xls. To create a frequency distribution incorporating information about the mean and standard deviation, it is first necessary to calculate those values for the HDI. This can be done using the =AVERAGE() and =STDEVP() functions. (Because this data set represents virtually all countries of the world for which the requisite data are available, it is being treated as a population rather than as a sample.) The actual mean of the HDI is 0.684, and the standard deviation is 0.181.

Using the Mean and Standard Deviation to Create a Frequency Distribution

The use of the mean and standard deviation in creating a frequency distribution is shown in Figure 6.8. In Figure 6.8, column B contains the countries of the world ranked by HDI number. There are actually 162 countries ranked in column B, but only the first 13 are shown in the figure. Column C contains the HDI score for the top 13 countries. The maximum score (for Norway) is 0.939. The minimum score (which is not shown and is for Sierra Leone) is 0.258. The mean of the HDI score across countries is shown in cell E2 as 0.684, and the standard deviation is shown in cell E3 as 0.181. Beginning in cell E6 is the sequence of numbers $-3, -2, \ldots 3$. This sequence represents a distance from the mean in numbers of standard deviations ranging from -3 to 3. These distances are actually calculated in cells F6:F12. The equation that is used to calculate the distances is shown for F6 in the formula line as =$E$2+E6*$E$3.

	F6	▼	=	=$E$2+E6*$E$3		
	A	B	C	D	E	F	G
1	HDI Rank, 1999		HDI99				
2	1	Norway	0.939	Mean	0.684		
3	2	Australia	0.936	StDev	0.181		
4	3	Canada	0.936				
5	4	Sweden	0.936		StDevs	Bin Values	Frequency
6	5	Belgium	0.935		-3	0.140	0
7	6	United States	0.934		-2	0.321	5
8	7	Iceland	0.932		-1	0.502	32
9	8	Netherlands	0.931		0	0.684	25
10	9	Japan	0.928		1	0.865	70
11	10	Finland	0.925		2	1.046	30
12	11	Switzerland	0.924		3	1.227	0
13	12	Luxembourg	0.924				162
14	13	France	0.924				

Figure 6.8 Frequency distribution with mean and standard deviation, HDI data

This formula notation means that when the formula is copied from cell F6 to cells F7 through F12, the formula will refer to the relevant consecutive cells from E7 to E12 but will always refer to cell E2 (the mean) and cell E3 (the standard deviation).

Table 6.2 shows the formulas for Figure 6.8.

Creating a Frequency Distribution Using the =FREQUENCY() Function

The frequency distribution is shown in G6:G12; it was calculated using the =FREQUENCY(C2:C163,F6:F12) function. You will recall that it is always necessary to use Ctrl+Shift+Enter to get the =FREQUENCY() function to work correctly because it is one of the functions that compute a value for more than one cell at a time. Two things might be noted about the frequency distribution. First, the sum of the frequency distribution given in cell G13 as 162 (=SUM(G6:G12)) confirms that all of the countries are included in the frequency distribution. Second, the HDI value for every

Table 6.2 Formulas for Figure 6.8

Cell	Formula
E2	=AVERAGE(C2:C163)
E3	=STDEVP(C2:C163)
F6	=$E$2+E6*$E$3. Cell F6 is copied down to cell F12.
G6	=FREQUENCY(C2:C163,F6:F12) Note: Remember to use Ctrl+Shift+Enter.
G13	=SUM(G6:G12)

country is contained in the range from 3 standard deviations below the mean to 2 standard deviations above the mean. (Remember that the Bin value refers to the top of a particular range so that −2 contains all countries with HDI scores between 0.140 and 0.321.)

The histogram created by this frequency distribution of the HDI data is also of interest; it is shown in Figure 6.9. Several things might be mentioned in regard to this figure. First, the histogram includes data only for the range from −3 to +3 standard deviations. Typically, most of the observations in almost any data set will be in the ±3 standard deviation range. A second point of interest is that column I contains Bin labels that were not used in the calculations in any way but were used to label the horizontal dimension of the graph. This was discussed in Chapter 4 in the section on construction of graphs. It should be remembered that the Bin values actually used in the =FREQUENCY() formula represent the top of the BIN range. For example, the −2 in cell E7, which is associated with the value 0.321 in cell F7, actually refers to the range from −3 to −2 standard deviations. Column H represents the percentage of countries in each BIN range.

The histogram itself shows a distribution of the frequencies that is not atypical for many distributions. The observations tend to cluster near the mean and be fewer further from the mean. Ninety-five of the 162 countries (58 percent) have HDI scores within 1 standard deviation of the mean. When one counts the number of countries within 2 standard deviations of the mean, there are 157 of the 162 (97 percent). This type of distribution of individual cases around the mean is typical of many distributions found in the real world. In many cases, data are distributed approximately in what is known as a *normal distribution*. The normal distribution was introduced in Chapter 5. There, it was indicated that the normal distribution is symmetrical with an equal number of

Figure 6.9   Histogram (graph) of HDI values

observations above and below the mean. A second characteristic of the normal distribution is that approximately 68 percent of the observations are within ±1 standard deviation of the mean and 95 percent of the observations are within ±2 standard deviations. The distribution in Figure 6.9 is not actually symmetrical (70 countries are in the range of 1 standard deviation above the mean, whereas only 25 are within the range of 1 standard deviation below). Still, the percentages of 58 percent at ±1 standard deviation and 97 percent at ±2 standard deviations are not far from the normal distribution percentages of 68 percent and 95 percent.

The Normal Distribution

The normal distribution was introduced in Chapter 5 and discussed briefly in the previous section. This section provides additional detail on the normal distribution and the importance of the mean and standard deviation in the normal distribution.

A normal distribution is one that is symmetrical and that has approximately 68 percent of its observations within ±1 standard deviation of the mean and 95 percent within ±2 standard deviations. In addition, a normal distribution has about 99 percent of its observations within ±3 standard deviations of the mean. Excel provides a number of options for constructing and visualizing a normal distribution. Figure 6.10 shows a normal distribution generated by Excel, one that shows the classic form of normal distribution. The distribution is symmetrical and takes on what has been called the *"bell-shaped" curve* because it looks somewhat like the side view of a bell.

Figure 6.10 Normal distribution

	C2		=	=1/SQRT(2*PI()*1)*EXP((-1/2)*((A2-0)/1)^2)	
	A	B	C	D	E	F
1	StDev	Normal Dist	Normal Dist2			
2	-4	0.0001338	0.0001338			
3	-3.9	0.0001987	0.0001987			
4	-3.8	0.0002919	0.0002919			
5	-3.7	0.0004248	0.0004248			
6	-3.6	0.0006119	0.0006119			
7	-3.5	0.0008727	0.0008727			
8	-3.4	0.0012322	0.0012322			
9	-3.3	0.0017226	0.0017226			
10	-3.2	0.0023841	0.0023841			
11	-3.1	0.0032668	0.0032668			
12	-3	0.0044318	0.0044318			
13	-2.9	0.0059525	0.0059525			
14	-2.8	0.0079155	0.0079155			
15	-2.7	0.0104209	0.0104209			
16	-2.6	0.013583	0.0135830			
17	-2.5	0.0175283	0.0175283			
18	-2.4	0.0223945	0.0223945			

Figure 6.11 Calculations for normal distribution

Constructing a Normal Distribution: The =NORMDIST() Function

The way in which the normal distribution in Figure 6.10 was constructed in Excel tells us a lot about the kinds of information that can be obtained from Excel. Figure 6.11 shows a portion of the spreadsheet that was used to produce the normal distribution shown in Figure 6.10. Column A, labeled StDev, represents the distance from the mean in standard deviation units. Cell A2 is shown as −4, which means that the cell represents 4 standard deviation units below the mean. Cell A3, with the value −3.9, represents 3.9 units below the mean, and so on. The values in column A increase to 4 in cell A82 (not visible in the figure). Column B is labeled Normal Dist. The value in cell B2 is produced by the =NORMDIST() function and represents the proportion of the normal distribution that falls at the point represented by −4. The proportion of the normal distribution falling at any single point is given in Equation 6.8. The values in column C, labeled Normal Dist2, represent the normal distribution values calculated by the formula shown in Equation 6.8. The way in which the formula is expressed in Excel is shown in the formula line in Figure 6.11.

$$f(x) = \frac{1}{\sqrt{2\pi}\sigma} e^{-\left(\frac{1}{2}\right)\left(\frac{x-\mu}{\sigma}\right)^2} \tag{6.8}$$

The syntax of =NORMDIST(), which is not shown in Figure 6.11, is =NORMDIST(Cell Ref,0,1,0). The =NORMDIST() function takes four arguments: (1) the cell reference (Cell Ref) for which the point proportion of the normal distribution is desired (e.g., 24, 23.9, etc.), (2) the mean of the distribution (in this case, 0), (3) the standard deviation of the distribution (here given as 1), and (4) a value of 0, indicating that the distribution desired is the normal probability density function and *not* the cumulative normal distribution. The cumulative normal distribution will be discussed later.

Characteristics of the Normal Distribution

Looking at Figure 6.10, it should be recognized that there is a very small proportion of the observations in a normally distributed data set that lies outside the range −3 to +3 standard deviations. In fact, a normal distribution has about 99 percent of its observations in the −3 to +3 range on either side of the mean. However, some proportion of a normal distribution (albeit a very small proportion) is out beyond 4 standard deviations, 5 standard deviations, and even 20 standard deviations. The probability of its being out at those extremes is finite, but very, very small. Although it is not obvious from Figure 6.10, about 68 percent of the observations lie in the range from −1 to +1 standard deviations and about 95 percent lie in the range from −2 to +2 standard deviations.

It is basically correct to say that 68 percent of all observations in a normal distribution are within 1 standard deviation on either side of the mean value. It is also true that approximately 95 percent of all observations are within ±2 standard deviations of the mean. In addition, around 99.7 percent of all observations lie within ±3 standard deviations of the mean. But an interesting characteristic of normal distributions is that they are based on scales that are continuous rather than discrete. For example, if one were measuring the height of U.S. adult men, the recorded measurement would be limited by the measuring device itself. A standard ruler probably has no units smaller than quarters of an inch. Therefore, one could measure a person's height to the nearest quarter inch only.

For a normal distribution it can be said that around:

- 68 percent of all observations are within +1/−1 standard deviation of the mean.

- 95 percent of all observations are within +2/−2 standard deviations of the mean.

- 99.7 percent of all observations are within +3/−3 standard deviations of the mean.

However, a more sophisticated measuring technique might make it possible to measure with more precision. In fact, it might be discovered that someone who was measured as being 5 feet, 10 and 1/2 inches tall might actually be 5 feet, 10 and 7/16th inches tall. A still more sophisticated measurement tool might measure that person as actually 5 feet, 10 and 455/1,000th inches tall.

By continuing to increase the precision of the measurement, we are able to measure things on what might be considered a true scale of infinite possibilities A consequence of this theoretical ability is that the probability of any given observation at any one specific spot in the normal distribution (e.g., exactly 1 standard deviation above the mean) is actually zero. We then have a finite number of objects distributed over an infinite number of sites (points in the scale). In turn, the probability that any one object will fall on any specific site will be the number of observations divided by infinity, which will always come out to zero. The consequence of this is that the actual proportion of observations between two points in a normal distribution (say, 2 standard deviations below to 2 standard deviations above the mean) cannot be calculated from the formula in Equation 6.8. Instead, the actual proportion of observations within any interval in the normal distribution must be taken from the cumulative normal distribution. This distribution is discussed in detail in the following subsection.

Cumulative Normal Distributions and Excel

The cumulative normal distribution sums all the probabilities of the normal distribution up to a given specific value. For example, suppose the mean weight of newborns is 3,600 grams (about eight pounds) and the standard deviation is 850 grams. If the weight of newborns is normally distributed, the cumulative normal distribution, then, using Excel, could tell us that we would expect that just under 10 percent of all newborns should be under 2,500 grams, the cutoff for low birth weight. This could be calculated with the =NORMDIST() function as =NORMDIST(2500,3600,850,1). In the function, 2,500 equals the low birth-weight level, 3,600 is the mean weight in grams, 850 is the standard deviation, and 1 indicates that the cumulative distribution is desired.

The value of the cumulative normal distribution is that it allows the determination of the exact probability of any observation when a normal distribution is assumed. Figure 6.12 shows a graph of the cumulative normal distribution based on standard deviations from the mean. The figure shows that the cumulative normal distribution starts at zero in the range to the left of 3 standard deviations below the mean. It increases (because it accumulates all previous percentages) to a maximum approaching one (100 percent) in the range to the right of 3 standard deviations above the mean.

Figure 6.12 Cumulative normal distribution

The actual value of any point on the cumulative normal distribution can be found by using the =NORMDIST() function, with the first argument being the value of the point of interest, the second being the mean of the distribution, the third being the standard deviation, and the fourth being the value 1, to denote that the cumulative normal distribution is being requested. The values of the cumulative normal distribution represent the area under a normal curve to the left of any number. We can also estimate the probability of being greater than or less than a certain value. For example, by subtracting =NORMDIST(5000,3600,850,1) from 1, we can predict that only about 5 percent of all newborns will weigh more than 5,000 grams (about 11 pounds).

Approximating the Area under a Normal Curve

The actual value we obtain is the integral of the area under the curve from $-\infty$ to the number in question, but it can be approximated using one of several methods. The formula in Equation 6.9 is the way the area under the cumulative normal distribution is calculated by Excel, and it duplicates the result of the Excel =NORMDIST(x,mean, stdev,1) function. This formula is an approximation, rather than an exact solution, but its results are far more readily obtained than any exact solution.

$$p(x) = 1 - Z(x)(b_1 t - b_2 t^2 - b_3 t^3 - b_4 t^4 - b_5 t^5) \qquad (6.9)$$

where

$$Z(x) = \frac{1}{\sqrt{2\pi\sigma^{-\frac{x^2}{2}}}} \qquad t = \frac{1}{1+px}$$

$$p = 0.2316419$$

$$b_1 = 0.319381530 \quad b_2 = -0.356563782$$

$$b_3 = 1.781477937 \quad b_4 = -1.821255978$$

$$b_5 = 1.330274429$$

Equation 6.9 works for values of x greater than 0. If the value of x is less than 0, it is necessary to subtract $p(x)$ from 1 in order to get the probability from ∞ to the value of x less than 0. For example, to obtain the cumulative proportion at -1, as shown in Figure 6.12 (approximately 15 percent, by the graph), it would be necessary to find the cumulative proportion at the value of 1, as shown in Figure 6.12, and subtract that value from 1 to get the cumulative proportion at -1.

There is no particular reason why you, as a user of this book, will need to know the formulas in Equation 6.8 or those in Equation 6.9. But we are always interested in how things happen. If Excel provides a value for the cumulative normal distribution, we like to know, if possible, where Excel got the value. Thus the equations are given. You may use them as you wish.

Understanding the Cumulative Normal Distribution in Excel

Figure 6.13 shows the values generated by a cumulative normal distribution based on the assumption that U.S. newborns average 3,600 grams and that the distribution of the weight of newborns has a standard deviation of 850 grams. Column A shows 0.5 standard deviation unit from the mean

C3		fx	=NORMDIST(B3,$E$3,$E$4,1)		
	A	B	C	D	E
1		Weight of Newborns			
2		Weight	Probability		
3	-3.5	625	0.000233	Mean	3600
4	-3	1050	0.001350	StDev	850
5	-2.5	1475	0.006210		
6	-2	1900	0.022750		
7	-1.5	2325	0.066807		
8	-1	2750	0.158655		
9	-0.5	3175	0.308538		
10	0	3600	0.500000		
11	0.5	4025	0.691462		
12	1	4450	0.841345		
13	1.5	4875	0.933193		
14	2	5300	0.977250		
15	2.5	5725	0.993790		
16	3	6150	0.998650		
17	3.5	6575	0.999767		

Figure 6.13 Cumulative normal probabilities for the weight of newborns

of 3,600. Column B shows the weight in grams that corresponds to each standard deviation unit from the mean, assuming a mean of 3,600 grams and a standard deviation of 850 grams. Column C is the probability that was obtained, as the formula line indicates, with the =NORMDIST() function. The first argument is the weight given in column B, the second is fixed as the mean given in cell E3, the third is the standard deviation given in cell E4, and the final argument is the 1 denoting cumulative distribution.

To understand the logic and use of the cumulative normal distribution, suppose there is an interest in knowing what proportion of newborns will weigh less than 2,000 grams (2 standard deviations below the mean). To determine this, given the assumption that the average is 3,600 grams and the standard deviation is 850 grams, it is necessary only to look at the probability given in cell C6 in Figure 6.13. According to that cell, fewer than 3 percent of newborns would weigh as little as 2,000 grams. What if the interest were in knowing what proportion of newborns would weigh more than some amount at birth—say, 4,875 grams? Still, assuming a mean of 3,600 and a standard deviation of 850, it is possible to see that the probability associated with 4,875 grams (cell C13) is approximately 0.93. But this is the proportion of newborns who will weigh 4,875 or less. To get the proportion that will weigh 4,875 or more, it is necessary to subtract the proportion at 4,875 from 1; so, the actual proportion who will weigh more than 4,875 grams at birth is $1 - 0.93$, or approximately 0.07.

Finding the probability of any occurrence that can be described by a normal distribution with a known mean and standard deviation can be accomplished with the use of the =NORMDIST() function. Suppose the weight of 13-year-old girls is normally distributed with a mean of 100 pounds and a standard deviation of 15 pounds. What is the likelihood of finding a 13-year-old girl who weighs less than 70 pounds? The answer can be found in Excel with =NORMDIST(70,100,15,1), which returns the result of about 0.02. Suppose the body temperature of healthy adults is normally distributed with a mean of 98.6 degrees Fahrenheit and a standard deviation of 0.5 degrees. What is the probability of observing a healthy adult with a temperature of 101 degrees Fahrenheit or more? The answer can be found using Excel's =NORMDIST(101,98.6,0.5,1) function, which produces 0.9999 to four decimals. We do not want to know the probability of finding a healthy adult with a temperature below 101. Rather, we want the probability of finding a healthy adult with a temperature of 101 or above. That would be found as $1 - 0.9999$, or 0.0001 at four decimal places. Because the probability of finding a healthy adult with a temperature of 101 is so small, we would typically conclude that such a person could not be healthy.

EXERCISES FOR SECTION 6.2

1. Use the Hospital charges worksheet in the file Chpt 4-1.xls.

   a. Based on the mean and standard deviation for LOS, generate a frequency distribution in terms of 1 standard deviation unit around the mean.

   b. Develop the Excel chart to show the frequency distribution generated in (a).

2. Use the SWC worksheet in the file Chpt 4-1.xls.

   a. Based on the mean and standard deviation for IMR, generate a frequency distribution in terms of 1 standard deviation unit around the mean.

   b. Develop the Excel chart to show the frequency distribution generated in (a).

3. Use the data set in Chpt 6-1.xls, and do the following:

   a. Calculate the mean and standard deviation of the HDI.

   b. Generate a frequency distribution for the HDI in terms of 1 standard deviation unit from the mean.

   c. Develop an Excel chart to show the frequency distribution generated in (b).

   d. Compare the result with the graph shown in Figure 6.9.

4. Use the mean and standard deviation for LOS as used in Exercise 1.

   a. Develop the probability distribution in terms of 1 standard deviation unit that would be expected if LOS were normally distributed. Include at least 3 standard deviations on each side of the mean.

   b. Develop an Excel chart to show the frequency distribution generated in (a).

5. Assume that the height of U.S. males is normally distributed with a mean of 70 inches and with a standard deviation of 3 inches.

   a. Generate the normal distribution probabilities for the height of adult males in one-inch units, including at least 3 standard deviations on each side of the mean.

   b. Develop an Excel chart to show the frequency distribution generated in (a).

6. Assume that adult diastolic blood pressure is normally distributed with a mean of 75 mm hg and a standard deviation of 5 mm hg.

   a. Generate the normal distribution probabilities for the diastolic blood pressure in one-mm hg units, including at least 3 standard deviations on each side of the mean.

   b. Develop an Excel chart to show the frequency distribution generated in (a).

7. Assume the mean and the standard deviation of the height of adult males as given in Exercise 5. Use the =NORMDIST() function to determine the following:

   a. The proportion of men who are less than 65 inches tall

    b. The proportion of men who are less than 69 inches tall

    c. The proportion of men who are greater than 71 inches tall

    d. The proportion of men who are greater than 68 inches tall

    e. The proportion of men between 67 and 70 inches tall

8. Assume the mean and standard deviation of diastolic blood pressure as given in Exercise 6. Use the =NORMDIST() function to determine the following:

    a. The proportion of people who have diastolic blood pressure less than 76 mm hg

    b. The proportion of people who have diastolic blood pressure less than 72 mm hg

    c. The proportion of people who have diastolic blood pressure greater than 73 mm hg

    d. The proportion of people who have diastolic blood pressure greater than 79 mm hg

    e. The proportion of people who have diastolic blood pressure between 72 and 78 mm hg

9. Assume that waiting time in an emergency room is normally distributed with a mean of 38 minutes and a standard deviation of 10 minutes. Using the =NORMDIST() function, determine the following:

    a. The proportion of people who wait less than 30 minutes

    b. The proportion of people who wait less than 20 minutes

    c. The proportion of people who wait more than 40 minutes

    d. The proportion of people who wait more than 50 minutes

    e. The proportion of people who wait between 25 and 45 minutes

6.3 The Sampling Distribution of the Mean

The previous subsection discussed the variance and the standard deviation as measures of dispersion that apply both to populations and to samples taken from populations. The discussion was concerned with the dispersion of the individual entities that make up the population or sample. So, for example, when waiting time for patients was discussed, it was the dispersion of the waiting times for individual patients that was the subject of the variance or standard deviation calculation. In this section we take up a somewhat different concept—the sampling distribution of the mean.

The Standard Error with a Known Variance

Consider a population made up of all discharges from a hospital for the past year. The hospital has 200 beds and an average LOS of 5.2 days. The total number of hospital discharges over the year is approximately 12,000.

Figure 6.14 Length of stay for one year of discharges from a 200-bed hospital

The standard deviation calculated for all stays is 4.12 days (the formula used is that in Equation 6.5, because this is the population of all discharges for the year). These 12,000 discharges are distributed as shown in Figure 6.14. As the figure shows, the length of stay for the 12,000 discharges is skewed to the right, as would be expected, because the length of stay can never be less than zero days, and the standard deviation is large, relative to the mean length of stay. If the distribution were not skewed, approximately 47.5 percent of a normally distributed variable would be within 2 standard deviations below the mean. So, although the standard deviation can be readily calculated for these hospital discharges, it must be remembered that the meaning of standard deviation is not what it would be if the length of stay were actually normally distributed.

We know the actual mean length of stay of the population of discharges. It is 5.2 days. But suppose we did not know the mean length of stay, and the only way we could get an estimate of it was to draw successive samples from all discharges. To keep the discussion relatively simple, we will say that it is possible to draw only samples of size 100. So we will be drawing successive samples of 100 discharges in order to estimate the true mean. Suppose we draw a first sample of 100 discharges and the mean for the sample is 5.76 days. This is an estimate of the true population mean, but, clearly, it is not the true mean. But we do not know this, because all we have at this point is the one sample estimate. So we draw a second sample of 100 to estimate the true mean. This time we get a value of 5.17 as an estimate of the mean of the total population. We continue to draw samples of size 100 from the discharges until we have 250 separate samples.

Calculating and Interpreting the Means of the Samples

Because we now have 250 sample means, we decide that the value we will accept for the true mean of the population will be the mean value of the

250 samples. When we calculate the mean of the 250 sample means, we discover that it is 5.22. So 5.22 becomes the estimate to represent the true mean of the population. But that is not the end of the story. Clearly, the mean values from our 250 samples have a distribution of their own. What can we say about that distribution? To look at that distribution, we are going to graph it in standard deviation units from the mean. But we are not going to use population, or even sample standard deviation units. We are going to use the standard deviation units of the sample means.

The standard deviation of the sample means is 0.402. The largest sample mean in the set of 250 was 6.45, and the smallest was 4.29. Given the standard deviation of 0.402, we would expect that about 95 percent of the sample means would be between 4.42 and 6.02, which is 2 standard deviations on either side of the mean of the samples, if the 250 means are normally distributed. The distribution of the 250 sample means is shown in Figure 6.15.

Figure 6.15 shows a very different picture when compared with Figure 6.14. Although the actual discharges as shown in Figure 6.14 are heavily skewed to the right, the means of 250 samples selected from that original data, shown in Figure 6.15, are almost normal in their distribution. It is not totally obvious from Figure 6.15, but about 70 percent of all sample means are within one *standard error* of the mean of all samples (the normal distribution has 68 percent). Also, about 97 percent of the mean values are within 2 standard deviations of the mean of all samples (the normal distribution has 95 percent). So the distribution shown in Figure 6.15 is seen to be a fairly close approximation of a normal distribution.

This finding that the means of 250 samples approximate a normal distribution reveals an interesting characteristic of sampling—or, rather, the means of samples. When the sample size is relatively large (30 or more in the sample is usually considered relatively large), the distribution of sample

Figure 6.15 Distribution of 250 sample means

means tends to be normal, regardless of the nature of the distribution of the actual values. This characteristic of the distribution of sample means will be very useful when the notion of confidence limits is examined in Chapter 7.

The Concept of Standard Error

In an examination of the distribution of sample means, a relatively new notion was introduced. This is the standard deviation of the sample means. Up until this time, the discussion of standard deviations has focused on the individual observations. When the standard deviation of actual lengths of stay was calculated for the hospital data, it was 4.12 days. But when the standard deviation of the 250 sample means was calculated, it turned out to be only 0.402 days. A question that might now be asked is whether there is any defined relationship between the standard deviation of the individual observations and the standard deviation of the sample means. This leads to the introduction of the concept of the standard error. The standard error is the standard deviation of the sample means for samples of a given size.

The standard error is the standard deviation of the sample means for samples of a given size.

If the true population variance is available, the standard error is given as shown in Equation 6.10. This shows that there is a very specific relationship between the standard deviation of the population and the standard error of the means of samples drawn from the population. This relationship is precisely that the standard error of the means is the standard deviation of the individual observations divided by the square root of the sample size.

$$S.E._{\bar{x}} = \frac{\sigma}{\sqrt{n}} \qquad (6.10)$$

The formula in Equation 6.10 provides an interesting comparison. However, let's go back for a moment to variance rather than the standard deviation. From Figure 6.4 it can be seen that the mean of the variance of all possible samples of size two from a population of four will be exactly equal to the variance of the four actual observations. Similarly, the standard deviation of all four observations divided by the square root of the sample size of two will be exactly the same as the standard deviation of the means from all possible samples of size two taken from the population of four. This is demonstrated in Figure 6.16, which is the same as Figure 6.4. However, Figure 6.16 now shows the population standard deviation divided by the square root of the sample size (cell B10) and the standard deviation

F20	▾	≡ =STDEVP(F2:F17)				
	A	B	C	D	E	F	G
1		Population	Sample	First	Second	Mean	Variance
2		2	1	2	2	2	0
3		4	2	2	4	3	2
4		5	3	2	5	3.5	4.5
5		7	4	2	7	4.5	12.5
6			5	4	2	3	2
7			6	4	4	4	0
8	Mean	4.50	7	4	5	4.5	0.5
9	Variance	3.25	8	4	7	5.5	4.5
10	StDev/sqrt(2)	1.27475	9	5	2	3.5	4.5
11			10	5	4	4.5	0.5
12			11	5	5	5	0
13			12	5	7	6	2
14			13	7	2	4.5	12.5
15			14	7	4	5.5	4.5
16			15	7	5	6	2
17			16	7	7	7	0
18							
19					Overall average	4.5	3.25
20					Standard Deviation of Means	1.27475	
21							

Figure 6.16 Comparison of the population variance divided by two and the variance of the mean of all samples of size two

of the means of all samples of size two (cell F20). These two values are exactly the same. (It should be noted that the standard deviation of the means of all samples is calculated using the population standard deviation function =STDEVP (). This is appropriate, because this set of means is the population of all mean values.)

Now let us return to our 250 samples of size 100. The standard error of the mean for samples of size 100 using Equation 6.10 is 4.12 divided by the square root of 100, or 0.412. This is close to the standard deviation of the means that was calculated from the 250 samples we selected (0.402) but is not identical. Why the difference? It is simply because we do not have all the possible samples of size 100 that could be selected from the 12,000 discharges. If we sampled with replacement, there would be $12{,}000^{100}$ such samples—a very large number indeed. However, if we did have the means of all those samples, they would be equal to the standard error as calculated in Equation 6.10, or exactly 0.412.

The Standard Error with an Estimated Variance

Equation 6.10 is fine if the population variance is known. In general, however, the population variance is not known. Typically, unlike the example previously discussed, we would have only one sample—with one sample mean and one sample standard deviation. How, then, would we be able to determine the standard error (the standard deviation of the sampling distribution of the means of all samples)? The best estimate of the standard deviation of the population when we have only one sample is the standard deviation of the sample values. So the standard error is typically estimated as given in Equation 6.11. More about the importance of the standard deviation of individual samples in calculating the standard error of the mean is provided in Chapter 7.

$$S.E._{\bar{x}} = \frac{s}{\sqrt{n}} \qquad (6.11)$$

The Standard Error When Sample Size Is Large, Relative to Population Size

Virtually all populations that we may have any interest in are finite; that is, they have a countable number of elements. The number of all hospital admissions for a year is a finite population. The infant mortality rate for all the countries of the world represents the infant mortality rate of a finite population. All the health departments in a state represent a finite population. But in some cases, a sample is large relative to a finite population, and in some cases it is not. A sample of 20 health departments from all those in a state is a large sample relative to the population if there are only 65 health departments in the entire state. A sample of 200 hospital discharges from all discharges for a year is not large relative to the population if the hospital has 15,000 discharges per year. However, in the former case, it is appropriate to reduce the standard error calculated by Equation 6.11 by multiplying times a value that is commonly called the *finite population correction*, or fpc.

The fpc is given by the formula in Equation 6.12. As the equation shows, the fpc is the square root of the population size minus the sample size divided by the population size minus 1. With a population of 15,000 discharges and a sample of 200, it is easy to confirm that the value of the fpc would be about 0.99, and probably not worth bothering with. However, for a sample of 20 health departments from a population of 65, the fpc would be about 0.84 and probably small enough to make a useful difference in the standard error.

$$fpc = \sqrt{\frac{(N-n)}{N-1}} \qquad (6.12)$$

If the finite population is to be used in the calculation of a standard error, the entire formula would be as shown in Equation 6.13.

$$S.E._{\bar{x}} = \frac{s}{\sqrt{n}} \sqrt{\frac{(N-n)}{N-1}} \qquad (6.13)$$

Drawing Multiple Samples of Any Size: Random Number Generation

The random number generation add-in that is part of the Data Analysis package in Excel provides a way to draw multiple random samples from a population. Although this would never be done in a real research project, it is useful as a learning device, particularly in regard to understanding the way in which the means of a large number of samples are distributed.

To see how Excel can be used to draw a large number of separate samples from a defined population, suppose we have a population of women who have come for prenatal visits. We will assume that this is a very large population. The distribution of the visits and the probability of their making a specific number of visits are shown in Figure 6.17. As the figure shows, there is about a 6 percent chance of their making one visit, an 11 percent chance of their making two visits, a 17 percent chance of their making three visits, and so forth. No woman made more than 15 prenatal visits.

Drawing Samples Using Excel's Data Analysis Add-In

We will draw a large number of samples of size 30 from this population using the Data Analysis add-in. The Data Analysis add-in is found in the Data ribbon in the Analysis tab. Selecting the Data Analysis menu in the

	A	B
1	Prenatal Visits	Proportion of Women
2	1	0.0588
3	2	0.1104
4	3	0.1710
5	4	0.1981
6	5	0.1702
7	6	0.1175
8	7	0.0795
9	8	0.0418
10	9	0.0237
11	10	0.0121
12	11	0.0068
13	12	0.0045
14	13	0.0030
15	14	0.0019
16	15	0.0007
17		

Figure 6.17 Probabilities of prenatal visits

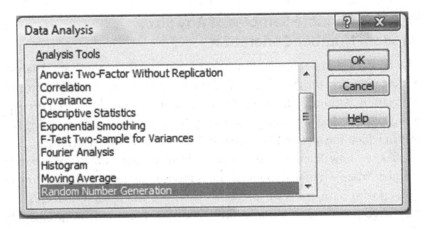

Figure 6.18 Data Analysis dialog box

Analysis tab will invoke the Data Analysis dialog box shown in Figure 6.18. In the Data Analysis dialog box we select Random Number Generation.

Selecting Random Number Generation will invoke the Random Number Generation dialog box, shown in Figure 6.19. This dialog box (shown along with the part of the spreadsheet that contains prenatal visits and the proportion of women making those visits) contains several items.

Figure 6.19 Random Number Generation dialog box

The first category of information that needs to be supplied is the number of samples desired, here labeled Number of Variables. We are going to generate 100 separate random samples, so we enter 100 in the Number of Variables field. Each sample we generate will include 30 observations, so we enter 30 in the Number of Random Numbers field. Figure 6.19 shows a dotted line from cell A2 to cell B16, the range that is put into the value and probability input range. Column A represents the discrete visits (from 1 to 15), and column B represents the probability of any woman making each number of visits during her pregnancy. In the Random Seed field we enter 3,275, which was generated using the =RAND() function, dropping the decimal point and taking only the first four digits. The last piece of information required by the Random Number Generation dialog box is where the output will go. We want it on a new sheet, so we click the New Worksheet Ply radio button.

Calculating the Measures of Central Tendency and Dispersion for the Sample

When we click OK in the Random Number Generation dialog box, Excel generates 100 samples of prenatal visits of size 30, based on the probabilities given in column B. The result of the generation of these 100 samples is shown in Figure 6.20. This figure shows only a portion of the spreadsheet in which the random numbers have been generated. Each column in the spreadsheet shown in Figure 6.20 represents a separate sample. The numbers in each column represent the number of visits made by the women selected to be part of each sample of 30. The first woman selected as part

	A	B	C	D	E	F	G
1	3	4	2	2	2	6	3
2	4	3	4	5	5	9	1
3	3	3	3	7	7	2	5
4	2	4	4	2	4	4	4
5	4	4	7	4	4	4	7
6	3	4	1	5	3	3	2
7	5	5	6	2	5	5	5
8	4	4	4	7	3	5	3
9	4	3	9	4	6	6	4
10	2	2	4	4	7	11	7
11	7	6	11	3	2	5	6
12	3	13	3	3	6	9	10
13	4	11	4	7	3	6	5
14	5	5	10	5	1	4	4
15	4	3	2	2	6	6	3
16	8	4	4	2	2	4	1

Figure 6.20 Random samples of visits

of the first sample (cell A1) made three visits to the clinic. The second woman selected for the first sample made four visits to the clinic, and so on. Because there are 30 observations in each sample, the numbers in each column actually run to row 30. Because there are 100 samples, the numbers in the columns run to column CV.

Given these 100 samples of size 30, we can calculate the mean, standard deviation, and standard error of each sample, as shown in Figure 6.21. In this figure, a first column has been added to the spreadsheet to provide a place to put the labels for mean, standard deviation, and standard error. This figure shows the last six numbers selected in the first six samples, and row 32 displays the mean of the number of visits for the 30 women in each sample. Row 33 shows the standard deviation as estimated by this sample, and row 34 shows the standard error. The calculation for the standard error for column B—the first sample—is shown in the formula bar.

Let us now look at the distribution of means from a large number of samples. Figure 6.22 shows the distribution of sample means from 250 samples of size 100 taken from the population of women who have come

B34	▼	=	=B33/SQRT(30)				
	A	B	C	D	E	F	G
25		5	4	5	4	4	5
26		6	3	3	3	3	5
27		6	8	3	3	7	4
28		3	4	1	3	4	3
29		9	3	6	12	5	9
30		3	6	6	6	8	1
31							
32	Mean	4.533333	4.933333	5.033333	4.2	4.433333	5.1
33	St Dev	1.995397	2.504249	2.697168	2.21904	1.851064	2.577756	2.5:
34	St Error	0.364308	0.457211	0.492433	0.405139	0.337956	0.470632	0.∕
35								

Figure 6.21 Example of calculations of means, standard deviations, and standard errors for 100 samples

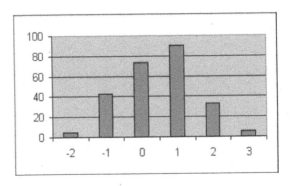

Figure 6.22 Distribution of means from 250 samples of size 100

for prenatal visits. The x-axis represents standard deviation units from the mean. The designation −2 shows those samples with mean values from −3 to −2 standard deviations from the mean. The designation −1 shows those samples with mean values from −2 to −1 standard deviations from the mean, and so on. It is clear from this figure that sample means from relatively large samples approximate a normal distribution, even though the original data may not.

This section discusses the use of Excel to generate a large number of samples with given attributes. It is important to remember, however, that, in general, one never draws more than one sample. The discussion here is presented solely for the purpose of helping the reader understand the use of the discrete sampling option in the random number generation add-in. This example is referred to again in Chapter 7, which discusses the calculation of confidence limits.

EXERCISES FOR SECTION 6.3

1. Determine the standard error of the mean for each of the following:

    a. A random sample of 100 persons whose blood pressure has been measured when the known standard deviation is 2.5 mm hg

    b. A random sample of 38 men when the known standard deviation for height is three inches

    c. A random sample of 65 persons who are waiting in an ER when the known standard deviation for waiting time is 10 minutes

    d. The LEB for 16 countries randomly selected from the SWC sheet of the file Chpt 4-1.xls when the countries on the sheet represent the entire population of countries (consider using the finite population correction)

    e. The IMR for 20 states randomly selected from the 50 states given on the U.S. IMR worksheet of the file Chpt 4-1.xls (consider using the finite population correction)

2. Determine an estimate of the standard error of the mean for the following:

    a. Waiting time in an emergency room for a random sample of 36 people selected from the Emergency Room Wait worksheet of the file Chpt 6-2.xls, assuming that the records shown represent the population of emergency room visits for a month

    b. U5MR for a random sample of 20 countries selected from the SWC worksheet of the file Chpt 4-1.xls (consider using the finite population correction)

    c. BP for a random sample of 42 persons selected from the BP worksheet of the file Chpt 6-2.xls, assuming that the records shown represent the population of persons who have had their blood pressure checked at a single clinic in the past month

   d. Number of prenatal visits for a sample of 60 women selected at random from the population of women shown in Figure 6.17

3. Using the Emergency Room Wait worksheet of the file Chpt 6-2.xls, do the following:

   a. With the discrete sampling option, select 100 samples of size 30 from the population of waits. (It is necessary to assign a probability of 1/832 to each of the 832 waits before drawing the samples. This probability should appear in column C.) Be sure to generate a random seed using =RAND().

   b. Calculate the mean, standard deviation, and standard error of each of the 100 samples.

   c. Generate a frequency distribution of the means of the 100 samples, based on 1 standard deviation unit around the mean of all sample means.

   d. Display the resulting frequency distribution in a column graph, and give some interpretation as to whether the distribution looks approximately normal.

   e. Save this file for later use.

4. Using the prenatal visits for the women shown in Figure 6.17 (Visits worksheet of Chpt 6-3.xls), do the following:

   a. With the discrete sampling option, select 250 samples of size 100 from the population of women. Be sure to generate a random seed using =RAND().

   b. Calculate the mean, standard deviation, and standard error for each of the 250 samples.

   c. Generate a frequency distribution of the means of the 250 samples, based on 1 standard deviation unit around the mean of all sample means.

   d. Display the resulting frequency distribution in a column graph, and give some interpretation as to whether the distribution looks approximately normal.

   e. Save this file for later use.

6.4 Mean and Standard Deviation of a Discrete Numerical Variable

The introduction of the prenatal visits shown in Figure 6.17 gives an opportunity to briefly discuss the mean and standard deviation of a *discrete numerical variable*. Discrete numerical variables can take on only whole number values. With a variable that takes on only whole number values, it is possible to introduce a different definition of the mean and standard deviation. These definitions are given in Equations 6.14 and 6.15.

$$\mu = \sum_{k=1}^{T} x_k p(x_k) \qquad\qquad (6.14)$$

and

$$\sigma = \sqrt{\sum_{k=1}^{T} (x_k - \mu)^2 p(x_k)} \qquad (6.15)$$

where k designates each separate value of x, T represents the total of all different values of x, and p represents the probability associated with each value of x.

What the formulas in Equations 6.14 and 6.15 say is that the population mean of a discrete numerical variable is given as the sum of all values that the variable takes on, multiplied by the probability of any one of those values. The population standard deviation is the square root of the sum of the difference between each value that the variable takes on and the population mean multiplied by the probability of any one of the values.

Calculating Mean and Standard Deviation of a Discrete Variable

A demonstration of the calculation of both the mean and standard deviation of a discrete numerical variable is shown in Figure 6.23. Columns A and B represent the number of visits made by women and the proportion of women making each number of visits, respectively, as originally shown in Figure 6.17. These columns have been renamed to indicate that they

	D2		= =(A2-$C$18)^2*B2	
	A	B	C	D
1	Visits (x)	Proportion (p(x))	x*p(x)	(x-mu)^2*p(x)
2	1	0.0588	0.0588	0.7499
3	2	0.1104	0.2208	0.7298
4	3	0.1710	0.513	0.4221
5	4	0.1981	0.7924	0.0646
6	5	0.1702	0.851	0.0313
7	6	0.1175	0.705	0.2399
8	7	0.0795	0.5565	0.4690
9	8	0.0418	0.3344	0.4915
10	9	0.0237	0.2133	0.4649
11	10	0.0121	0.121	0.3566
12	11	0.0068	0.0748	0.2810
13	12	0.0045	0.054	0.2483
14	13	0.0030	0.039	0.2131
15	14	0.0019	0.0266	0.1689
16	15	0.0007	0.0105	0.0761
17				
18			4.5711	5.0071
19				2.2377

Figure 6.23 Calculation of the mean and standard deviation of a discrete numerical variable

represent the variable x (column A) and the probability of the value of x, $p(x)$ (column B). Column C represents the multiplication of each value of x by the probability of x. The sum of column C is given in cell C18, with the formula =SUM(C2:C16). This is the population mean. Column D represents the square of the difference between each value of x and the mean of x (in cell C18), multiplied by the probability of x. The sum of values in column D is given in cell D18 with the formula =SUM(D2:D16). This is the population variance. The standard deviation—the square root of the variance—is given in cell D19, or with the formula =SQRT(D18).

It should be recognized that the results obtained by the formulas in Equations 6.14 and 6.15 produce exactly the same results as the formulas in Equations 6.1 and 6.5. The difference lies in the fact that the latter formulas treat each observation individually, whereas the former deals with the values of the variable and the proportion of times the values appear in the data set.

EXERCISES FOR SECTION 6.4

1. Using the data shown in Figure 6.17 (Visits worksheet in Chpt 6-3.xls), replicate the figure to calculate the mean and standard deviation for prenatal visits.

2. Chapter 5 discussed the probabilities of having zero through seven children (Figure 5.3) in a population of 2,556 women. Using those data (or the Births worksheet in Chpt 6-3.xls), calculate the mean and standard deviation of this population of 2,556 women by using the appropriate formulas from this section.

3. A local health department does an audit of 600 of its records and discovers the distribution of recording errors as shown on the Errors worksheet in Chpt 6-3.xls. Use these data to calculate the mean and standard deviation of the errors in records, using the appropriate formulas in this section.

4. A hospital knows that 0.646 percent of the persons coming to the emergency room come for true emergencies. Using the formulas in this section and the binomial distribution, calculate the mean and standard deviation for any 10 arrivals at the emergency room.

6.5   The Distribution of a Proportion

The binomial distribution, discussed in Chapter 5, is the distribution that describes the way in which a sequence of events, all independent of one another and each having two possible outcomes, will be distributed. One example that introduced the binomial distribution was the probability of arrival at an emergency clinic of any given number of emergencies out of

43 arrivals. When the number of observations is relatively large (say, 30 or more) and when the probability associated with either outcome of the observations is in the range 0.2 to 0.8, the binomial distribution can be relatively effectively approximated by the normal distribution.

Calculating Population Proportions

Recall from Chapter 1 the home health agency that wanted to estimate the proportion of correctly completed Medicare forms. It wanted a proportion estimate for all 800 clients from a sample of 80 forms taken at random. If fewer than 85 percent of the sample forms were filled out correctly, this would signal the need for relatively costly training to ensure that the forms were henceforward filled out correctly. The sample of 80 forms showed that only 60 (or 75 percent) had been filled out correctly. The immediate result of this would probably be to alert the agency to the need to initiate this costly remedial training. But before it proceeds, it might be interested in the probability that the true population proportion could be 85 percent. To determine this probability, the agency can treat the distribution of the proportion as if it is normal with a mean at 0.75 and a standard error as given in Equation 6.16.

$$S.E._p = \sqrt{\frac{p \times (1-p)}{n}} \tag{6.16}$$

The value of Equation 6.16 would be exactly the same if =STDEVP()/SQRT(n) were applied to a series of ones and zeros in which 75 percent were ones (or zeros). This idea is demonstrated in Figure 6.24. The figure shows a determination of whether the Medicare

Figure 6.24 Portion of correctly and incorrectly completed forms

forms were filled out correctly for the first nine forms (cells A5:A13). There are actually 80 forms represented in column A (cell A3 is provided by =COUNT(A5:A84)). The 0.75 in cell A1 represents the average for all 80 forms, which is the same as the proportion. The standard error of the distribution is given in cell A2 as calculated using =STDEVP() divided by the square root of 80. Notice that in calculating this standard error, it is assumed that the sample actually represents the entire population, thus the =STDEVP(). If this were not done, the standard error calculated using Equation 6.16 would not equal the result using the actual observations. The standard error calculated using Equation 6.16 is shown in cell B2.

Calculating Population Proportions via the =NORMDIST() Function

Now the probability that the true population proportion of correct forms could be 0.85, given that the sample yielded a proportion of 0.75, can be calculated using the =NORMDIST() function. Recall that in Chapter 5 this probability was calculated using the actual binomial distribution as either 2.2 percent or 1.3 percent, depending on whether the distribution around 0.75 or around 0.85 was considered. Figure 6.25 shows the result of the use of the =NORMDIST() function to determine this same probability. It turns out to be quite similar: 1.9 percent. The difference from the other two values is due to the fact that the binomial distribution is not exactly symmetrical.

Suppose, now, that the home health agency was concerned that if the true population value was 70 percent or less correct, a training event would not be sufficient. In turn, the entire process of keeping the home health records would have to be wholly reorganized. How might the agency determine the probability that the true proportion was 70 percent or less, given a sample value of 75 percent? Again, the agency would use the

Figure 6.25 Calculation of probability of 85 percent correct

C5	▼	= =NORMDIST(0.7,A1,B2,1)		
	A	B	C	D	E
1	0.75				
2	0.048412	0.048412			
3	80				
4	Correct		0.019433		
5	1		0.15085		
6	1				
7					

Figure 6.26 Probability of 70 percent or less

=NORMDIST () function, as shown in Figure 6.26. As this figure shows, the probability that the true population value could be as low as 70 percent or less, given a sample value of 75 percent, is 0.15. On the basis of this result, it is unlikely that the home health agency will decide to restructure its entire process of record keeping.

Why Subtract the Normal Distribution from 1.0?

In determining the probability of being at 0.85 or higher, we subtracted the =NORMDIST () function from 1 (0.019433 in Figure 6.25). In determining the probability of being at 0.7 or lower, we did not subtract the =NORMDIST () function from 1. How was that decision made? In general, it is important to realize what the magnitude of a desired probability is likely to be. If we realize that the distribution around 0.75 is essentially normal, we know that the further from 0.75 we go, the smaller will be the likelihood of our finding the true mean value there. If we are interested in the probability of being away from 0.75 on either side, either higher or lower, we must expect that the probability will be less than 0.5. If we did not subtract the =NORMDIST () function from 1 in Figure 6.25, the probability would have been about 0.98. Clearly that is not less than 0.5, and therefore it must be incorrect. Conversely, when we look at the calculation as being below 0.7, we see that it is away from 0.75 on the other side. Again, the result must be less than 0.5, and so =NORMDIST () alone is the appropriate function. Let's say we had been interested in knowing the probability that the true mean of the population would have been 0.85 or less, given a sample value of 0.75. Once again we would have used the =NORMDIST () function alone, which would have yielded about 98 percent. Because we are now interested in a range that actually includes the sample proportion, we can see that the probability must be more than 0.5—which it is.

Rule of Thumb: When to Subtract the Normal Distribution from 1.0

But if you are interested in a foolproof way of knowing whether to subtract the =NORMDIST() function from 1, here is a general rule: If you wish to know the probability that the true population value is above proportion $p1$, given a sample proportion p_s, subtract the =NORMDIST() function from 1. This is regardless of whether the hypothesized true population value is above or below the sample value. If you wish to know the probability that the true population value is below proportion $p2$, given a sample proportion p_s, do not subtract the =NORMDIST() function from 1. This is demonstrated in Figure 6.27. As the figure shows, when the inequality sign points to the right, one subtracts =NORMDIST() from 1. When the inequality sign points to the left, one does not subtract the =NORMDIST() function from 1.

It was said earlier that the normal distribution when used with a proportion is an approximation of the binomial distribution, which actually applies to a proportion, because a proportion is inevitably a dichotomous outcome. We have seen, in comparing the discussion of the correct forms in Chapter 5 with the discussion here, that the binomial distribution and normal distribution produce similar values but not exactly equal values. Why, then, would we use the normal distribution to find the binomial probabilities?

The reason resides primarily in the difficulty of finding the result. Until the advent of computer programs like Excel, figuring the actual binomial distribution for a probability was much more difficult than obtaining the normal distribution probabilities. Even now, with the use of Excel, it is not possible to obtain binomial distribution probabilities for more than 1,029 observations. This is because the factorial calculations that are involved in the binomial distribution formula result in numbers too large for Excel to handle. In consequence, it is often impossible to use exact binomial probabilities to determine the likelihood of binomial events.

	A	B	C
1			
2	Sample	Population	Formula
3	0.75	>.85	=1-NORMDIST()
4		<.85	=NORMDIST()
5		>.7	=1-NORMDIST()
6		<.7	=NORMDIST()
7			

Figure 6.27   Use of the =NORMDIST() function

EXERCISES FOR SECTION 6.5

1. Use the formula in Equation 6.16 to determine the following standard errors:

    a. $p = 0.3, n = 80$

    b. $p = 0.5, n = 80$

    c. $p = 0.3, n = 250$

    d. $p = 0.5, n = 250$

2. A practice of 18 dentists upgraded their electronic medical records (EMR) system and suspects that in the process they lost information on recalls for many of their patients. They drew a simple random sample of 200 patient records and discovered that 22 of those had follow-up calls that were not included in the new EMR system. Use the =NORMDIST() function to determine the following:

    a. The probability that the true proportion of missed follow-up calls is less than 10 percent among all records

    b. The probability that the true proportion of missed follow-up calls is greater than 20 percent among all records

3. A local health department is concerned about full immunization among children in its state. They draw from state birth records a sample of 150 children born between one and two years before and follow up on the children to determine if they are fully immunized. They discover that 90 of the children are fully immunized. Use the =NORMDIST() function to determine the following:

    a. The probability that the true proportion of fully immunized children is 90 percent or more

    b. The probability that the true proportion of fully immunized children is less than 50 percent

6.6   The *t* Distribution

The normal distribution has been the subject of several sections in this chapter. The normal distribution is a distribution that is based on the notion of an infinite number of observations. Thus far, whenever the normal distribution has been discussed in this book, it has been stated that a distribution tends to be normal—or that the data are approximately normally distributed. This, in part, has been because the normal distribution assumes an infinite number of observations. An important distribution for statistics is a distribution that approximates the normal distribution but does not assume infinite observations. This distribution is called the *t distribution*.

What Is the *t* Distribution?

Whereas the normal distribution assumes an infinite number of observations, the *t* distribution assumes a finite number of observations. Because the normal distribution assumes an infinite number of observations, there is a single normal distribution. Because the *t* distribution depends on the number of observations in question, there is a whole family of *t* distributions. Each *t* distribution corresponds to a separate number of observations—or, more precisely, to a separate degree of freedom.

> The *t* distribution assumes a finite number of observations, whereas the normal distribution assumes an infinite number of observations.

Degrees of Freedom

The concept of *degrees of freedom* will arise a number of times in our discussion of statistics. The discussion of degrees of freedom is central to the probability of an outcome. Before discussing the *t* distribution in more detail, it is desirable to clarify what the concept of degrees of freedom means. Suppose we have a set of four numbers that we know will add to 10. We are going to select those four numbers any way we choose, but at the end they have to add to 10. If we think about the first number, it could be anywhere on the number scale, from $-\infty$ to $+\infty$. For our example, let's say that the first number we choose is 4. We can now select the second number, and it, too, is limited only by $+\infty$ to $-\infty$. But let us say that the second number is -5. Now the third number can be selected, again with no limitations—but imagine that we select 8 as the number. What happens now?

The scenario so far is shown in Figure 6.28. We have selected the numbers 4, -5, and 8 as the first three numbers, and we now wish to select the fourth number. But the total must be 10. For this to be true, we have no choice for the fourth number. It must be 3. Because we wished to choose four numbers that all added to 10, we had three degrees of freedom. We could choose any numbers we wished for the first three numbers (thus the degrees of freedom), but we were constrained to pick the only number that would make the four numbers add to 10 as the fourth number. Here we have seen that the degrees of freedom are the number of values under

	A	B
1	Number	Value
2	1	4
3	2	-5
4	3	8
5	4	?
6	Sum	10

Figure 6.28 Degrees of freedom

consideration less 1. In a very large number of statistical applications, the degrees of freedom will be the number of observations less 1, or as it is often given, $n - 1$.

The t Distribution Approximates the Normal Distribution

Let us go back now to the *t* statistic. The *t* distribution, which approximates the normal distribution, depends on the degrees of freedom. A *t* distribution with 100 degrees of freedom (a sample of size 101) will be more nearly normal in shape than a distribution with 4 degrees of freedom (a sample of size 5). Figure 6.29 shows two different *t* distributions. The white distribution is the *t* distribution for degrees of freedom equal to 100. The dark gray distribution is the distribution for degrees of freedom equal to four. The horizontal axis shows standard deviations from the mean.

The distribution for 100 degrees of freedom is nearly normal. The proportion of cases within 1 standard deviation on either side of the mean

Figure 6.29 Two *t* distributions

is 0.68, and the proportion within 2 standard deviations is 0.95. The distribution for degrees of freedom equal to four appears approximately normal (and it is), but as can be seen from the figure, there are fewer observations in the middle of the distribution and more at the extremes. With the distribution for four degrees of freedom, only about 63 percent of the distribution is within 1 standard deviation of the mean and about 88 percent is within ± 2 standard deviations.

Finding the Exact Percentage of Observations at Any Point on the *t* Distribution

At many times in the course of a statistical analysis, it will be important to know what proportion of a *t* distribution is beyond, for example, 2 standard deviations from the mean, or 3 standard deviations from the mean. One of the capabilities provided by Excel is that of finding the exact probability associated with any portion of a *t* distribution, given the degrees of freedom. In the past, before the widespread availability of computer programs that would do statistics, and particularly before the advent of Excel, the only way to determine this probability was from a table of probabilities of the *t* distribution. Most statistics books, even today, have such tables. The use of the tables is generally described along with the tables themselves at some point in the body of the book.

Using the = TDIST Function

Excel eliminates the need for such tables. Take a look at the two distributions shown in Figure 6.29. We wish to know the exact probability of being outside the range of 2 standard deviations from the mean with 100 degrees of freedom (the white distribution) and with 4 degrees of freedom (the dark gray distribution). The answer can be found with the =TDIST() function. Figure 6.30 shows the exact probability of being outside one, two, and three standard deviations of the mean for 100 degrees of freedom and for 4 degrees of freedom. The formula bar shows the =TDIST() function, which takes three arguments. The first is the number of standard deviations from the mean (column A). The second argument is the number of degrees of freedom (given in B2 and C2). The third argument is the number of tails to consider in the distribution. The number of tails can be 1 if the exact probability of being either above or below a particular standard deviation number is desired (i.e., in only one tail of the distribution). The number of tails will be two if the exact probability of being both above *or* below a

Figure 6.30　Exact probabilities of *t* distributions

certain number of standard deviations is desired (i.e., in both tails of the distribution). Rows 4, 5, and 6 show the two-tail probabilities, whereas rows 8, 9, and 10 show the one-tail probabilities. As Figure 6.30 demonstrates, for example, only about 5 percent of the distribution with 100 degrees of freedom is beyond 2 standard deviations (two-tail), whereas nearly 12 percent of the distribution is beyond 2 standard deviations (two-tail) with 4 degrees of freedom.

Using the =TINV Function

Excel also provides another useful function related to the *t* distribution, the =TINV() function. The =TINV() function will return the exact value of *t* (i.e., the number of standard deviations from the mean) for any probability. So, for example, if one wishes to know the number of standard deviations, it is necessary to go out from the mean in order to include 95 percent of all observations in a *t* distribution with 100 degrees of freedom; that number can be found with =TINV(0.05,100). The result of the =TINV() function, written as in the last sentence, will be 1.98. This means that it is necessary to go out 1.98 standard deviations on either side of the mean to find the interval within which 95 percent of the observations will fall.

One important point about the =TINV() function is that it always returns the two-tail distance from the mean in standard deviation for any probability. For example, if one wanted the one-tail probability distance for a probability of 0.05 and degrees of freedom equal to 100, it would be necessary to use the function =TINV(0.1,100).

EXERCISES FOR SECTION 6.6

1. What is the number of degrees of freedom in each of the following?

    a. A sample of 10 observations

    b. A sample of 100 observations

    c. A sample of 250 observations

    d. A sample of 1,000 observations

2. What is the two-tail probability in each of the following?

    a. $n = 10$, S.E. from the mean = 2

    b. $n = 10$, S.E. from the mean = 3

    c. $n = 100$, S.E. from the mean = 2

    d. $n = 100$, S.E. from the mean = 3

    e. $n = 250$, S.E. from the mean = 2

    f. $n = 250$, S.E. from the mean = 3

3. What is the one-tail probability in each of the following?

    a. $n = 10$, S.E. from the mean = 2

    b. $n = 10$, S.E. from the mean = 3

    c. $n = 100$, S.E. from the mean = 2

    d. $n = 100$, S.E. from the mean = 3

    e. $n = 250$, S.E. from the mean = 2

    f. $n = 250$, S.E. from the mean = 3

4. How many standard errors from the mean are the following assuming two-tail results?

    a. $p = 0.05, n = 10$

    b. $p = 0.12, n = 10$

    c. $p = 0.05, n = 100$

    d. $p = 0.12, n = 100$

5. How many standard errors from the mean are the following assuming one-tail results?

    a. $p = 0.05, n = 10$

    b. $p = 0.12, n = 10$

    c. $p = 0.05, n = 100$

    d. $p = 0.12, n = 100$

KEY TERMS

=AVERAGE()	degrees of freedom
=FREQUENCY()	discrete numerical variable
=MEDIAN()	dispersion
=MODE()	finite population correction
=NORMDIST()	HDI
=RAND()	mean
=SQRT()	median
=STDEV()	mode
=STDEVP()	normal distribution
=TDIST()	population
=TINV()	standard deviation
=VAR()	standard error
=VARP()	*t* distribution
"bell-shaped" curve	variance
central tendency	

PART 2

CHAPTER 7

CONFIDENCE LIMITS AND HYPOTHESIS TESTING

*In ancient times they had no statistics so they had to
fall back on lies.*

—Stephen Leacock

One of the most important functions of statistics, and the
one to which the remainder of this book is devoted, is the
determination of whether two *variables* could be considered to be independent of each other. This is a determination that is made on a sample of observations but is understood to apply to an entire population. The central task of
determining independence is the establishment of confidence limits and the testing of hypotheses about the data.

7.1 What Is a Confidence Interval?

A confidence interval is the range within which we
expect a true population value (e.g., a mean) to lie.

A *confidence interval* is the range within which we
expect a true population value (e.g., a mean) to lie.
Confidence intervals are established from samples and
are used to predict a population value when it is not
possible (e.g., because of high cost or limited time) to
measure the true value directly. For example, suppose
a hospital financial officer wishes to know the average cost of services provided to the hospital's inpatients. But the only record that the hospital maintains
for most hospital stays is information about the insurance-reimbursable amount and total charges. Both of these items

LEARNING OBJECTIVES

- Understand the definition of confidence intervals and confidence limits

- Understand how to calculate confidence limits for multiple samples and the AND ( ) functions

- Understand the concepts associated with hypothesis testing

- Understand and define the types of errors that can be committed when hypothesis testing

- Understand the processes associated with determining and selecting sample sizes are based primarily on length of stay and diagnosis. The only way to get the actual cost of services for any inpatient stay is to examine the specific hospital record, determine which services were provided, and assign a cost to each of these services. In addition, an average-sized hospital might have 10,000 to 15,000 discharges in a given year. If the financial officer were to try to examine each of these to determine the average cost of services provided to inpatients, the magnitude of the task would be prohibitive.

Using a Representative Sample to Infer a Mean

So what is that financial officer to do? The financial officer might reasonably expect that such an assessment could be made for a sample of hospital discharges (e.g., 100). Let's say the financial officer selected a random sample of 100 hospital discharges from all discharges for the past year. It could then be possible to estimate, on the basis of this sample, the true mean cost of services for inpatients. In doing this, the financial officer would calculate a mean value for the sample and infer that this is the mean for all discharges. But as we saw in Chapter 6, the mean value for one sample would not necessarily be the same as the mean value of a second sample. In fact, we learned that if we selected many samples, the means from those many samples would tend to be normally distributed around the mean of all samples (and also around the true mean of all discharges).

Now, the financial officer should be very interested in this point estimate (i.e., the sample mean) of costs per discharge. However, he might also be interested in the range within which the true population mean of costs for all discharges might lie if he were able to measure the cost of all discharges. To examine this question, he would have to begin integrating the mean with a measure of dispersion. To do this we need to return to the data from the 12,000 hospital discharges examined in Chapter 6. But this time, instead of looking at length of stay, we are going to look at hospital costs. In turn, we must look at both a point estimate of the sample mean and the dispersion around that mean to create a confidence interval. How to get from point estimates to confidence intervals is discussed next.

From Point Estimates to Confidence Intervals

As was previously discussed, it is infeasible for the hospital financial officer to get the true mean cost of discharges for the year. However, for the sake of discussion in this book, let us assume that we have accomplished this and that the mean cost of a discharge is $5,905.75. The distribution of costs in standard deviation units is shown in Figure 7.1. Column A shows standard deviation units above and below the actual mean of $5,905.75. Column B shows the actual dollar amount at the top of each standard deviation range.

	A	B	C
1	Stand Dev	Cost	Proportion
2	-2	$ (3,655.16)	0.0000
3	-1	$ 1,125.29	0.0080
4	0	$ 5,905.75	0.6530
5	1	$ 10,686.20	0.2335
6	2	$ 15,466.66	0.0575
7	3	$ 20,247.11	0.0275
8	4	$ 25,027.56	0.0110
9	5	$ 29,808.02	0.0045
10	6	$ 34,588.47	0.0020
11	7	$ 39,368.93	0.0015
12	8	$ 44,149.38	0.0010
13	9	$ 48,929.84	0.0005
14			

Figure 7.1 Distribution of costs for 12,000 discharges

Column C shows the proportion of discharges in the range up to the dollar amount shown in column B. For example, the value $5,905.75 in column B represents those discharges that cost between $1,125.29 and $5,905.75. All other cells in column B are interpreted similarly.

It appears, then, from Figure 7.1, that just over 65 percent of all hospital discharges have costs in the range of 1 standard deviation below the mean (those in cell C4). Twenty-three percent of all discharges have costs in the range of 1 standard deviation above the mean (those in cell C5). Only 0.8 percent of discharges have costs below 1 standard deviation below the mean (cell C3). The remaining discharges have costs ranging from 1 standard deviation above the mean to 9 standard deviations above the mean. Clearly, actual costs are not normally distributed. However, based on what was learned in Chapter 6, we can have some confidence that if samples of a large enough size are taken, the means of those samples will be approximately normally distributed. This assumption is valid in that it is the mean that we wish to estimate rather than any one individual discharge cost.

Integrating the Sample Mean and Standard Error

So, for example, suppose the financial officer chose a random sample of 100 discharges from among all the hospital discharges for the year in question. In turn, let's say he determined after an examination of the records that the mean for the 100 discharges was exactly $6,586.30. He might then infer that the true average cost of hospital stays was $6,586.30. However, the financial officer must keep in mind that this is only an estimate about the population mean based on a sample.

Now, because the officer had a graduate course in statistics he decides to determine a confidence interval for this mean value. The financial officer remembers that sample mean values are distributed approximately as a t distribution, with degrees of freedom (df) equal to the sample size minus 1—for our example, $df = 100 - 1 = 99$. He also remembers that having two standard errors on either side of the mean gives the approximate range in which he will have a 95 percent likelihood of finding the true mean of the population. (In fact, 1.98 standard deviations on either side of the mean will give him the exact 95 percent likelihood of finding the true mean, but 2 is close enough in most applications.)

Calculating Confidence Limits

The financial officer calculates the standard error of the mean by using the formula in Equation 6.11 and determines that the standard error is $526.27. Based on this, he determines that there is a 95 percent likelihood that the true mean cost per hospital stay lies between $5,533.75 and $7,638.84. In other words, the 95 percent confidence limits are $5,533.75 and $7,638.84. Equation 7.1 displays the calculations. As the equation indicates, the limits are the sample mean plus or minus the appropriate value of t times the standard error of the mean. The exact 95 percent value of t is 1.98 for a sample of 100 observations, but 2 is close enough. The exact percentage of the means expected to fall within two standard errors of the mean with a sample of size 100 is 95.2 percent.

$$CL = \bar{x} \pm t \times S.E._{\bar{x}} \tag{7.1}$$

where CL designates the confidence limits and t represents the number of standard errors on either side of the mean required to encompass a desired proportion of the t distribution (generally 95 percent). Note: Refer to Equation 6.11 for the definition of $S.E._{\bar{x}}$.

Finding Confidence Level t Values

Finding the exact t values for any level of confidence can be done by using the =TINV() function in Microsoft Excel. To find the exact t value for a 95 percent confidence limit and a sample of 100, for example, the function would be =TINV(.05,99), where 0.05 is the confidence level desired (this is usually called *alpha*) and 99 is the degrees of freedom for a sample of size 100 (i.e., 100 minus 1, or 99). If you wanted to find the t value for a 99 percent confidence limit with a sample of 30, the function would be =TINV(.01,29) and would produce a t value of 2.76. The range 2.76 standard deviations on both sides of a mean from a sample of 30 would produce the 99 percent confidence limits.

One-Tail versus Two-Tail t Values

It should be recognized that the =TINV() function always returns the two-tail value for t. If you wanted to know the t value for a one-tail test, it would be necessary to double the value of alpha. For example, the one-tail value for t of the 95 percent probability below which the mean value for the population would lie given a sample of 100 is as follows: Take 100% less 95% = 5% (i.e., the alpha value), next take 5% and double it (i.e., 2 * 5% = 10%), then find the degrees of freedom (100 − 1 = 99), and in turn the appropriate statement in Excel would be TINV(0.1,99). The formula in Excel produces a t value of 1.66.

It is important to discuss briefly the one-tail test. When both upper and lower confidence limits are found (such as are pictured in Figure 7.2), the 5 percent of all possible sample means that are outside the 95 percent limits could be either above the upper limit or below the lower limit. Frequently, the interest is in establishing 95 percent (or other percentage value) limits relative only to a single direction from the mean. For example, suppose the hospital financial officer is interested only in determining what the highest value of true hospital charges could be, based on the sample mean of $6,586.30 and a standard error of $526.27. What is the upper limit below which he is 95 percent confident that the true average hospital cost will lie?

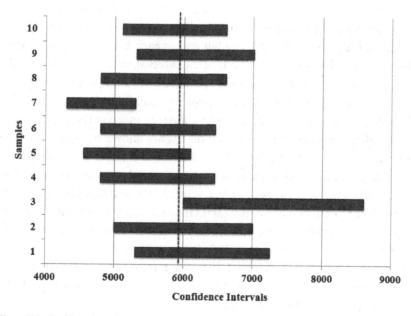

Figure 7.2 Confidence limits from 10 samples

In this case, the financial officer is not interested in the lower limit of the distribution. The consequence of this lack of interest in the lower limit of the distribution signifies that the 5 percent of possible mean values outside the limits $(1 - .95)$ must all be at the top end of the distribution. With the limits at both ends, 2.5 percent of $1 - .95$ is at each end of the continuum. If it is desired to have 5 percent at the top end of the continuum only, it is not necessary to go out as far from the sample mean in terms of standard errors. For a sample of size 100, the upper limit (the only limit of interest) would be $6,586.30 + $526.27 × 1.66$, or $7,459.91$. In other words, the financial officer can be 95 percent certain that the true average hospital cost lies below $7,459.91$.

What Does the 95 Percent Confidence Limit Mean?

Having determined the 95 percent confidence limits for the cost of cases discharged from the hospital, what has the financial officer actually found? He has not found limits within which the true mean has a 95 percent likelihood of falling. The true mean is either in his 95 percent range or it is not. If it is, the probability that the mean is in the range (which it is, given that the true mean is 5905.75) is 1. If it is not, the probability that the true mean is in the range is 0. So what does the 95 percent confidence limit actually mean?

To understand, we must look at Figure 7.2, which shows the confidence intervals calculated for the mean of cost per discharge. The confidence interval is created for 10 samples of 100 discharges drawn from the population of 12,000 hospital discharges. The left end of each bar representing a confidence interval is at the lower limit of the interval, and the right end of the bar is at the upper limit of the interval. The bar itself represents the range within which the true mean has a 95 percent likelihood of being found. The dashed vertical line at $5,905$ represents the true mean of the population.

Confidence limits for 10 sample means are shown in Figure 7.2. The confidence limits for samples 1, 2, 4, 5, 6, 8, 9, and 10 actually contain the true sample mean. The confidence limits for samples 3 and 7 do not. If we were to draw many samples of a given size (here, $n = 100$) and calculate the 95 percent confidence limits for each (approximately two standard errors on either side of the sample mean), 95 percent of the confidence intervals would contain the true mean. This is what is meant when 95 percent confidence limits are constructed. If a large number of samples were taken and the confidence limits were calculated, 95 of 100 of them would be expected to contain the true mean.

EXERCISES FOR SECTION 7.1

1. Using =TINV() and Equation 7.1, calculate the exact 95 percent upper and lower confidence limits for the following:

    a. $n = 40$, mean = 32, *S.E.* = 1.23

    b. $n = 40$, mean = 32, *S.E.* = 3.23

    c. $n = 140$, mean = 32, *S.E.* = 1.23

    d. $n = 140$, mean = 32, *S.E.* = 3.23

2. Using $t = 2$ and Equation 7.1, calculate approximate 95 percent upper and lower confidence limits for the following:

    a. $n = 40$, mean = 32, *S.E.* = 1.23

    b. $n = 40$, mean = 32, *S.E.* = 3.23

    c. $n = 140$, mean = 32, *S.E.* = 1.23

    d. $n = 140$, mean = 32, *S.E.* = 3.23

3. How well do the values in Exercise 2 approximate those in Exercise 1?

4. Using =TINV() and Equation 7.1, calculate the exact 99 percent upper and lower confidence limits for the following:

    a. $n = 40$, mean = 32, *S.E.* = 1.23

    b. $n = 40$, mean = 32, *S.E.* = 3.23

    c. $n = 140$, mean = 32, *S.E.* = 1.23

    d. $n = 140$, mean = 32, *S.E.* = 3.23

5. Using =TINV() and Equation 7.1, calculate the exact 95 percent upper confidence limit only (95 percent of observations below the upper limit) for the following:

    a. $n = 40$, mean = 32, *S.E.* = 1.23

    b. $n = 40$, mean = 32, *S.E.* = 3.23

    c. $n = 140$, mean = 32, *S.E.* = 1.23

    d. $n = 140$, mean = 32, *S.E.* = 3.23

6. Use the Infants worksheet in the file Chpt 2-2.xls. Assume that this is a random sample of weights of one-year-olds from a much larger defined population, and calculate the exact 95 percent upper and lower confidence limits for the weight of one-year-olds in the population.

7. Use the Hospital charge worksheet in the file Chpt 4-1.xls. Assume that the data represent a random sample from a larger population, and do the following:

    a. Calculate the exact 95 percent upper and lower confidence limits for the population mean of LOS.

    b. Calculate the exact 95 percent upper and lower confidence limits for the population mean of charges.

    c. Calculate the exact 95 percent upper limit only for the population mean of charges—that is, the value below which 95 percent of all sample means will be expected to fall.

    d. Calculate the exact 95 percent upper and lower confidence limits for the population proportion, which is female.

8. Use the Emergency room wait worksheet in the file Chpt 6-2.xls and =RAND() to draw a random sample of 60 records from the 832 on the sheet. Calculate the exact 95 percent upper and lower confidence limits for the population mean.

7.2 Calculating Confidence Limits for Multiple Samples

Section 7.1 discussed the drawing of numerous samples of a given size. This was also discussed in the third subsection of Section 6.3. In that subsection, we generated 100 samples of size 30 from a file that contained the probability of having a specified number of prenatal visits, from 0 to 15, for a population of women. Selected numbers from the first 7 of the 100 samples were shown in Figure 6.20, and the calculation of the mean, standard deviation, and standard error for the first 6 samples was shown in Figure 6.21. We will use these 100 samples to calculate the upper and lower 95 percent confidence limits for each sample and determine what proportion of the limits contain the actual mean value for the population.

Calculating Confidence Limits

The calculation of the upper and lower confidence limits is shown for the first 6 samples of the 100 in Figure 7.3. The number of prenatal visits for the last six women in the first six samples is shown in cells 25 through 30 in columns B through G. A new column has been inserted at A to allow labels to be put in rows 32 to 39. The mean value of the first sample (cell B32) is 4.533, the mean of the second is 4.933, and so on. The standard deviation of the first sample (cell B33) is 1.995, and the standard error of the mean (cell B34, the standard deviation divided by the square root of 30) is 0.364.

B39	▼	=	=AND(B37>$B$35,B38<$B$35)				
	A	B	C	D	E	F	G	H
25		5	4	5	4	4	5	
26		6	3	3	3	3	5	
27		6	8	3	3	7	4	
28		3	4	1	3	4	3	
29		9	3	6	12	5	9	
30		3	6	6	6	8	1	
31								
32	Mean	4.533333	4.933333	5.033333	4.2	4.433333	5.1	
33	St Dev	1.995397	2.504249	2.697168	2.21904	1.851064	2.577756	2.534
34	St Error	0.364308	0.457211	0.492433	0.405139	0.337956	0.470632	0.46
35	mu	4.5711						
36	t	2.045231						
37	Upper limt	5.278427	5.868436	6.040473	5.028604	5.124532	6.062551	5.646
38	Lower limit	3.788239	3.998231	4.026194	3.371396	3.742134	4.137449	3.753
39	Contain mu?	TRUE	TRUE	TRUE	TRUE	TRUE	TRUE	TRU
40		91						
41								

Figure 7.3 Calculation of means and limits

Mu (μ, cell B35) is the true mean of the population and was calculated in Figure 6.23. Cell B36 contains the exact 95 percent value for t calculated by Excel, using =TINV(0.05,29). Row 37 is the upper limit and row 38 is the lower limit for the 95 percent confidence interval. The values in these two rows are calculated as given in Equation 7.1. Row 39, labeled "Contain mu?," is a logical statement that tests whether the true mean of the population (cell B35) is between the upper and lower limits. The logical statement is as that shown in the formula line in Figure 7.3 and uses the =AND() function. Table 7.1 contains the exact Excel functions for Figure 7.3.

Table 7.1 Formulas for Figure 7.3

Cell	Formula	Notes
B32	=average(B1:B30)	Copied to cells C32 and down the row
B33	=stdev(B1:B30)	Copied to cells C33 and down the row
B34	=B33/(sqrt(30))	Copied to cells C34 and down the row
B35	=average(B1:CW30)	
B36	=TINV(0.05,29)	95% confidence is a 5% t value and 29 is the degrees of freedom (e.g., df $= n - 1$ or $30 - 1 = 29$)
B37	=B32+$B$36*B34	Copied to cells C37 and down the row
B38	=B32−$B$36*B34	Copied to cells C38 and down the row
B39	=AND(B37>$B$35, B38<$B$35)	Copied to cells C39 and down the row; also note the $ in the formula to lock the column and row. Make sure TRUE is spelled and capitalized exactly.
B40	=COUNTIF(B39:CW39, TRUE))	

Use of the =AND ( ) Function

The =AND ( ) function takes two arguments, as the formula line indicates. The =AND ( ) function returns a value of TRUE if both statements in the arguments are true, and it returns a value of FALSE otherwise. So if the true mean as given in cell B35 is either above or below any one of the sample limits, the =AND ( ) function will return FALSE. The 91 in cell B40 is produced by the =COUNTIF ( ) function that was used to count the number of TRUE entries in row 39. It turns out that for this series of 100 samples, 91 samples had upper and lower 95 percent limits that contained the true mean. In general, we would have expected 95 of 100 samples to have upper and lower limits that contained the true mean. But these are probabilities, and for a series of 100 samples, it is not likely that the actual true value of 95 of 100 will be generated.

This section discusses the use of Excel to determine upper and lower confidence limits for a large number of samples with given attributes as a means of demonstrating the meaning of the notion of confidence limits. It is important to remember, however, that, in general, one never draws more than one sample. The discussion here is presented solely for the purpose of helping you understand what confidence limits actually are.

EXERCISES FOR SECTION 7.2

1. Use the file generated by selecting 100 samples of 30 waiting times (see Exercise 3 of Section 6.3).

    a. Calculate the exact 95 percent upper and lower confidence limits for each sample.

    b. Use the =AND ( ) statement, as given in Figure 7.3, to determine whether the confidence limits for each sample contain the true population mean.

    c. Use =COUNTIF ( ) to determine whether the proportion of samples of the 100 actually contains the true mean of the population within the 95 percent limits.

    d. Can you account for the result you got in (c)?

2. Use the file generated by selecting 250 samples of 100 from the prenatal visits for women (see Exercise 4 of Section 6.3).

    a. Calculate exact 95 percent upper and lower confidence limits for each sample.

    b. Use the =AND ( ) statement, as given in Figure 7.3, to determine whether the confidence limits for each sample contain the true population mean.

    c. Use =COUNTIF ( ) to determine whether the proportion of samples of the 250 actually contains the true mean of the population within the 95 percent limits.

    d. Can you account for the result you got in (c)?

7.3   What Is Hypothesis Testing?

In a statistical context, *hypothesis* testing is the process of determining from a sample whether something could be true of a population—in other words, inferring from a sample what may be true in a population, hence what statisticians refer to as inferential statistics. In particular, the something is usually a mean value or a proportion for the population. For example, suppose a county public health nurse is concerned about whether children in her county are growing at the normal rate for all children in the United States. She decides to collect some data and test the hypothesis that children in her area of responsibility are normal in height relative to all U.S. children. Rather than assess all children of all ages, she decides to assess a specific age and sex group and use that to provide an indicator of all children in her county. She decides to assess the height of six-year-old boys as her yardstick for assessing all children.

Inferring from a Sample to a Population

The public health nurse knows that height-for-age scales indicate that the national average height for six-year-old boys is approximately normally distributed, with a mean of 48 inches and a standard deviation of 10 inches. That is essentially the same as saying that 95 percent of all six-year-old boys are between 28 and 68 inches tall (i.e., $48 \pm 2 \times 10$). The public health nurse knows that she has the resources to select a random sample of 100 six-year-old boys from the schools in her county and measure the height of each of the boys. She will compare the results of this sample with what is known for the overall population of six-year-old boys to determine if the children in her county are growing at the expected rate.

> Inferential statistics is the act of converting information about a sample into intelligent guesses about a population.

Creating Hypothesis Statements

To do this, the public health nurse will be looking at the results of the sample to see if those results could have come from a population of six-year-old boys in which the true average height was 48 inches. Implicitly, the nurse might say, "I will take a sample of six-year-old boys to see if I can support the view that the average height of the entire population in the county is 48 inches." From the standpoint of hypothesis testing, however, the nurse would be saying that her initial hypothesis is that six-year-old boys in her county are 48 inches tall. This hypothesis might be stated formally as:

H0: The average height of six-year-old boys (h) is equal to 48 inches

or

H0: $h = 48$.

This is sometimes called the null hypothesis—thus, the designation *H0*. And H0 is often pronounced not "H zero" but "H naught."

Every null hypothesis has an accompanying alternative hypothesis, usually designated H1, against which it is being tested. In general, the most frequently posited alternative is simply:

H1: The average height of six-year-old boys (h) is not equal to 48 inches

or

H1: $h \neq 48$.

Every hypothesis test is a test of whether H0, the null hypothesis, is consistent with the data that come from a sample. If the data that come from the sample are of such a nature that H0 is consistent with the data, then H0 is retained. If the data that come from the sample are of such a nature that H0 is not consistent with the data, then H0 is rejected and the alternative hypothesis, H1, is accepted by default. A statistical test is never a direct test of H1 but is always a test of H0.

Acceptance or Rejection of the Initial Hypothesis

But how can we tell if the data are or are not consistent with the null hypothesis, H0? In the first subsection of Section 7.1, we calculated confidence limits for sample values. In regard to hypothesis testing, if the H0 value that we have posited (i.e., the value we expect the population mean or proportion to be) is contained within specified confidence limits about the sample mean, we will retain H0. If the H0 value we have posited is not within the confidence limits determined for the sample mean, we will reject H0. As has already been stated, the rejection of H0, our null hypothesis, automatically means the acceptance of H1, our alternative hypothesis.

Suppose, then, that the nurse has taken a sample of 100 six-year-old boys from the population of six-year-old boys in the schools in her county. When she did so, she discovered that the mean height of the boys in her sample was 49 inches, with a standard deviation of 10 inches. She wishes to set the confidence limits at approximately 95 percent, and she can use the formula proposed in Equation 7.1. Therefore, with a sample of 100, her confidence limits will be:

CL lower limit = $(49 - [2 * 10/\sqrt{(100)}]) = 47$ inches

and

CL upper limit = $(49 + [2 * 10/\sqrt{(100)}]) = 51$ inches

Because her originally hypothesized value of 48 inches is contained within the 95 percent confidence limits of her sample average height of 49 inches, the public health nurse will not reject the null hypothesis. Thus, she will conclude that the average height for six-year-old boys in her county is the same as the national average (48 inches).

Another Example of Acceptance and Rejection

But let us consider another example. Suppose the sample that the public health nurse took had a mean value of 45 inches, still with a standard deviation of 10 inches. On the basis of these data, she would calculate 95 percent confidence limits for her sample mean as:

CL lower limit = $(45 - [2 * 10/\sqrt{100}]) = 43$ inches

and

CL upper limit = $(45 + [2 * 10/\sqrt{100}]) = 47$ inches

Now, the value of the null hypothesis, 48 inches, is no longer contained in the confidence interval the nurse has calculated. As a consequence, from the standpoint of hypothesis testing, she would reject the null hypothesis of 48 inches. In turn, she would accept the alternative hypothesis, which is that the average height of six-year-old boys in her county was *not* 48 inches. In fact, because her sample result was less than the initially hypothesized mean, she would probably decide that the average height for six-year-old boys in her county was less than the national average.

EXERCISES FOR SECTION 7.3

1. Suppose the 20 people who have made clinic visits, as represented on the Visits sheet of Chpt 3-1.xls, are considered to be a random sample of all the people who have ever come or will ever come to the clinic in question.

   a. Test the null hypothesis at the 95 percent level of confidence that the average Visit Time for the population is 37 minutes (H0: $VT = 37$) against the alternative hypothesis that the Visit Time is not 37 minutes (H1: $VT \neq 37$), and state your conclusion.

b. Test the same hypothesis at the 99 percent level of confidence, and state your conclusion.

c. Test the null hypothesis at the 95 percent level of confidence that average Charges for the population is $75 (H0: $C = \$75$) against the alternative hypothesis that Charges is not $75 (H1: $C \neq \$75$), and state your conclusion.

d. Test the same hypothesis at the 99 percent level of confidence, and state your conclusion.

2. Suppose the 100 hospital discharges on the Hospital charges worksheet in Chpt 4-1.xls represent a random sample of all Medicare-eligible persons discharged from a specific hospital.

a. Test the null hypothesis at the 95 percent level of confidence that average Charges for the population is $6,000 (H0: $C = \$6,000$) against the alternative hypothesis that average Charges is not $6,000 (H1: $C \neq \$6,000$), and state your conclusion.

b. Test the same hypothesis at the 99 percent level of confidence, and state your conclusion.

c. Test the null hypothesis at the 95 percent level of confidence that average LOS for the population is 7.5 days (H0: $LOS = 7.5$) against the alternative hypothesis that LOS is not 7.5 (H1: $LOS \neq 7.5$), and state your conclusion.

d. Test the same hypothesis at the 99 percent level of confidence, and state your conclusion.

3. Use the Emergency room wait spreadsheet in file Chpt 6-2.xls.

a. Draw a simple random sample of 60 records, using any method you choose.

b. Test the null hypothesis at the 95 percent level of confidence that the average wait time is 38.4 minutes (H0: $W = 38.4$) against the alternative that the average wait time is not 38.4 minutes (H1: $W \neq 38.4$), and state your conclusion.

c. Test the same hypothesis at the 99 percent level of confidence, and state your conclusion.

7.4   Type I and Type II Errors

What Are Type I and Type II Errors and Why Do We Care?

Two types of errors can be committed when hypothesis testing: Type I and Type II.

- The Type I error is the error of concluding that the null hypothesis is false when it is, in fact, true. This is referred to as a False Positive.

- The Type II error is the error of concluding that the null hypothesis is true when it is, in fact, false. This is referred to as a False Negative.

In arriving at the decisions previously discussed, the public health nurse runs the risk of making two types of errors. When she concluded on the basis of the sample mean of 45 inches that the average height for six-year-old boys in her county was not 48 inches, she ran the risk of making the *Type I error*, the error of concluding that the null hypothesis is false when it is, in fact, true. When she concluded on the basis of the sample mean of 49 inches that the average height of six-year-old boys in her county was 48 inches, she ran the risk of making the *Type II error*, the error of concluding that the null hypothesis is true when it is, in fact, false. Let us look further at both the Type I and the Type II error.

To begin with, consider the possibility that the true mean height of six-year-old boys in the public health nurse's county is really 48 inches and that the standard deviation is 10 inches. If the nurse were to draw an infinite number of samples of size 100 from this population of six-year-old boys, the resulting distribution of the mean values of those samples might be as shown in Figure 7.4.

Type I Error

In looking at Figure 7.4, it is possible to see that it depicts a normal distribution with the midpoint (and the mean) at 48 inches. There is a vertical dotted line at 46 inches and one at 50 inches. These two lines represent the cutoff point for two standard errors on either side of the mean, or the 95 percent confidence limits. The figure represents the following fact:

Figure 7.4 Distribution of sample means around 48 inches

"If the nurse drew an infinite number of samples of size 100 from the population of six-year-old boys in her county, assuming that the true mean is 48 inches, the mean of 95 percent of those samples would be between 46 and 50 inches."

The mean of 5 percent of the samples would be either above or below the dotted cutoff lines in Figure 7.4, or outside the 95 percent limits. Thus, when the nurse draws her one sample to assess the hypothesis that the true mean of the height of six-year-old boys in her county is 48 inches, she has 5 chances in 100 of drawing a sample that will have a mean value greater than 50 inches or less than 46 inches. It should be noted that this would happen even when the true mean is 48 inches. Any result outside the upper limit of 50 inches or the lower limit of 46 inches will result in her rejecting the null hypothesis and consequently making the Type I error of concluding that the true mean height of six-year-old boys in her county is not 48 inches. The probability of making the type I error is called alpha (α), and in this case it is set by the public health nurse at 5 percent by her decision to use the 95 percent confidence limits.

Consider again the two possible samples that the nurse might have drawn—one with a mean of 49 inches and the other with a mean of 45 inches. In the first case, she would conclude that the true mean was 48 inches and would be making no error (still assuming that the true mean is 48 inches). In the second, she would conclude that the true mean is not 48 inches and would have made the Type I error.

Type II Error

Now consider the alternative possibility, the Type II error. Figure 7.5 shows the distribution of the sample means for all possible samples of size 100 from a population in which the true mean is 48 inches (i.e., Figure 7.4). Figure 7.5 also shows the distribution of the means for all possible samples of size 100 from a population in which the true mean is actually 49 inches. Figure 7.5 also shows the vertical dashed lines that represent the 95 percent confidence limits for a true mean of 48 inches.

Now suppose the true mean of the population of six-year-old boys in the county in which the public health nurse is working is actually 49 inches. Admittedly, this is not greatly different from 48 inches. But it is different. The question that is now raised is, "Could the nurse detect this difference on the basis of her sample of 100 boys?" Based on her 95 percent criteria, she would reject the null hypothesis of 48 inches when the true mean was 49 inches, with only about a 20 percent likelihood. This 20 percent comes from the portion of the distribution around 49 inches that is to the right

Figure 7.5 Distribution of sample means for 48 inches and 49 inches

of the right-most vertical dashed line in Figure 7.5. She would have about an 80 percent likelihood (the portion of the distribution being around 49 inches to the left of the right-most vertical dashed line in Figure 7.5) of accepting the initial hypothesis of 48 inches when, in fact, the true mean is not 48 inches but 49 inches. In this case, she has an 80 percent chance of making the Type II error of accepting the null hypothesis when it is not true. The probability of making the Type II error is known as *beta* (β), and in this case, it is about 0.8.

But what of the sample in which she got a mean of 45 inches? She could not make the Type II error, because she rejected the initial hypothesis of 48 inches. But if the true mean of the population were, in fact, 45 inches, there still is the possibility of her making the Type II error relative to the null hypothesis. To illustrate this, consider the distribution of the sample means from a population in which the true sample mean is 45 inches. This distribution is shown, along with the distribution around 48 inches, in Figure 7.6. Again, the two dashed vertical lines representing the 95 percent confidence limits for a true mean of 48 inches are also shown in Figure 7.6.

Now, an examination of Figure 7.6 shows that perhaps 30 percent of the distribution of the sample means around a true mean of 45 inches will be to the right of the left-most vertical dashed line. This is the region in which the null hypothesis is accepted. In this case, then, even when the true mean is 45 inches, there is approximately a 30 percent likelihood, β, of making the Type II error. In other words, there is a 30 percent chance of accepting the initial hypothesis of 48 inches when the null hypothesis is false.

Figure 7.6 Distribution around true means of 45 and 48 inches

The Mutual Dependence of Alpha and Beta

In Figure 7.6, the confidence limits around the true mean of 48 inches are set at 95 percent, thus making alpha equal 0.05. In setting alpha equal to 0.05, and assuming a population standard deviation of 10 and a sample size of 100, the lower confidence limit is at 46 inches. This means that beta for a true population mean of 45 inches—the portion of the distribution around 45 inches that is right of 46 inches—is about 30 percent, or 0.30. It is possible to reduce β for a true mean value of 45 inches by increasing α for a mean of 48 inches. For example, instead of decreeing α to be 0.05, suppose we were willing to have alpha be equal to 0.32. This level of α is equivalent to saying that we are willing to take a 0.32 percent risk of making a Type I error (i.e., rejecting H0 when it is true). That would mean that we would put the upper and lower confidence limits only one standard error from the mean. The result is shown in Figure 7.7.

In Figure 7.7, the vertical dashed lines are now at 47 and 49 inches. Any sample result to the left of the left-most dashed line or the right of the right-most dashed line will now lead to the rejection of the initial hypothesis that the mean value is 48 percent. But look also at what has happened to beta for a true mean of 45 inches, relative to the initial hypothesis of 48 inches. The portion of the distribution around 45 inches that is to the right of the left-most vertical dashed line probably represents only about 10 percent of the total distribution around 45. Thus, by increasing α, we have decreased β. This is a general result. Increasing α will always lead to a decrease in β, all other things being equal.

Figure 7.7 Sixty-eight percent confidence limits for a distribution around 48 inches

The Reality of Many Betas

In Section 7.3, the null hypothesis was introduced as h = 48 inches and the alternative hypothesis was introduced as h ≠ 48. If the null hypothesis is rejected, it means that the height of six-year-old boys in the county in which the public health nurse is working could be anything other than 48 inches. It could be 39 inches, it could be 49 inches, it could be 50 inches, or it could be 55 inches. What does this mean in terms of beta or Type II error?

A general notion of what many alternative realities regarding the true height of six-year-old boys may mean is shown in Figure 7.8. This figure shows the distribution around a true mean of 48 inches, a true mean of

Figure 7.8 Distributions around three true means

50 inches, and a true mean of 52 inches. The figure also shows the 95 percent confidence limits for a true value of 48 inches as the vertical dashed lines at 46 and 50 inches. If the null hypothesis is that the true mean is 48 inches and the alternative is that the true mean is not 48 inches, the true mean might be 50 inches or it might be 52 inches (or any other value).

If the true mean is 50 inches, then the value of β for the null hypothesis of 48 inches is exactly 50 percent. That is, half the distribution of sample means around a true mean of 50 are left of the right-most dashed line in Figure 7.8. In turn, these values will fall in the region in which H0 will be falsely accepted. If the true mean is 52 inches, then the value of β for the null hypothesis of 48 inches is probably in the region of 3 percent. Only about 3 percent of the distribution of sample means around a true mean of 52 inches is to the left of the vertical dashed line at 50 inches. The point of this discussion is that there is an infinite set of beta values. Each β is associated with one of the infinite number of possible values that an alternative hypothesis of h $\neq$ 48 inches could take on.

Specifying α and β

It is increasingly common to wish to specify both α and β in current statistical applications. Frequently, one might encounter a statement in a report of a statistical analysis such as "$\alpha = \beta = 0.05$." As we have seen, there is an infinite set of beta values, each associated with a different real alternative possibility for the value being assessed as the null hypothesis. Harking back to the example of Medicare charges, we can relate the following: If the null hypothesis says that the Medicare case total charges across all hospitals in a state come to $5,300, then the alternative hypothesis that the average is not $5,300 would have a β value for every other possible average case charge imaginable. In order to set a β value equal to any specific probability, it is necessary to state the alternative hypothesis as a specific value rather than as simply not H0.

Consider again the public health nurse interested in the height of six-year-old boys. She might be interested in this because she wants to assure herself and the appropriate county authorities that growth among children in her county is normal, relative to the rest of the United States. If six-year-old boys in her county were smaller in stature than six-year-old boys in general, it might signal the need for efforts to ensure adequate nutrition, such as school lunch programs. If local six-year-old boys are taller in stature than six-year-old boys in general, this might not be a cause for concern, but it might lead to a question of why this may have occurred. It is likely that the nurse's main concern, however, would be that the six-year-old boys in her county not be found to be smaller in stature than six-year-old boys in general.

Determining β

Suppose the nurse wished to make sure that she could test the null hypothesis that the height of six-year-old boys in her county was 48 inches against an alternative hypothesis that would allow her to set the Type II error (β) at some predetermined level. If that were the case, she would have to determine ahead of time how different an alternative height might be before it would be important enough to lead to a decision to institute an intervention. The nurse knows that the average height of U.S. six-year-old boys is 48 inches and that the standard deviation is approximately 10 inches. So she would not be concerned if six-year-old boys in her county averaged somewhat less than 48 inches—say, as little as 46 inches. But she has decided from her experience that if she finds that six-year-old boys in her county average as little as 44.6 inches, some intervention is indicated.

So the public health nurse restates her null and alternative hypotheses as follows:

H0: The average height of six-year-old boys (h) is equal to 48 inches.

or

H0: $h = 48$.

and

H1: The average height of six-year-old boys (h) is equal to 44.6 inches.

or

H1: $h = 44.6$.

β and the One-Tail Test

Now two things have happened. First, the public health nurse has determined that she will accept H0 for any value of height greater than some lower limit around 48 inches, because she has specified an alternative value below 48 inches, thus creating what is known as a one-tail test. A one-tail test is a test in which the null hypothesis can be rejected only in one end of the normal distribution, in this case the lower end. Second, the nurse has provided a specific value for the alternative hypothesis so that she can assess the value of beta, the likelihood of making a Type II error.

To consider the one-tail test first, in the statement of the original alternative hypothesis, H1: $h \neq 48$, h could be greater or less than 48. Thus the region in which H0 would be rejected would be at either end of the distribution around 48 inches. So it is necessary to have half the region of rejection (2.5 percent of the distribution around 48 inches) at the upper tail of the curve, and half (again 2.5 percent) at the lower tail of the curve. Because the alternative hypothesis H1: $h = 44.6$ now specifies that the alternative is less than 48, any value at the upper end of the distribution around 48 will be irrelevant to rejecting H0. Thus it is reasonable and accepted by most statisticians to determine that all of the 5 percent region of rejection will be in the lower half of the distribution around 48 inches. In a normal distribution, about 1.7 standard errors on either side of the mean will cut off about 5 percent of the distribution on either side (the exact number of standard errors required can be found with =TINV(0.1,d.f.)). So the lower limit for rejecting H0 (the only limit of interest relative to the present alternative hypothesis) is approximately calculated as follows:

$$\text{CL lower limit} = (48 - [1.7 * 10/\sqrt{100}]) = 46.3 \text{ inches}$$

This value is used rather than the previous 46 inches because we are now using a one-tailed test.

Consider the second point, specifying the actual value of β. By specifying the alternative hypothesis as H1: $h = 44.6$, it is possible to say that the upper 5 percent region in which we will accept H0 when, in fact, H1 is true will be about 1.7 standard errors above the value of 44.6, or about 46.3 (i.e., $44.6 + 1.7 \times 10/\sqrt{(100)}$). So now it is possible to say that $\alpha = \beta = 0.05$ for the test:

$$\text{H0: } h = 48$$

$$\text{H1: } h = 44.6$$

This concept is illustrated in Figure 7.9, which shows the sampling distribution of the means around a true population mean of 48 inches (the distribution to the right) and the sampling distribution around a true

Figure 7.9 Distributions around 48 and 44.6 inches

mean of 44.6 inches (the distribution to the left). The vertical dashed line representing the lower 95 percent limit for the distribution around 48 inches is now at about 46.3 inches, or 1.7 inches below the mean of 48. The vertical dashed line is also about 1.7 inches above the alternative mean of 44.6 inches. The two distributions now overlap in such a way that the probability of making a Type I error, of rejecting H0 when it is true, is equal to the probability of making a Type II error, of accepting H0 when it is false (or alternatively of rejecting H1 when it is true). The probability of a Type I error and/or a Type II error is approximately 5 percent. It must be remembered, however, that the ability to specify alpha and beta depend on the exact specification of a value for the alternative hypothesis.

Controlling Beta

Again, one must take note that the ability to specify $\alpha = \beta = 0.05$ as shown in Figure 7.9 depends on the specification of the alternative hypothesis. In this case, it was posited as being exactly that alternative which would create the results desired. It was also based upon the given standard deviation of the height of six-year-old boys as approximately 10 inches and a sample of 100.

Now let's suppose the public health nurse had decided that if the six-year-old boys in her county averaged 46 inches in height rather than 48, some intervention to assure adequate nutrition of schoolchildren was warranted. How could the nurse test the hypothesis, H0: $h = 48$, against the alternative hypothesis, H1: $h = 46$, and ensure that $\alpha = \beta = 0.05$? The solution to this problem lies in the fact that the standard error of the mean is inversely related to the sample size (i.e., the standard error formula is derived by dividing by the square root of the sample size). To see this, imagine that instead of selecting a sample of 100 six-year-old boys on which to test the null hypothesis, the nurse had selected a sample of 290 six-year-old boys. (This county is a large metropolitan area, so a sample of 290 six-year-old boys is not unreasonable.) With a sample of 290 six-year-old boys, the sampling error of the sampling distribution now becomes about 0.6, and 1.7 standard errors below the mean of 48 (the point below which H0 will be rejected) is at about 47 inches. Similarly, the region for the distribution around 46 inches, above which H0 will be accepted, also lies at 47 inches. Figure 7.10 shows this result. By comparing Figure 7.10 with Figure 7.9, you can see that the second set of distributions is now much more narrowly dispersed about the two means. Also, the vertical dashed line at 47 inches now cuts off about 5 percent of the lower end of the upper distribution and about 5 percent of the upper end of the lower distribution. Again, $\alpha = \beta = 0.05$ (approximately). Thus, if the alternative hypothesis is given as a specific

Figure 7.10 Two distributions for a sample of 290

number value and one knows the probable standard deviation of the data, it is possible to determine the size of the sample that will be required to ensure that $\alpha = \beta = 0.05$ (or any other confidence limit that may be deemed acceptable).

Calculating the Value of Beta for Any Alternative Hypothesis

So we assume that a researcher sets the value of α. If the researcher wishes to make sure that a Type I error will be no greater than 0.05, then the researcher can use 95 percent confidence limits to determine the sample values that will lead to the rejection of H0. In the case of the public health nurse we've been discussing, she can decide that she will reject H0 if the value found in her sample is more than approximately two standard errors (or approximately 1.7 standard errors if it's a one-tail test) away from the mean. When she got a sample value of 45 inches, she determined that the value of H0 of 48 inches was not contained in the 95 percent confidence limits for 45 inches, so she rejected H0. The likelihood that she was in error is 5 percent.

However, β is determined not by the level of confidence, but, as seen earlier, it is an artifact of the sample size, the standard deviation of the data, and the setting of a specific alternative hypothesis. So how can the researcher know what the value of β is for an assessment such as that carried out by the public health nurse? First and foremost, it is necessary to specify an alternative hypothesis before any determination of β can be made. As we have seen, there are an infinite number of values of beta, one for each of the infinite number of values other than that specified by H0. So the first step is to select an alternative hypothesis that is meaningful in practice.

Selecting an Alternative Hypothesis and Calculating a t Value

Suppose the alternative hypothesis was that the height of six-year-old boys in the county was 46 inches. This was discussed in the fourth subsection of Section 7.4. In addition, the public health nurse wished to know what the value of β would be if she were limited to a sample of 100. This continues to assume a standard deviation in height of six-year-old boys as 10 inches. Because she has decided that the alternative is less than 48 inches, she has automatically moved from a two-tail test to a one-tail test. She is interested in knowing only if the alternative is less than 48 inches. So her region of rejection of H0 would be only the lower end of the distribution around a true mean of 48 inches.

She then calculates the lower confidence limit for 48 inches as 46.34 inches $(48 - 10/\sqrt{(100)} * 1.67)$. Now she can subtract the value of H1 (46 inches) from the lower limit for H0 to get 0.34. When she divides this by the standard error $(10/\sqrt{(100)})$, she gets a value of 0.34 again, because the standard error is 1. But this now represents the value of t that the lower limit for H0 is above. She can now use this value in the =TDIST() function to determine the exact probability of β. The =TDIST() function in this case is written =TDIST(0.34,99,1), where 0.34 refers to the number of t units, 99 refers to the degrees of freedom ($df = 100 - 1 = 99$), and 1 refers to a one-tail probability.

The formula for finding the exact value of beta may be expressed as shown in Equation 7.2. Basically, the value of beta is found by subtracting the value of H1 from the relevant limit (upper or lower) for H0, dividing the result by the standard error to convert it to t units, and then using that t value to find the proportion of the distribution around H1 that lies within the limits of acceptance for H0, using the =TDIST() function. It should be noted, however, that this equation, as given, works only when H1 is less than the lower limit of H0—for example, if H1 actually specifies a lower value than H0, or when H1 is greater than the upper limit of H0 or if H1 specifies a higher value than H0. If H1 is closer to H0 than the limit of H0, however, it is always true that beta will be greater than 50 percent.

$$t_\beta = \frac{|H0(L) - H1|}{S.E.} \qquad (7.2)$$

and

$$\beta = TDIST(t_\beta, df, 1)$$

where $H0(L)$ is the upper or lower limit for $H0$, $H1$ is the value of $H1$, and $S.E.$ is the standard error that applies to $H0$ (assumed to apply to $H1$ as well).

Small Alpha or Small Beta and the Cost of Research and Intervention

In the best of all possible worlds, researchers (including the public health nurse) would not have to choose between a small α (traditionally set at 0.05 or 0.01) and a small β (generally hoped by the researcher to be equal to β). But, as the previous sections indicate, the size of α will depend both on the extent to which a specific alternative hypothesis differs from the null hypothesis and on sample size. If the difference between the null hypothesis and the alternative is small, relative to the standard deviation of the data, it will require a large sample to ensure that the values of both α and β are relatively small.

Consider again the public health nurse assessing the height of six-year-old boys. This time, however, assume that the public health nurse is not deciding whether there should be a supplemental nutrition program in the school but is instead trying to assess the effectiveness of a supplemental nutrition program for kindergarteners that has been in place in the county for some time. Six-year-old boys would generally be expected to be in the first grade, so they would have had the benefit of the program during the previous year. The nurse believes that if the nutrition program is effective, one result will be an increase in the stature of six-year-old boys. So she wishes to draw a sample to see if six-year-old boys in the county could be assessed as being taller on average than all six-year-old boys in the nation.

But the nurse is not optimistic enough to think that the supplemental nutrition program will make a great difference in the height of six-year-old boys. She believes that on average, the six-year-old boys in her county may be one inch taller than all U.S. boys. Couched in terms of hypothesis testing, her null hypothesis would not typically be that six-year-old boys in her county averaged 49 inches, $h = 49$. Rather, her hypothesis would be that there is no difference in the height of six-year-old boys in general. Thus her hypotheses would be:

$$H0: h = 48$$

$$H1: h = 49$$

It has already been shown in Figure 7.5 that for a sample of 100 six-year-old boys, the region of nonrejection for $H0$ extends from 46 to 50 inches (for a two-tail test at $\alpha = 0.05$). Furthermore, only about 20 percent of the distribution around a true mean of 49 inches lies above the region of rejection for H0. Thus, if she maintains an $\alpha = 0.05$ and even if the true average height of six-year-old boys in her county is 49 inches, confirming her belief that the supplemental nutrition program has made a difference, she is not likely to be able to demonstrate a difference. So, in order to have a reasonable likelihood of rejecting her null hypothesis ($h = 48$), if, in fact, it is false, she must draw a larger sample.

Sample Size and Hypothesis Testing

How large would the sample have to be to provide the public health nurse with $\alpha = \beta = 0.05$ for a null hypothesis of 48 inches and an alternative of 49? First, it should be remembered that the nurse has specified the alternative hypothesis as being $h = 49$ inches. Therefore, she is interested only in a statistical test of whether the average for six-year-old boys in her county is greater than 48. Thus, for an $\alpha = 0.05$, she need go only about 1.7 standard errors above 48 inches to set the limit. Now, if the standard deviation of the height of six-year-old boys remains 10 inches, she must draw a sample large enough so that the standard error of the distribution, multiplied by 1.7, will be equal to 0.5 inches. The logic of this is shown in Figure 7.11.

Figure 7.11 shows the distribution around 48 inches and the distribution around 49 inches for a sample large enough for the upper 95 percent (one-tail) limit for 48 inches to be 48.5 inches. In other words, this represents 5 percent of the distribution of mean values that fall above 48.5 inches if those samples are from a population with a true mean of 48 inches. Similarly, 5 percent of the mean values from samples in which the true mean of the population is 49 inches will fall below 48.5 inches. In this case, $\alpha = \beta = 0.05$. Still assuming a standard deviation of height in the

Figure 7.11 Upper limit for $\alpha = \beta = 0.05$

population of six-year-old boys as 10 inches, the nurse would have to select and measure a sample of about 1,150 six-year-old boys. A sample of 1,150! That seems very large.

It is certainly feasible for the public health nurse to measure 1,150 six-year-old boys. But it is a much bigger job than measuring 100 six-year-old boys. Moreover, the county health officer may not be willing to grant her the time and resources away from her other duties to carry out a survey this large. Suppose instead that the county health officer agrees with the nurse that it may be useful to assess the effectiveness of the supplemental nutrition program for kindergarteners. They agree that the nurse can have the time and resources to select and measure a sample of 500 six-year-old boys. What then can be said of her perception that the program might have increased the height of six-year-old boys by one inch on the average?

If the nurse follows the prevailing tenets of statistical testing, which is to try to ensure against making the Type I error (rejecting the null hypothesis when it is true), she will set the upper 95 percent limit at about 48.75 inches. This result will be as seen in Figure 7.12, which shows the dashed vertical line at about 48.75 inches, so that 5 percent of the region of rejection of H0 will be above that value. But because the nurse has a sample of only 500, about 40 percent of the distribution around the mean of 49 percent is to the left of the dashed line. So while the nurse has only a 5 percent chance of rejecting H0 when it is true (Type I error), she has about a 40 percent chance of accepting H0 when it is false, and, in fact, H1 is true (a Type II error).

Avoiding Type I and Type II Errors

Both science and conventional logic are on the side of allowing a 40 percent Type II error, in the event that the nurse can select only a sample of 500

Figure 7.12 Positioning $\alpha = 0.05$

six-year-old boys. It is generally deemed less unattractive to say nothing happened than to say that something happened when we are not absolutely sure that it did (unless we are absolutely sure that something did happen). Thus, both science and conventional logic place the greatest emphasis on avoiding the Type I error.

But let us leave the realm of science for a moment and enter the realm of evaluation. The supplemental nutrition program has been in place for several years and has, in fact, become a fixture in the county. County supervisors have allocated funds for the program (to supplement grant funds received from the federal government) for the next 10 years. In essence, the supplemental nutrition program is already paid for. Only if it were shown that the program did not make any difference would the county supervisors be inclined to take the politically unattractive steps necessary to discontinue it. The program essentially costs less money at this stage than no program.

Under these circumstances, the public health nurse would be most concerned about not making the Type II error, the error of accepting H0 when it is false, or in terms of the program, the error of assuming that it had no effect when it actually did. If this were the case, the nurse—given that she is constrained to a sample of 500—might consciously set α large enough so that the probability of the Type II error—β—would be low, say 0.05. She might do this even if it means that α must be larger than 0.05. If the nurse set β for H0: $h = 48$ and H1: h = 49 to 0.05, the result would be as that shown in Figure 7.13, wherein the area of acceptance of H0 has now been moved down to about 48.25 inches. Any sample value larger than that will be assumed to have come from a population in which the true mean value is 49 inches. In turn, the supplemental nutrition program will be deemed to have had an effect by its having increased the height of

Figure 7.13 Low beta value

six-year-old boys. In this case, it is α that is large, being about 0.4, whereas β is about 0.05.

Although the logic discussed here might be reasonable, it is, in fact, rarely the case that a researcher would be willing to accept a value of α as high as 0.4. Occasionally, α might be set as high as 0.1, or even 0.15. But higher levels of α, even to reduce β in situations such as those previously described, would be very unlikely.

EXERCISES FOR SECTION 7.4

1. What is a Type I error?

2. What is a Type II error?

3. What is the meaning of alpha (α) and of beta (β)?

4. Consider the hypothesis about adult men: H0: Diastolic BP = 86 and H1: Diastolic BP $\neq$ 86, to be tested at the 95 percent level of confidence.

    a. Is alpha known in principle? If yes, can its value be stated from the information given? If yes, what is alpha?

    b. Is beta known in principle? If yes, can its value be stated from the information given? If yes, what is beta?

5. Consider the following hypothesis. H0: average age at first birth for mothers in the United States is 23.7 years, and H1: average age for first-time mothers in the United States is 21 years, to be tested at the 99 percent level of confidence.

    a. Is alpha known in principle? If yes, can its value be stated from the information given? If yes, what is alpha?

    b. Is beta known in principle? If yes, can its value be stated from the information given? If yes, what is beta?

6. Consider the following hypothesis. H0: average cost per stay in a large hospital is $6,200, and H1: average cost per stay is $5,600, to be tested at the 95 percent level of confidence. A sample of 120 records has been selected and assessed for cost. The standard deviation of the costs is $3,100.

    a. Is alpha known in principle? If yes, can its value be stated from the information given? If yes, what is alpha?

    b. Is beta known in principle? If yes, can its value be stated from the information given? If yes, what is beta?

7. Consider the following hypothesis. H0: the average number of prenatal visits among women to county health department prenatal clinics in a state is seven, and H1: the average number

of prenatal visits is 5.5, to be tested at the 95 percent confidence level. A sample of records of 75 women with completed pregnancies has been randomly selected from among all those women coming to the health department clinics, and a standard deviation of 2.5 visits was found.

a. Is alpha known in principle? If yes, can its value be stated from the information given? If yes, what is alpha?

b. Is beta known in principle? If yes, can its value be stated from the information given? If yes, what is beta?

8. Consider the following hypothesis. H0: the proportion of nonemergency visits at an emergency room facility is 0.35, and H1: the proportion of nonemergency visits is 0.45, to be tested at the 95 percent confidence level. The sample that will be used to test this will be a random sample of 80 records from all emergency room records for the past three years.

a. Is alpha known in principle? If yes, can its value be stated from the information given? If yes, what is alpha?

b. Is beta known in principle? If yes, can its value be stated from the information given? If yes, what is beta?

7.5 Selecting Sample Sizes

In dealing with confidence limits and Type I and Type II errors, the issue of sample size has come up several times. In particular, it was noted that in order for the public health nurse to be able to distinguish between H0 = 48 and H1 = 49, she would have to have a sample of 1,150 six-year-old boys. How was that number derived?

Sample Size and Confidence Level

If you recall the formula in Equation 7.1, 95 percent confidence limits are set by multiplying the t value for 95 percent (approximately 2) by the standard error of the mean. This value is then added to or subtracted from the mean to get the upper or lower limits of the confidence interval. What can be effectively varied in this formulation is the size of the standard error. As the sample size increases, the standard error will decrease, because it is the standard deviation divided by the square root of the sample size. Let us see what this means in regard to the confidence limits for a sample of six-year-old boys.

Measurement Error and Sample Size

We have said that the standard deviation of the height of six-year-old boys is 10 inches. Given that standard deviation, we can calculate the standard error for any given sample size. Knowing the standard error, we can calculate the size of the interval on either side of the sample mean value that will include the true population mean in 95 percent of all the samples. Statistically speaking, half of the confidence interval will be called the measurement error, and it will be designated (ME). (ME) is defined as shown in Equation 7.3. As you can see, Equation 7.3 is just Equation 7.1 with the mean removed. It represents half of the total 95 percent confidence interval. In no case should (ME) be confused with the standard error.

$$(ME) = t \times S.E._{\bar{x}} \tag{7.3}$$

Figure 7.14 shows the effect of sample size on the standard error, the measurement error (ME), and the upper 95 percent limit for a mean of 48 inches, assuming a two-tail test (i.e., t in either Equation 7.1 or Equation 7.3 is 2; if a one-tail test were assumed, t would have to be approximately 1.7). For a sample of size 100, the standard error is 1 and (ME) is 2. For a sample of 500, the standard error is 0.447 and (ME) is 0.894. For 1,150, the standard error is 0.295 and (ME) is 0.590. Although it is not immediately obvious from Figure 7.14, the size of both the standard error and (ME) decreases as the square root of the increase in sample size. For example, 1,150 is 11.5 times larger than 100. The standard error for a sample of 1,150, 0.295, is 3.39 times smaller than the standard error for a sample of 100. The square root of 11.5 is 3.39. This is a general result. The size of the standard error, and hence the size of (ME), decreases as the square root of the increase in sample size. So if sample size doubles, (ME) decreases by 1.44. If sample size increases by a factor of 9, (ME) decreases by a factor of 3.

How to Determine Sample Size

If you know the standard deviation, you can set the standard error, and thus the confidence interval, virtually anywhere you like. You just need to have

C2		▼	= =$A$2/SQRT(B2)		
	A	B	C	D	E
1	StDev	Sample	StError	ME	Upper 48
2	10	100	1.000	2.000	50.000
3		500	0.447	0.894	48.894
4		1150	0.295	0.590	48.590

Figure 7.14 Effect of sample size on standard error and measurement error

the resources required to obtain the sample size needed. The actual formula for determining the sample size, given knowledge of the standard deviation and a good idea of how large (ME) should be, is given in Equation 7.4. This equation says that the sample size n is equal to the square of the value of t times the square of the standard deviation divided by the square of whatever the error of measurement, (ME), is expected to be.

$$n = \frac{t^2 s^2}{(ME)^2} \tag{7.4}$$

Equation 7.4 would seem to have an intellectually soothing quality. If you know how much measurement error you can tolerate, then you can set the sample size necessary for that error. For example, in the case of the public health nurse who wished to distinguish between an average height of 49 inches and an average height of 48 inches, measurement error required 0.5 inches. Apart from the problem that the sample size set may be quite large and therefore quite expensive, there is another problem. This is the problem of knowledge of the variance (s^2) in Equation 7.4. In general, it is necessary to collect some data and calculate the variance before the variance is known. So, in order to determine how large a sample is required, it is already necessary to have some sample data. This is in the nature of a statistical catch-22.

There is one realm, however, in which the standard deviation can be known before any data are collected. The variance of a proportion can be calculated directly from the proportion as the square root of the proportion times 1 minus the proportion. So, for example, if you have some general knowledge of the size of a proportion to be estimated, it is possible to determine the sample size necessary to be within some specified measurement error by Equation 7.5.

$$n = \frac{t^2 p(1-p)}{(ME)^2} \tag{7.5}$$

EXERCISES FOR SECTION 7.5

1. Calculate the approximate sample size required for each of the following at 95 percent confidence:

   a. Standard deviation = 10, (ME) = 0.5, two tail

   b. Standard deviation = 10, (ME) = 0.5, one tail

   c. Standard deviation = 10, (ME) = 1.5, two tail

   d. Standard deviation = 10, (ME) = 1.5, one tail

    e. Standard deviation = 35, (*ME*) = 5, two tail

    f. Standard deviation = 35, (*ME*) = 5, one tail

    g. Standard deviation = $3,200, (*ME*) = 400, two tail

    h. Standard deviation = $3,200, (*ME*) = 400, one tail

2. A hospital administrator wants to measure average cost per stay in his institution. He is willing to be within $200 of the true value with a probability of 95 percent. An initial investigation of a random sample of 10 records determined that the standard deviation of cost was $3,987. How large a sample will need to be taken to meet the administrator's needs?

3. After learning of the size of sample needed in Exercise 2, the administrator decided that he would be willing to be within $500. How big a sample does he need to reach this level of error?

4. A state public health worker wants to determine the average number of visits to prenatal health department clinics expectant mothers are making in the state. She believes that the standard deviation of visits is three visits. On the basis of her belief, how large a sample must she have to test H0: visits = 7 against the alternative H1: visits = 6 with *alpha* = *beta* = 0.05?

5. The proportion of true emergencies coming to an emergency room is believed to be 60 percent. How large a sample of visits would the emergency room administrator have to take to confirm this 60 percent with a measurement error (*ME*) of 0.05?

KEY TERMS

=AND()	confidence interval
=COUNTIF()	hypothesis
=TDIST()	Type I error
=TINV()	Type II error
alpha	variable
beta	

CHAPTER 8

STATISTICAL TESTS FOR CATEGORICAL DATA

It is the mark of a truly intelligent person to be moved by statistics.

—George Bernard Shaw

As indicated elsewhere in this book, a major part of statistical analysis is the assessment of the independence of two or more variables. The t test assesses the independence of two variables, one measured on a numerical scale and the other measured on a categorical scale that takes only two values. Analysis of variance (ANOVA) assesses the independence of two or more variables. With ANOVA, one variable is measured on a numerical scale and the others are measured on categorical scales that may take on any number of values, although typically the number of values will be limited to fewer than five or six. Regression assesses the independence of two or more variables, all of which can be measured on a numerical scale. The chi-square statistic (χ^2) is a statistical analysis that can be used to establish the independence of two or more variables, each of which is measured on a categorical scale.

8.1   Independence of Two Variables

Chapter 5 introduced the subject of independence of two variables. There it was noted that independence could be thought of as mathematical independence or alternatively as statistical independence. This chapter takes up these two topics again, with a more detailed discussion of statistical independence as a way of introducing the chi-square.

Mathematical Independence

The concept of mathematical independence has been discussed previously in Chapter 5. But, to reconsider that discussion here, suppose 100 persons visited the emergency room in the community hospital over the past 24-hour period. Thirty of those people came for true emergencies. Seventy of those people came for some condition that would not be considered a true emergency. Also, 60 of the people came during the day (say, from 6 a.m. to 6 p.m.), whereas the other 40 came at night. The marginal values of this joint distribution are shown in Figure 8.1. Now, if we had no other information about the people who came to the emergency room, how would we expect the people to be distributed in the four internal cells of the table—cells B2 : C3? Or, from another perspective, what is the most likely distribution of people in those four cells?

After a little thought, most people would conclude that the most likely distribution of people in the four cells—B2 : C3—would be as shown in Figure 8.2. It is possible that some people might not even know immediately why they arrived at the frequency distribution shown in cells B2 : C3. If questioned, however, they would probably come up with reasoning that involved the idea that, for example, total emergencies are 30 percent of all visits, so emergencies during the day should be 30 percent of all visits that occur during the day. Similarly, emergencies during the night should be 30 percent of all visits that occur during the night. Once either of those decisions is made, the rest of the cells are fixed by the marginal values.

When a person decides that the number of emergencies during the day should be 18, because 18 is 30 percent of 60, all other cells are fixed. If 18 is assigned to the Day/Emergency cell, 12 must be assigned to the Night/Emergency cell, because the sum of the two cells must be 30. Similarly, if 18 is assigned to the Day/Emergency cell, then 42 must be

	A	B	C	D
1		Day	Night	Total
2	Emergency			30
3	Other			70
4	Total	60	40	100
5				

Figure 8.1   Marginal frequencies

	A	B	C	D
1		Day	Night	Total
2	Emergency	18	12	30
3	Other	42	28	70
4	Total	60	40	100
5				

Figure 8.2   Marginal frequencies with most probable internal frequencies

assigned to the Day/Other cell, because the sum of the two cells must be 60. The 28 in the Night/Other cell is fixed in the same way. Because a decision can be made about the number of observations in only one cell of the table, given the marginal totals, a two-by-two table has only one degree of freedom. In general, any $r \times c$ (rows $\times$ columns) table will have $(r-1) \times (c-1)$ degrees of freedom. In the table in Figure 8.2, there are two rows and two columns, and thus $(r-1) \times (c-1)$ equals 1.

The distribution of observations shown in Figure 8.2 is one that is characterized by mathematical independence. Mathematical independence is defined as a situation in which the marginal probabilities in a table, such as that shown in Figure 8.2, are equal to the conditional probabilities.

> Mathematical independence is when marginal probabilities equal conditional probabilities in a joint probability table.

As we saw in Chapter 5, marginal probabilities are just the probabilities associated with the frequency distribution of a single variable. The table in Figure 8.2 has two marginal probabilities, one for the distribution of coming during the day or night, and one for the distribution of coming for an emergency or for another reason. Again, as seen in Chapter 5, a conditional probability for this example could be defined as a patient coming in for an emergency on the condition that the person came during the day.

Marginal and Conditional Probabilities: Link to Mathematical Independence

Figure 8.3 shows the marginal probabilities of a person coming for an emergency or coming for another reason as 0.3(30/100) and 0.7(70/100). Figure 8.3 also shows the conditional probabilities of a person coming for an emergency on the condition that (or given that) one came during the day— or during the night. For example, the conditional probability of a person coming for an emergency, given that one came during the day, is 0.3(18/60). In turn, the conditional probability of a person coming for another reason during the day is 0.7(42/60). If we designate the marginal probability of a person coming for an emergency as $p(E)$ and the conditional probability

	A	B	C	D
6		Day	Night	Total
7	Emergency	0.3	0.3	0.3
8	Other	0.7	0.7	0.7
9	Total	60	40	100
10				

Figure 8.3 Marginal and conditional probabilities

of a person coming for an emergency, given that one came during the day, as $p(E|D)$, then mathematical independence is defined as $p(E) = p(E|D)$. The tables shown in Figure 8.2 and Figure 8.3 have only one degree of freedom. Therefore, finding that any one of the conditional probabilities in the table equals any one of the marginal probabilities is equivalent to finding all conditional probabilities equivalent to all corresponding marginal probabilities.

It should be clear that this analysis has examined conditional and marginal probabilities in only one direction—by columns. We could equally well have looked at the marginal probability of a person coming during the day $p(D)$ or during the night $p(N)$. Take a look again at the example table in Figure 8.2. For example, the probability of a person coming during the day $p(D)$ is exactly equal to the probability of a person coming during the day, given that one came for an emergency $p(D|E)$. In most cases, though, it is conventional to examine conditional probabilities by columns rather than by rows.

As indicated here, the definition of mathematical independence for two categorical variables is that the marginal and corresponding conditional probabilities are equal. For a two-by-two table, it is necessary to examine only one conditional probability to make this determination. In a larger table, however, it may be necessary to examine more than one conditional probability to ensure mathematical independence. In general, it will be necessary to look at as many conditional probabilities as there are degrees of freedom in the table before declaring mathematical independence.

Statistical Independence of Two Variables

Before proceeding to discuss statistical independence of two variables, it is important to be sure that what was discussed in the first subsection of Section 8.1 is fully understood. Mathematical independence means that there is no relationship between the time of day (or night) that people arrive at the emergency clinic and whether they come for an emergency. Considered another way, knowing if a person arrived during the day or during the night does not improve any prediction of whether the person came for an emergency.

But consider now that the data examined in the first subsection of Section 8.1 were for only 100 emergency room visits. These visits might be chosen at random, or they might represent a single day's visits or several days' visits. But even if time of day is mathematically independent of arrival for an emergency, we might not always find the results we did. If we had examined a different sample—a larger or smaller sample, for example, or

	A	B	C	D
1	*Frequencies*	Day	Night	Total
2	Emergency	17	13	30
3	Other	43	27	70
4	Total	60	40	100
5				
6	*Probabilities*	Day	Night	Total
7	Emergency	0.283	0.325	0.3
8	Other	0.717	0.675	0.7
9	Total	60	40	100
10				

Figure 8.4 Different conditional probabilities

one taken at a somewhat different time—these differences might have led us to find that the conditional and marginal frequencies were very close but were not exact matches. What, then, might we conclude?

Let us posit that the data in Figure 8.4 represent a sample of 100 emergency room visits. These sample visits were taken from among those visits that occurred in the month following the one in which the data in Figure 8.2 were taken. Cells A1 : D4 give the actual frequencies for the 100 visits. These visits are divided, as before, into 30 visits for emergencies and 70 for other reasons, with 60 visits occurring during the day and 40 visits occurring at night. Cells A6 : D9 show the conditional and marginal probabilities by columns. Now, the conditional probability, for example, of a person coming for an emergency, given that one came during the day ($p(E|D) = 0.283$) is given in cell B7. This conditional probability is not exactly the same as the marginal probability of a person coming during the day ($p(D) = 0.3$). So one might conclude that the two variables are no longer independent mathematically. However, are they close enough to be considered independent statistically, and what might that mean?

Statistical Independence: The Chi-Square Test

Statistically, if we took many samples of size 100 of people who came to an emergency room, we would expect that the conditional probabilities would not match exactly the marginal probabilities for every sample. This would be true even if the variables, time of arrival, and arrival for an emergency were truly mathematically independent of one another. So we would like to have a statistical test to determine whether the two variables can be considered statistically independent of each other. We would like this test even if the two variables are not considered strictly mathematically independent for every sample we may examine. The test of statistical independence is the chi-square, or χ^2 test.

The chi-square test determines if two variables are statistically independent of each other.

The chi-square test is a test of independence between two variables. It is calculated as given in Equation 8.1. In Equation 8.1, r is the number of rows in the table and c is the number of columns. O is the observed frequency in each cell, and E is the expected frequency in the cell. The squared difference between each observed frequency and each expected frequency is divided by the expected frequency. These values are then summed across all $r \times c$ cells in the table. The result is the chi-square value. If the chi-square value is greater than some predetermined value, the two variables will be considered statistically independent.

$$\chi^2 = \sum_{i=1}^{rc} \frac{(O_i - E_i)^2}{E_i} \qquad (8.1)$$

Consider the data shown in cells B2:C3 in Figure 8.4 as the observed values. Based on the conditional probabilities shown in cells B7:C8, we know that the two variables shown in that table are not mathematically independent. But if we calculate the chi-square, will they be found to be statistically independent? To determine this, we need to know the expected values. But what are the expected values? It turns out that the expected values are the values we will expect to get if the marginal probabilities and the conditional probabilities are the same—in other words, what we decided should be the values in cells B2:C3 in Figure 8.2, based on the distributions of the marginal values. Given these expected and marginal values, the calculation of the chi-square statistic for the data shown in cells B2:C3 in Figure 8.4 is shown in Equation 8.2. The calculated chi-square value is 0.1984. The question then would be, what is the likelihood of finding a chi-square value that large if the null hypothesis that arriving for an emergency is independent of time of arrival is actually true?

$$\chi^2 = \frac{(17 - 18)^2}{18} + \frac{(13 - 12)^2}{12} + \frac{(43 - 42)^2}{42} + \frac{(27 - 28)^2}{28} = 0.1984 \quad (8.2)$$

The =CHIDIST() Function

The probability of a chi-square value as large as 0.1984, given that the null hypothesis of independence is true, is found with the =CHIDIST() function. The =CHIDIST() function takes two arguments: the value of the chi-square statistic and the number of degrees of freedom. The calculation of the =CHIDIST() function shown in Equation 8.3 is 0.656. This value means that there is about a 66 percent probability of finding a chi-square value as large as 0.1984 under the null hypothesis that arrival for an emergency is independent of time of arrival. In general, we would reject the null hypothesis only if the probability of the chi-square value were less than 0.05; so, in this case, we would conclude that the observed frequencies in cells B2:C3 in Figure 8.4 are not different enough from the expected frequencies. In turn, we would say that time of arrival and arrival for an emergency are statistically independent of each other.

$$p = \text{CHIDIST}(0.1984, 1) = 0.656 \tag{8.3}$$

The =CHIINV() Function

But how large must a chi-square be before one can conclude that the two events are statistically independent? The value of the chi-square required, referred to as the critical value of the chi-square, can be found using the =CHIINV() function. This function takes two arguments: the probability at which we will reject the null and the degrees of freedom. The critical value for the chi-square for a table with one degree of freedom (any table with two rows and two columns) is given in Equation 8.4. According to that equation, it is necessary to have a chi-square value of at least 3.84 before the null hypothesis of statistical independence is rejected at the 95 percent level of confidence.

$$Chi\text{-}square|crit = \text{CHIINV}(0.05, 1) = 3.84 \tag{8.4}$$

The Chi-Square Critical Value

What kind of difference would be necessary between observed and expected values in the table in Figure 8.4 before the critical value of chi-square would be reached? Figure 8.5 shows a template for the calculation of the chi-square statistic. The template also shows one of the smallest differences in the distribution of observed versus expected values that result in a chi-square that exceeds the critical value. Figure 8.5 deserves substantial explanation.

First, consider cell B2 of Figure 8.5. The value of 13 in the cell (13 people came for emergencies during the day) is the closest value to the expected (shown in cell B7) that can appear in that cell and produce a chi-square greater than the critical value. Because there is one degree of freedom in this example, 13 in cell B2 fixes all three other cells in B2:C3, given the marginal values in column D and row 4. The expected values for the given marginal values (cells B7:C8) are shown in Figure 8.2, but here, a simple way of calculating those expected values is given. The formula for cell B7 is

	B7	▼	=	=B$4*$D2/$D$4			
	A	B	C	D	E	F	
1	*Observed*	Day	Night	Total			
2	Emergency	13	17	30			
3	Other	47	23	70			
4	Total	60	40	100			
5							
6	*Expected*	Day	Night	Total			
7	Emergency	18	12	30			
8	Other	42	28	70			
9	Total	60	40	100			
10							
11	*Chi-square*	Day	Night	Total			
12	Emergency	1.388889	2.083333	30	Chi-square	4.960317	
13	Other	0.595238	0.892857	70	Prob	0.025935	
14	Total	60	40	100	Crit	3.841455	
15							
16	*Probabilities*	Day	Night	Total			
17	Emergency	0.217	0.425	0.3			
18	Other	0.783	0.575	0.7			
19	Total	60	40	100			
20							

Figure 8.5 Template for the chi-square

shown on the formula line above the spreadsheet. The formula uses the $ convention to fix appropriate rows and columns so that it can be copied to all four cells in which expected values are desired. To explain the formula, B$4 fixes the first term in row 4, which allows the formula to be moved to cell B8 without changing the reference to cell B4. $D2 fixes the second term in the equation in column D so that it is possible to move the equation to cell C7 without changing the reference to cell D2. Finally, $D$4 fixes cell D4 so that it is possible to move the equation to any of the cells without changing the reference to cell D4. With this formula in cell B7, it is possible to click the lower right corner of the cell and drag the formula across to cell C7, and then to drag both cells down to row 8. This produces the expected values for the marginal values observed.

The values shown in cells B12:C13 are the calculations of the chi-square statistic. Each cell represents one of the calculations $(O - E)^2/E$, shown in Equation 8.1. The chi-square value itself is shown in cell F12 and is the sum of cells B12:C13. The probability of the chi-square value is shown in cell F13 as 0.0259. Because this value is less than 0.05, we would reject the null hypothesis that the two variables—arrival for an emergency and time of arrival—are independent of each other.

The last table in Figure 8.5 shows the conditional probabilities of reason for arrival, given arrival during the day or during the night. These conditional probabilities show that about 22 percent of the people arriving during the day came for an emergency, whereas about 43 percent of those coming at night came for an emergency. In general, one of the best ways to interpret the results of a chi-square applied to any contingency table is to form the conditional probabilities by columns and interpret them by comparing rows. For our example, compare the conditional probabilities for those who came for an emergency during the day or during the night. This gives a succinct way of describing the differences in the observed values that produce the chi-square value large enough to reject the null hypothesis of independence.

Using the =CHITEST() Function

Microsoft Excel does not include a Data Analysis add-in to do the chi-square test, but it does include a function that will carry out the chi-square analysis. This function is =CHITEST(). The =CHITEST() function takes two separate arguments: the range represented by the observed data and the range represented by the expected data. The table in Figure 8.6 reproduces the observed and expected frequencies from Figure 8.5, but it now shows the calculation of the =CHITEST() function, in cell D11. The formula line in Figure 8.6 shows the two ranges B2:C3 and B7:C8, which are included as arguments of the =CHITEST() function. The =CHITEST() function produces not the chi-square value but the probability of finding that value, given the null hypothesis of independence. The actual chi-square value can be reproduced by using the =CHIINV() function with the value of the probability and one degree of freedom. This reproduced chi-square value is shown in cell D12. The =CHIINV() function will not always reproduce

Figure 8.6 The =CHITEST function

the chi-square value, however. If the probability of the chi-square is less than 3.0E-7, the =CHIINV() function returns #NUM!.

The Chi-Square and Type I and Type II Errors

Chapter 7 introduced the notion of Type I and Type II errors with regard to the t distribution. A few comments should be made about Type I and Type II errors with regard to the chi-square distribution. The chi-square distribution is not a "normal" distribution as the t distribution is, in the sense that it is symmetrical about some mean value. In fact, the chi-square distribution tends to be heavily skewed to the right. Figure 8.7 shows the chi-square distribution with one degree of freedom. This is the most extremely skewed chi-square distribution. As degrees of freedom increase, the distribution begins to take on a less skewed appearance, and if the degrees of freedom increase to 40 or 50, the distribution begins to look more and more normal. But most chi-square applications, particularly in regard to contingency tables, are limited to degrees of freedom in the range 1 (a two-by-two table) to less than 10 or 12 (a four-by-five table).

With one degree of freedom, the point in the distribution at which the null hypothesis of no relationship between two variables (as previously discussed) would be rejected at alpha = 0.05 would be at approximately 3.8 (as shown by the vertical dashed line in the figure). Any chi-square value that resulted in a probability to the right of the dashed line (i.e., any value greater than 3.8) would be expected to occur less than 5 percent of the time when the null hypothesis is true. Thus, any value in that range would lead to the rejection of H0 (no relationship between or independence of the two variables) and the acceptance of the alternative—that the two variables are not independent. The area to the right of the dashed line, then, which is usually set at 0.05, is the area of Type I error, or alpha.

Figure 8.7   The chi-square distribution for one degree of freedom

Type I Error

Let us consider the Type I error in another way. In the example analysis shown in Figure 8.5, the expected joint probability "and" for Day and Emergency is 18/100, or 0.18. Because the other probabilities in the table are fixed by 0.18, given the marginal values (the table has one degree of freedom), the expected probabilities for the other three cells are 0.12 for Night and Emergency, 0.42 for Day and Other, and 0.28 for Night and Other. Let's say we generate many samples—say, 1,000 samples of size 100—from a population in which these proportions are true. In turn, the distribution of chi-square values for these samples would be such that approximately 5 percent (about 50 out of the 1,000) would have chi-square values that exceed 3.8. So even though the null hypothesis of independence would be true, there would be some proportion of the samples for which we would reject H0.

Type II Error

But what now of beta or the Type II error? How can we conceive of the Type II error with this same example? To see this, consider the possibility that the true proportion of Day and Emergency visits is not 0.18 but 0.15 in the larger population (the other proportions change at the same time). Let's assume we again took many samples (1,000 samples of size 100) from a population in which the true proportion of Day and Emergency was 0.15. In turn, we would discover that about 70 percent of these samples had values of the chi-square that did not exceed 3.8 (the 0.05 level of significance). Thus, in the case of a true proportion for Day and Emergency of 0.15, we have about a 70 percent chance of making the Type II error (accepting the null hypothesis of independence, or Day and Emergency equals 0.18) when it is false.

In fact, one may ask, what if there were an even greater variation from 0.18? Suppose the actual probability of Day and Emergency in the population is 0.11. Do we now have any chance of making the Type II error? The answer is yes. Suppose we took many samples (1,000 samples of size 100) from a population in which the true proportion of Day and Emergency was 0.11. We would discover that about 10 percent of those samples would have values less than 3.8; so, in this case, we would have about a 10 percent chance of making the Type II error.

As with the Type II error associated with a normal or *t* distribution, we can reduce the Type II error associated with the chi-square by increasing the sample size. Again, suppose we were to take a large number of samples of a larger size (1,000 samples of size 200) from a population in which the true proportion of Day and Emergency was 0.15. We would discover that only about 50 percent of the samples would lead us to falsely accept H0 (Type II error), whereas the other 50 percent would lead us correctly to reject H0. The larger the sample we take, the lower the level of beta will be for any given divergence of the true value from that hypothesized by H0.

EXERCISES FOR SECTION 8.1

1. Calculate expected values for the following two-by-two tables:

a.

		25
		42
34	33	67

b.

		125
		230
200	155	355

c.

		33
		230
200	63	263

2. Calculate chi-square values for the following tables:

a.

18	7	25
16	26	42
34	33	67

b.

47	78	125
153	77	230
200	155	355

c.

21	12	33
179	51	230
200	63	263

3. Determine whether you would accept or reject the hypothesis of independence for the two variables in each of the tables in (a), (b), and (c) of Exercise 2.

4. Calculate conditional and marginal probabilities for the cross-tabulations in (a), (b), and (c) of Exercise 2, and give them an interpretation.

8.2 Examples of Chi-Square Analyses

Thus far the discussion has focused solely on contingency tables with one degree of freedom (two-by-two tables). This section will consider several examples of chi-square calculations taken from examples that have appeared in various journals and includes further discussion of not only two-by-two contingency tables but also larger contingency tables.

An Example of a Two-by-Two Table

To better understand the chi-square test and its interpretation, consider the example shown in Figure 8.8. That figure shows data taken from an article by Halpern et al. (2001), and the data shown in the table were taken from the second table in the article (p. 1682). Figure 8.8 contains data to address the question of whether an adolescent has experienced either physical or psychological violence from a partner in an opposite-sex romantic relationship. The supposition is that the violence is independent of whether the respondent is male or female. The implied null hypothesis is independence; the implied alternative is nonindependence.

In Figure 8.8, cells A1:D4 show the observed cell values and marginal values. Cells A6:D9 show the expected values based on the calculations shown in cell B7 in Figure 8.6. Cells A11:D14 show the calculation of the chi-square values for each cell, and cell F12 shows the total chi-square value. The probability of this chi-square value under the null hypothesis of independence is shown in cell F13 as 0.0076. Because this value is less than 0.05, we reject the null hypothesis of independence and conclude that experiencing violence is not independent of sex.

	A	B	C	D	E	F
1	*Observed*	Male	Female			
2	Violence	1130	1239	2369		
3	No Violence	2275	2849	5124		
4		3405	4088	7493		
5						
6	*Expected*	Male	Female			
7	Violence	1076.531	1292.469	2369		
8	No Violence	2328.469	2795.531	5124		
9		3405	4088	7493		
10						
11	*Chi-Square*	Male	Female			
12	Violence	2.655715	2.212014	2369	Chi-Square	7.118246
13	No Violence	1.227828	1.022689	5124	Prob	0.00763
14		3405	4088	7493	Crit	3.841455
15						
16						
17	*Probabilities*	Male	Female			
18	Violence	33%	30%	32%		
19	No Violence	67%	70%	68%		
20		100%	100%	100%		
21						

Figure 8.8 Example from the Halpern et al. (2001) article

Interpreting the Chi-Square Statistic: Statistical versus Practical Significance

Saying that experiencing violence is not independent of sex implies that either male adolescents or female adolescents are more likely than the other gender to experience violence in an opposite-sex romantic relationship. But by looking at the observed values in cells A1:D4, it is difficult to tell which sex is more likely to experience such violence. Consequently, the easiest way to interpret the results of a chi-square test is by looking at the conditional probabilities of experiencing violence. Cells A17:D20 show the conditional probabilities of having experienced violence, given sexual identity. Perhaps somewhat surprisingly, 33 percent of males said that they had experienced violence, whereas 30 percent of females said the same. These percentage differences are not large, but the fact that there are 7,493 respondents in the study gives this relatively small percentage difference *statistical significance.*

Having seen the results from Figure 8.8, it is useful to say a few words about the difference between statistical significance and practical signifi-cance. The notion of statistical significance is associated with the rejection of the null hypothesis, whether that hypothesis is explicit or implied. So, in the case of the data examined in Figure 8.8, "statistical significance" refers to the fact that the chi-square value is large enough to reject the null hypoth-esis. But "practical significance" refers to the importance of a result found in a statistical test. Because the number of respondents is relatively large, as shown in Figure 8.8, a relatively small percentage difference results in statistical significance. Whether this relatively small percentage difference has practical significance is not a question that can be addressed by statistics. It is a question that can be addressed only by knowledge of the subject, experience, and understanding. Consequently, statistics can address statistical questions, but the value placed on the results of statistical analysis remains with the observer, who must assess the importance of these results.

An Example of an n-by-Two Table from the Literature

The extension of the chi-square statistic to tables with more than four cells is direct. The original data reported in the article referenced for Figure 8.8 were presented for the experiencing of physical violence, psychological violence, or no violence. The tables in Figure 8.9 show the data in both categories of violence and no violence. Cells A1 : D5 are the observed values for the data, whereas cells A7 : D11 are the expected values. Again, the expected values are calculated by multiplying the row total for each cell times the column total for the cell and dividing by the grand total. The formula used and replicated by dragging to each cell, B8 : C10, is shown in the formula bar in Figure 8.9. Cells B14 : C16 are the chi-square values for

Figure 8.9 An n-by-two chi-square

each individual cell, and the overall chi-square value is shown in cell F14. The probability of the chi-square value in cell F14, under the implied null hypothesis of independence, is given in cell F15. The value in cell F15 is now determined with =CHIDIST() with two degrees of freedom. The critical value for a chi-square with two degrees of freedom is given in cell F16.

Notice that the critical value is 5.99, which is very close to six. The data being analyzed in Figure 8.9 are presented in a three-by-two table. Each table contains six internal cells. The data analyzed in Figure 8.8 were in a two-by-two table. A two-by-two table has four cells, and the critical value was 3.8. A three-by-two table has six cells, and the critical value is about 6. In general, one can be fairly certain that if the chi-square value is as large as the number of cells in a table, it is likely that the null hypothesis of independence will be rejected at the 0.05 level.

In general, if the chi-square value is as large as the number of cells in the contingency table, it is likely that the null hypothesis of independence will be rejected at the 5 percent level.

Again, the question of how the interpretation of the data is to be made arises. The interpretation is best based on the conditional probabilities of experiencing different types of violence or no violence, given that the recipient is male or female. Cells B20:C22 show these differences. The major difference in the experiencing of violence between males and females is that 21 percent of males reported experiencing psychological violence, whereas 18 percent of females reported such violence. There is no difference in the percentages for physical violence.

An Example of a Two-by-n Table from the Literature

An example of a two-by-n variable is also available from the literature. The data in Figure 8.10 came from a study of 3,158 women in the Sudan with at least one child. The study was reported in *Studies in Family Planning* ("Sudan 1989/1990" 1992). The women were asked if they wanted another child. Their answers were tabulated with the number of children they currently had in categories from one to five and six or more. The observed frequencies are given in cells A1:H4. The expected frequencies are given in cells A6:H9. The formula for the calculation of expected frequencies is shown for cell B7 in the formula line at the top of the figure. The chi-square values for the individual cells are shown in cells A11:H14, and the overall chi-square, 531.72, is given in cell J12. The probability of the chi-square is

B7		= =B$4*$H2/$H$4									
	A	B	C	D	E	F	G	H	I	J	K
1	Observed	1 Child	2	3	4	5	6+	Total			
2	Want More	512	426	398	320	233	482	2371			
3	Do not want more	21	37	54	104	114	457	787			
4	Total	533	463	452	424	347	939	3158			
5											
6	Expected	1 Child	2	3	4	5	6+	Total			
7	Want More	400.172	347.617	339.358	318.336	260.525	704.993	2371			
8	Do not want more	132.828	115.383	112.642	105.664	86.4753	234.007	787			
9	Total	533	463	452	424	347	939	3158			
10											
11	Chi square	1 Child	2	3	4	5	6+	Total			
12	Want More	31.2504	17.6746	10.1336	0.0087	2.90801	70.534	2371	Chi-Square	531.7207	
13	Do not want more	94.1481	53.2483	30.5295	0.02622	8.76099	212.498	787	Prob	1.1E-112	
14	Total	533	463	452	424	347	939	3158	Crit	11.07048	
15											
16	Probabilities	1 Child	2	3	4	5	6+	Total			
17	Want More	96%	92%	88%	75%	67%	51%	75%			
18	Do not want more	4%	8%	12%	25%	33%	49%	25%			
19	Total	100%	100%	100%	100%	100%	100%	100%			

Figure 8.10 Number of children and desire for more

given in cell J13. You should recognize that the chi-square value in this case is very large and the probability is very small. Because the number of cells in the table is 12, the critical value of the chi-square is about 12 (actually 11.07). Any value of the chi-square larger than this would lead us to reject the implied null hypothesis of independence between the number of children and the desire for an additional child. In short, we reject that implied null.

The conditional probabilities of wanting an additional child, given the number of children a woman already has, are shown in cells A16 : H19. Ninety-six percent of women with only one child want an additional child. Only 51 percent of women with six or more children want an additional child. Between these two extremes there is a monotonic decrease in the percentage of women who want another child. The conclusion is quite clear: Among these women from the Sudan, the more children a woman has, the less likely she is to desire an additional child. Although this is not unexpected, the data from this study confirm the expectation.

An n-by-n Example from the Literature

The extension of the chi-square statistic from n-by-two or two-by-n to n-by-n tables is also direct. Consider, for example, the data shown in Figure 8.11. These data represent the results of a study carried out by Brook and Appel (1973) on the assessment of the quality of medical care. Each of three physicians reviewed 296 case records for patients who had been treated for urinary tract infection (UTI), hypertension (Hyper), or ulcer. The treatment of the case was judged adequate or inadequate by each of the three physicians. On the adequacy dimension the data are displayed

B14	▼	=	=(B2-B8)^2/B8			
	A	B	C	D	E	F	G
1	*Observed*	UTI	Hyper	Ulcer	Total		
2	Adequate by 2+	13	31	25	69		
3	Adequate by 1	17	29	12	58		
4	Adequate by 0	77	54	38	169		
5		107	114	75	296		
6							
7	*Expected*	UTI	Hyper	Ulcer	Total		
8	Adequate by 2+	24.943	26.574	17.483	69		
9	Adequate by 1	20.966	22.338	14.696	58		
10	Adequate by 0	61.091	65.088	42.821	169		
11		107	114	75	296		
12							
13	*Chi-square*	UTI	Hyper	Ulcer	Total		
14	Adequate by 2+	5.718133	0.73705	3.2319	69	Chi-Squar	19.49331
15	Adequate by 1	0.750296	1.986961	0.494567	58	Prob	0.000629
16	Adequate by 0	4.142812	1.888834	0.542761	169	Crit	9.487728
17		107	114	75	296		
18							
19	*Probabilities*	UTI	Hyper	Ulcer	Total		
20	Adequate by 2+	12%	27%	33%	23%		
21	Adequate by 1	16%	25%	16%	20%		
22	Adequate by 0	72%	47%	51%	57%		
23		100%	100%	100%	100%		

Figure 8.11 Adequacy of treatment of three conditions

in three categories: judged adequate by two or three physicians (*Adequate by 2+*), judged adequate by one (*Adequate by 1*), or judged adequate by none (*Adequate by 0*).

Cells A1 : E5 show the observed data for the 296 cases. Cells A6 : E11 show the expected values for each of the cells by the convention column total × row total/grand total. The chi-square calculations for each individual cell are shown in cells A13 : E17, and the overall chi-square value of 19.49 is shown in cell G14. The actual probability of obtaining a chi-square value that large under the null hypothesis that adequacy of treatment is independent of diagnosis is given in cell G15 as 0.0006, or 6 times out of 10,000. Because the probability is so small, we conclude that we must reject the null hypothesis, which is equivalent to saying that judged adequacy of treatment depends on the initial diagnosis.

To see which diagnosis is more likely to be judged to be treated adequately, it is useful to form the table of conditional probabilities shown in cells A19 : E23. Here it can be seen that 12 percent of UTI cases are judged adequately treated by two or three physicians, whereas 27 and 33 percent of hypertension and ulcer, respectively, are similarly judged. However, 72 percent of UTI cases are judged adequately treated by not a single one of the three physicians. Clearly, the dependence between judgment of adequacy and diagnosis rests primarily in the difference between UTI cases and the other two.

EXERCISES FOR SECTION 8.2

Pivot tables were covered in Chapter 4. Please refer to Chapter 4 for assistance with creating pivot tables.

1. Use the data on worksheet Violence 1 of Chpt 8-1.xls to replicate the analysis given in Figure 8.8.

2. The data on the SWC worksheet of Chpt 8-1.xls show the countries of the world, with the countries of Africa indicated as 1 on the variable Africa, and countries with under-five mortality less than 100 indicated by 1 on the variable Child Friendly.

   a. Use the pivot table capability of Excel and the chi-square to test the hypothesis of independence between being a country in Africa and being child-friendly.

   b. Use conditional probabilities to provide an interpretation of the result.

3. The data on the Hospital Stay worksheet of Chpt 8-1.xls show a sample of 100 hospital stays by Sex and LOS. Stays > three days are coded as Long; those three days or less are coded Short.

   a. Use the pivot table capability of Excel and the chi-square to test the hypothesis of independence between Sex and Stay as coded Long or Short.

   b. Use conditional probabilities to provide an interpretation of the results.

4. Use the data on worksheet Violence 2 of Chpt 8-1.xls to replicate the analysis given in Figure 8.9.

5. The MS-DRG worksheet of Chpt 8-1.xls shows Sex and four MS-DRG categories (MS-DRG Categ) for 300 hospital admissions.

   a. Use the pivot table capability of Excel and the chi-square to test the hypothesis of independence between Sex and MS-DRG category as coded in four categories.

   b. Use conditional probabilities to provide an interpretation of the results.

6. Use the data from the Brook and Appel (1973) example located on the Adequacy of Treatment worksheet, cells A1:E5, in Figure 8.11 to replicate the analysis given in Figure 8.11.

7. The Late Delivery worksheet of Chpt 8-1.xls shows the reason for late delivery of the noon meal in three wards of a hospital to be problems with personnel, the facility, or the patient.

   a. Use the pivot table capability of Excel and the chi-square to test the hypothesis of independence between ward and the reason for lateness.

   b. Use conditional probabilities to provide an interpretation of the results.

8.3   Small Expected Values in Cells

The use of the chi-square statistic assumes relatively little about the data. There is no underlying assumption, for example, that the data need be normally distributed. Any data in a contingency table will be acceptable. There is one limitation, however, about the magnitude of the expected value in any cell in the contingency table. In general, small expected values in any table cell tend to inflate the value of the chi-square and increase the likelihood of rejecting the null hypothesis when it should not be rejected. There are several ways of dealing with this possibility, and these alternatives depend, in part, on the number of cells in a table.

Small Expected Values When $df = 1$

If the expected value in any cell of a two-by-two table is less than about 10, one way of dealing with the small expected values is to apply what is known as *Yates's correction*. Yates's correction is applied using the formula shown in Equation 8.5, which indicates that the absolute value of the difference between the observed and expected frequencies is reduced by 0.5 before the value is squared. To see how the application of this equation works, consider the example shown in Figure 8.12.

$$\chi^2 = \sum_{i=1}^{rc} \frac{(|O_i - E_i| - 0.5)^2}{E_i} \tag{8.5}$$

Figure 8.12 shows data comparable to that in Figure 8.2, except that in the case of Figure 8.12 there are only 50 observations rather than 100. The consequence of this difference, given the same marginal probabilities, is that the expected values for cells B7 and C7 are less than 10. In this case, the chi-square formula given in Equation 8.1 is not strictly appropriate, because it produces a chi-square value larger than it should be. For the observed data seen in cells A1 : D4, the chi-square using Yates's correction (Equation 8.5) is shown in cells A11 : F14. The comparison chi-square using the standard formula (Equation 8.1) is shown in cells A16 : F19. Although the decision one would reach does not differ in either of these computations, it can be seen that the Yates's corrected chi-square is a more conservative test. It is less likely than the standard formula to result in a rejection of the null hypothesis when expected cell values are small.

When expected cell values fall below 5, Yates's correction is also no longer considered appropriate. In such a case, the statistical test recommended is the Fisher exact test. The calculation of the Fisher exact test,

B12		= =(ABS(B2-B7)-0.5)^2/B7			
A	B	C	D	E	F
1 Observed	Day	Night	Total		
2 Emergency	5	10	15		
3 Other	25	10	35		
4 Total	30	20	50		
5					
6 Expected	Day	Night	Total		
7 Emergency	9	6	15		
8 Other	21	14	35		
9 Total	30	20	50		
10					
11 Yates'	Day	Night	Total		
12 Emergency	1.361111	2.041667	15	Chi-square	4.861111
13 Other	0.583333	0.875	35	Prob	0.027469
14 Total	30	20	50	Crit	3.841455
15					
16 Standard	Day	Night	Total		
17 Emergency	1.777778	2.666667	15	Chi-square	6.349206
18 Other	0.761905	1.142857	35	Prob	0.011743
19 Total	30	20	50	Crit	3.841455
20					

Figure 8.12 Yates's correction

although not difficult using Excel, is complicated and difficult to understand, and so it is not presented here. In general, the decision reached by the Fisher exact method, although statistically correct, will not be different from the decision reached using either the chi-square or the chi-square with Yates's correction. One reasonable approach to the issue of very small cells would be to base the decision on the probabilities derived from the Yates's correction. This will be, in general, more conservative than the Fisher exact test, in that the null hypothesis of independence is slightly less likely to be rejected. But, at the same time, the probability of making the Type I error will not be greater than the probability level that has been set.

Small Expected Values When df > 1

When degrees of freedom are greater than one, or in other words tables are larger than two rows by two columns, there is no equivalent to Yates's correction or the Fisher exact method. In such tables, two strategies might be used. One is to try to increase the number of observations in general, so that the expected cell frequencies in all cells are at least 5 and preferably 10. Another strategy is to collapse cells where doing so might make logical sense in order to increase the expected values in cells. To illustrate this latter approach, consider again the data shown in Figure 8.11. Those data

	J	K	L	M	N
1	Assessment	UTI	Hypert	Ulcer	Total
2	adequate by 3	2	19	8	29
3	adequate by 2	11	12	17	40
4	adequate by 1	17	29	12	58
5	adequate by 0	77	54	38	169
6	Total	107	114	75	296
7					
8	Assessment	UTI	Hypert	Ulcer	Total
9	adequate by 3	10.483	11.169	7.348	29
10	adequate by 2	14.459	15.405	10.135	40
11	adequate by 1	20.966	22.338	14.696	58
12	adequate by 0	61.091	65.088	42.821	169
13	Total		107	114	75	296
14					

Figure 8.13 Small expected values in $df > 1$

were originally given in the form of the table shown in Figure 8.13. The two rows adequate by 3 and adequate by 2 were collapsed into a single row, adequate by 2+, to avoid the small expected value in cell M9.

It is worth noting that in the case of the data shown in Figure 8.13, numerous researchers would not bother to collapse the two rows adequate by 3 and adequate by 2. This could be considered to be justified because the expected value in cell M9 is not all that small and there is only one such cell smaller than 10. This logic could change had there been several cells with expected values smaller than 10, or if any of the cells had been less than 5. Collapsing the cells or increasing the overall number of observations in the study would have been most advisable from the standpoint of the appropriateness of the chi-square value.

EXERCISES FOR SECTION 8.3

1. Use the Emergency worksheet in Chpt 8-1.xls to replicate the analysis in Figure 8.12.

2. The data in the Satisfaction worksheet in Chpt 8-1.xls represent the responses of a random sample of 35 people to a satisfaction question about a primary care clinic.

    a. Use the pivot table capability of Excel and Yates's correction for the chi-square to test the hypothesis of independence between Sex and Satisfaction.

    b. Use conditional probabilities to provide an interpretation of the results.

KEY TERMS

#NUM!

=CHIDIST()

=CHIINV()

=CHITEST()

statistical significance

Yates's correction

t TESTS FOR RELATED AND UNRELATED DATA

Definition of Statistics: The science of producing unreliable facts from reliable figures.

—Evan Esar

The chi-square discussion in Chapter 8 provides a means of assessing whether two or more categorical variables are statistically independent of one another. This chapter takes up the *t* test. The *t* test is a means of assessing whether a numerical variable—either continuous or discrete—is independent of a categorical variable that takes on only two values. The *t* test provides another capability. It provides the ability to assess whether a value found from a sample could have come from a population in which a hypothesized value is true. This chapter addresses both of these issues, beginning with the latter.

9.1 What Is a *t* Test?

To begin with a discussion of the *t* test, recall the question addressed by the hospital financial officer in Chapter 7. The CFO wished to know the true average cost of a hospital discharge. He decided to take a sample of 100 discharge records. He then calculated the true cost of each hospital stay. In turn, he used the mean cost of this sample of discharges as the mean cost for all 12,000 hospital stays. Suppose that before the financial officer had taken the sample and determined the cost of each, the chief executive officer of the hospital had said to him, "If the average cost of a discharge is $6,000, our charges schedule is fine. If the average cost is more than $6,000, we are going to have to renegotiate our charges schedule with all our payers, and that will be a big hassle. On the other hand, if our cost is less than $6,000, our payers are going to demand that we renegotiate our charges schedule, and that is going to be a hassle also. So I want you to use your sample to determine if our average cost per discharge is $6,000 or not. But I want your best estimate of the true situation, because if it is not $6,000, we need to get to work."

If the financial officer has had some statistics in graduate school (which, of course, he has), he could tell the CEO that there is no way to determine from a sample if the average cost per discharge is exactly $6,000. He can get an estimate of only the average cost. But the financial officer decides to try to answer the CEO's question in the best way he can, using statistical analysis.

The *t* test can produce a result that may range from $-\infty$ to ∞, although practically speaking it is usually in a more finite range. The =TDIST() function works only with positive values of *t*. Therefore, when using the =TDIST() function to determine the true probability of a negative *t* value, it is necessary to change the negative value to a positive one. Because the *t* distribution is symmetrical with regard to the probability of being at $-t$ or t, the conversion makes no difference. Consequently, if the two-tail probability of a value of -2.3 were desired, the way to determine this would be by using =TDIST(2.3,df,2).

t Tests: Setting Up the Hypotheses

The financial officer posits the CEO's concern in the following two hypotheses:

> H0: The average cost per discharge is $6,000.
>
> or
>
> H0: $c = \$6,000$
>
> and
>
> H1: The average cost per discharge is not $6,000.
>
> or
>
> H1: $c \neq \$6,000$

The financial officer knows that the sample mean he obtains for the cost of hospital discharges will be only one of many means he could have gotten, had he taken other samples instead of the one he took. He also knows that the distribution of the means from all those other samples will be approximately a *t* distribution, with degrees of freedom equal to the sample size minus 1. Can he use this information to test whether the mean cost he discovers from the one sample he gets would lead him to accept or reject H0? The answer is yes. The way this test is carried out is given in Equation 9.1.

$$t = \frac{\bar{x}_s - \mu_H}{S.E._{\bar{x}_s}} \qquad (9.1)$$

where $\bar{x}_s$ is the sample mean, μ_H is the population value hypothesized by H0, and $\bar{x}_s$ is the standard error of the sample mean.

Chapter 7 discussed a sample of 100 discharges drawn from the hospital discharge records. The average cost per discharge was exactly \$6,586.30. Although not mentioned there, the standard deviation for the sample was \$5,262.73. The estimate of the *standard error* of the means, based on a sample size of 100, is then \$5,262.73/sqrt(100), or \$526.27. Using this sample information, the t test can be used to assess the probability that the true cost per case is \$6,000, as shown in Equation 9.2.

$$t = \frac{6586.30 - 6000}{526.27} = 1.11 \qquad (9.2)$$

Finding t Values in Excel: The =TDIST() Function

The value of $t = 1.11$ can now be assessed using the =TDIST() function in Microsoft Excel. The =TDIST() function takes three arguments: the t value, the number of degrees of freedom, and a 1 or a 2. The last argument depends on whether the test is a one-tail test or a two-tail test. Because the CEO is interested in whether the true population mean cost per case is either greater or less than \$6,000, a two-tail test is appropriate. If the CEO had cared only if the true cost per case was greater than \$6,000, we would have conducted a one-tail test.

> Two-tailed tests are always associated with a hypothesis that is testing whether something is either greater or less than a value. One-tailed tests are always associated with a hypothesis that is testing whether something is solely greater than a value or solely less than a value.

The result of the =TDIST() function is shown in Equation 9.3.

$$= TDIST(1.11, 99, 2) = 0.268 \qquad (9.3)$$

where 1.11 is the value of t, 99 is the degrees of freedom ($100 - 1$), and 2 indicates the two-tailed test.

Interpreting the *t* Test Results

The result found in Equation 9.3 indicates that there is a 0.268 probability that H0 is true (i.e., the true cost per case is $6,000), given that the sample mean was $6,586.30 with a standard error of the mean of $526.27. Stated another way, there is a 0.268 probability that we could have gotten a sample value of $6,586.30 from a population in which the true average cost per case is $6,000. As was discussed in Chapter 7, it is usually the case that we are interested in having a small *Type I error*—or the likelihood of rejecting H0 when it is true. In this case, we would want a small likelihood of rejecting the belief that the cost-per-case average is $6,000 if that belief were true. Usually, we would want the result of the *t* test to produce a probability of 0.05 or less before we would reject H0. And this is exactly what we will do in this case. Because the probability that H0 is true is as large as 0.268, we will not reject it (even though, having all the data, we know that the true mean is $5,905 and change). This is a *t* test.

Where Does a *t* Test Come From?

Where does the *t* test come from and what does it mean? To try to answer these questions, let us consider another example. Suppose the CEO had said that if the true cost per case is not $5,905.75, change must occur in the hospital. Now we know the true mean is $5,905.75. But the financial officer doesn't know this. He still has to take a sample, calculate the true average cost of the sample, and run a *t* test to see if the sample mean was likely to have come from a population in which the true mean is $5,905.75. But it is highly unlikely that he will find the sample mean equal to $5,905.75. As was discussed earlier, one possible sample outcome is $6,586.30.

Now, it is essential to remember that in real life, one ever takes only a single sample and one must be satisfied, in general, with the results of that single sample. However, in our case, instead of taking a single sample, let's take a large number of samples—say, 250. We can do this by using the Data Analysis add-in in Excel as was presented earlier in the text. In turn, we can calculate estimates of the mean and standard error for each of these samples and conduct a *t* test by the formula in Equation 9.1.

The Shape of the *t* Distribution

It was indicated earlier that the *t* test results are distributed as a *t* distribution. If we examined the results of 250 *t* tests, we would expect a large number of those to produce values in the range of −1 to +1.

(This corresponds to 1 standard deviation on each side of 0, the value that would be generated if there were no difference between the sample mean and H0.) In fact, we would expect that 68 percent of the results of the *t* tests from our 250 samples would lie between −1 and +1. Furthermore, we would expect 95 percent to lie between −2 and +2, for the same reason.

Figure 9.1 is a graph showing the distribution of the 250 *t* tests, based on the samples taken from the 12,000 hospital discharge records. Exactly 68 percent of the *t* tests provide results in the range −1 to +1. Ninety-three percent (rather than the expected 95 percent) of *t* tests provide results in the range −2 to +2. Seven percent of the results are outside the range −2 to +2 for the means of these 250 samples when H0 is the true mean. So for a perfect *t* distribution, this means that when H0 is the true mean, there is about a 5 percent probability of rejecting H0 when it is true. However, in this example, there is a 7 percent probability of rejecting the null hypothesis, H0. But, in general, the probability of rejecting H0 when it is true is small. The consequence of this is that if the *t* test produced a value outside the range −2 to +2, we would typically conclude that the sample did not come from a population in which H0 was true (even though we recognize that there is a small likelihood that it could have).

What Does the *t* Test Mean? The Link to Type I and Type II Errors

Let us look at this result from another perspective. Suppose H0 had been $4,500. That is, suppose the CEO had said, "If the average cost of a hospital stay is not $4,500, we are going to have to make some changes." Now, when we draw the 250 samples and carry out the *t* tests, the distribution of the *t* values is as shown in Figure 9.2. This figure shows that the distribution of

Figure 9.1 Distribution of 250 *t* tests when H0 = $5,905

Figure 9.2   Distribution of 250 *t* tests when H0 = $4,500

t values is centered on 3.5. A *t* value greater than 2 would lead us to reject H0 and accept the alternative. Thus, we would (correctly) conclude that the population mean is not $4,500.

But the calculation of the 250 *t* tests and their distribution as shown in Figure 9.2 also gives us one other type of information of interest. In general, we would accept H0 for any value of *t* within the range −2 to + 2. Looking at Figure 9.2, it is possible to see that some of the *t* tests produced *t* values of less than 2 (the column labels in Figures 9.1 and 9.2 reflect the Excel =FREQUENCY() function convention of putting the frequency between two values at the point of the higher value). In fact, about 1 percent of the 250 *t* tests produced values of less than 2. In testing the null hypothesis, H0: $c = \$4,500$, [that] 1 percent of samples would have led us to accept H0, producing the Type II error of accepting H0 when it is false. So, in this case (where cost is posited to be $4,500), beta is about 0.01.

One-Tail and Two-Tail *t* Tests

The *t* test that is discussed in the previous section is a two-tailed test. As was discussed in Chapter 7, assessments of hypotheses can be one-tailed or two-tailed. In a two-tailed test, the region of rejection of H0 can be at either end of the continuum of possible *t* values. In a one-tailed test, the region of rejection of H0 is at only one end of the continuum. In regard to the question of cost per hospital stay discussed earlier, the discussion is of a two-tail test. This is because the CEO indicated he was concerned about the possibility that the mean value might be either more or less than H0 (in either case, adjustments would have to be made).

But suppose, for example, that the CEO is not interested in knowing whether the true cost is less than $6,000. His only concern is that if the true costs are greater than $6,000, he will have to take steps to renegotiate charges to bring them into line with true costs. So, in this case, the hypotheses posed by the financial officer would be as follows:

H0: The average cost per discharge is $6,000 or less.

or

H0: $c \leq \$6,000$

and

H1: The average cost per discharge is greater than $6,000.

or

H1: $c > \$6,000$

Now the initial hypothesis and the alternative hypothesis are stated in such a way that the null will be rejected only if the sample mean is greater than $6,000. Any sample mean less than $6,000 produces a t test value that will *never* be in the region of rejection of H0. This is logical, because any sample value less than $6,000 cannot be used to reject H0. The t test to assess H0 and H1 is given in Equation 9.1. But, now, the number of standard deviation units required for rejection of H0 will not be approximately 2 (depending on sample size) but will be closer to 1.7. The lower number of standard deviation units is due to the one-tail nature of the test.

Figures 9.3 and 9.4 show the comparative regions of rejection for a two-tail test (Figure 9.3) and a one-tail test (Figure 9.4). The region of rejection for the two-tail test is outside the two vertical dashed lines at -2 to $+2$. If the t test result falls outside -2 to $+2$, H0 will be rejected. The region of rejection for the one-tail test is to the right of the dashed line in Figure 9.4 at about 1.7. Any t value larger than 1.7 (but not smaller than -1.7) will lead to the rejection of H0. In the one-tail test, any value lower than 1.7, no matter how low it may be, will not lead to the rejection of H0.

It is important to keep in mind the direction of H0 when interpreting the result of a one-tail t test. In the case of the hypothesis H0: $c \leq \$6,000$, any value of t in the negative range will not lead to the rejection of H0. However, if H0 had been stated as $c \geq \$6,000$, then any value of t in the positive range would not lead to the rejection of H0.

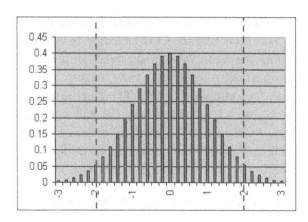

Figure 9.3 Region of rejection for two-tail test

Figure 9.4 Region of rejection for one-tail test

EXERCISES FOR SECTION 9.1

1. Calculate the *t* value for the following hypotheses, given the sample outcomes indicated.

    a. H0: $\mu = 11$, H1: $\mu \neq 11$, $\bar{x} = 12.2$, standard deviation = 8.9, $n = 40$.

    b. H0: $\mu = 11$, H1: $\mu \neq 11$, $\bar{x} = 14.0$, standard deviation = 8.9, $n = 40$.

    c. H0: $\mu = 11$, H1: $\mu \neq 11$, $\bar{x} = 13.7$, standard deviation = 8.9, $n = 40$.

    d. H0: $\mu = 234$, H1: $\mu \neq 234$, $\bar{x} = 228.4$, standard deviation = 40.53, $n = 120$.

    e. H0: $\mu = 234$, H1: $\mu \neq 234$, $\bar{x} = 226.4$, standard deviation = 40.53, $n = 120$.

    f. H0: $\mu = 234$, H1: $\mu \neq 234$, $\bar{x} = 226.4$, standard deviation = 40.53, $n = 120$.

2. Determine the probability of t in each example in Exercise 1, and decide for each whether you would accept or reject H0.

3. Use the Hospital charges worksheet in Chpt 4-1.xls. Assume that the 100 records represent a random sample from all hospital discharges for a year and test the hypothesis H0: *Charges* = $6,000 against the alternative H1: *Charges* $\neq$ $6,000, and indicate your conclusion.

4. Use the BP worksheet in Chpt 6-2.xls and the Uniform distribution option in Data ribbon ➤ Data Analysis with a random seed of 7375 to draw a sample of 60 blood pressure readings. Test the hypothesis H0: BP = 83 mm hg against the alternative H1: BP $\neq$ 83 mm hg, and indicate your conclusion.

5. Use the ER Wait worksheet in Chpt 6-2.xls and Uniform distribution option in Data ribbon ➤ Data Analysis with a random seed of 2538 to draw a sample of 40 waiting times. Test the hypothesis H0: waiting time = 35 minutes against the alternative H1: waiting time <35 minutes, and indicate your conclusion.

9.2   A t Test for Comparing Two Groups

Thus far, we have discussed a t test concerned with comparing a sample mean with an a priori hypothesized value. With that in mind, we tested whether the result of a sample could have been taken from a population in which the true mean was H0. But t tests can also be used to compare samples from two potentially different groups to determine if, statistically, they can be seen as different or not.

For example, suppose the financial officer of our hypothetical hospital were asked by the CEO to determine whether the costs of a hospital discharge differed between males and females. Although it may not be possible to negotiate differing charges on the basis of sex, it might still be important for the CEO to know if actual costs differed. So now, the financial officer might be addressing the following two hypotheses:

H0: The average cost per discharge is equal between men and women.

or

H0: $c_m = c_w$

and

H1: The average cost per discharge is not equal between men and women.

or

H1: $c_m \neq c_w$

Selecting the Groups to Test: A Stratified Sampling Approach

Now, the financial officer must be somewhat careful about how he selects his sample of discharges. If the selection is done strictly randomly, there is a small possibility that either no men or no women might be selected for the sample, making it impossible to assess the hypotheses. Luckily, the financial officer knows that he can divide the total 12,000 records into those for men and those for women, so that he can take a sample of each group. This is what is known as a stratified sample, because he will be stratifying the population into men and women before taking a sample from each group.

In general, with a stratified sample, it is best to take samples of equal size from each stratum. This is true if the desire is to compare the two strata and if there is no perception that the variances of the two strata differ. There is no particular reason, a priori, for the financial officer to expect that the costs for men are more or less variable than the costs for women (even though the means may differ). Therefore, the best decision is to take equal-sized samples of men and women. The financial officer believes he can still muster the resources to ascertain the true costs of hospital stays for a total of 100 discharges. Therefore, he decides to take a sample of discharges for 50 men and another for 50 women.

Using a t Test to Compare Two Means

To determine if the cost for men and women is the same (the assessment of H0), it will first be necessary to determine the average cost for each sample of 50. It will then be necessary to use the appropriate t test to determine whether the means of the two samples could have come from two populations in which the true mean of costs was the same. The t test that will be used to determine this when sample sizes are the same is given in Equation 9.4.

$$t = \frac{\bar{x}_1 - \bar{x}_2}{\sqrt{\frac{s_1^2 + s_2^2}{n}}} \tag{9.4}$$

where $\bar{x}_1$ is the sample mean for men, $\bar{x}_2$ is the sample mean for women, s_1^2 is the sample variance for men, s_2^2 is the sample variance for women, and n is equal to the sample size in either group.

Assume that the financial officer has taken a sample of 50 men and 50 women and has recorded an average cost of $6,460.04 for men and $6,177.30 for women, with variances (the square of the standard deviation, or s^2) of 23837156 and 24477861. The t test to compare men and women is then found by the formula in Equation 9.5.

$$t = \frac{6460.04 - 6177.30}{\sqrt{\frac{23837156 + 24477861}{50}}} = 0.288 \qquad (9.5)$$

Using the =TDIST Function: Finding the Probability of a *t* Value

The *t* value of 0.288 given in Equation 9.5 will not lead to rejection of H0. In general, if the level of the Type I error (a) is set at 0.05, H0 will be rejected only when the absolute value of *t* is approximately 2 or greater. (Recall that *t* can be a negative or a positive number.) However, the exact probability of finding a *t* as large as 0.288 can be determined by using the =TDIST() function. For this *t* test, because there are actually 100 ($2n$) observations, and because one degree of freedom is used up for each sample, there are $2n - 2$ degrees of freedom. With $2n - 2$ degrees of freedom, the exact probability of finding a *t* value as large as 0.288 or larger is given by Equation 9.6. The interpretation of the probability given in Equation 9.6 is as follows:

• We initially believe that the population mean for cost per discharge was exactly the same for both men and women, and

• In turn, the *t* value calculated for a large number of samples of discharges for 50 men and 50 women would be as large as 0.288 in about 77 percent of the samples selected.

Because the probability of getting a *t* value as large as 0.288 is very high, H0 is accepted and the financial officer reaches the conclusion that there is no cost difference between men and women.

$$p_t = \text{TDIST}(0.288, 98, 2) = 0.774 \qquad (9.6)$$

Type I and Type II Errors in Comparing Means

Let us consider further what it means to say that there is no difference in the cost between men and women. For the 12,000 hospital discharges, there are 4,560 men and 7,440 women. The true mean of cost for men is $5,825.63, and for women it is $5,954.85. So, in fact, there is a real difference in the mean cost between men and women, although the difference is only $129.22. This is a real difference, but is it an important difference? Such a question is not one that statistics can answer. The question of what may be an important difference must be left to the CEO to decide. However, we still can use statistics to assist in the decision-making process.

Type I Error

But suppose there were truly no population-level difference between the cost for men and the cost for women. Suppose the true mean for men were exactly equal to the true mean for women, which would then both be equal to $5,905.75. Suppose we were to select a large number of samples of size 50 for men and size 50 for women from these two populations. Next we calculated the *t* value for each sample by using Equation 9.4. In turn, the distribution of those mean values would be a *t* distribution with 98 degrees of freedom. Furthermore, the distribution would look identical to that shown in Figure 9.3. Similarly, we would expect that about 5 percent of all *t* values calculated by using Equation 9.4 would have values outside the range −2 to + 2. These would be the *t* values that would lead us to reject H0, even when it was true and would represent a Type I error.

Type II Error

Consider now the Type II error. Rather than look at the real average difference between the two populations, which is only $129.22, assume that the true population mean for men was $5,000 and the true population mean for women was $7,000. Let's also assume the same variance as that which is true of the actual data. Therefore, the distribution of the *t* test values from a large number of samples would look very much like the distribution shown in Figure 9.5. In Figure 9.5, about half the distribution is to the left of the dashed vertical line. That is the region in which we would reject H0 and conclude, in fact, that the true cost is different between men and women.

To the right of the dashed vertical line, which also includes about half the distribution, is the region in which we will erroneously accept H0, even when the true average difference between the two groups is as large

Figure 9.5 Type II error for true means of $5,000 and $7,000

Figure 9.6 Type II error for true means of $5,000 and $7,000 and sample size 150 for each group

as $2,000. In this case, then, the Type II error is about 0.5. As previously discussed, the only way to reduce the Type II error in this setting is to increase the size of the sample.

If we had the resources to increase the sample size to, for example, 150 for men and 150 for women, then the pooled standard error would be reduced considerably over a sample of 50 each. That would produce a graph of all possible *t* test values as shown in Figure 9.6. In this figure, the bulk of the *t* distribution is to the left of the vertical dashed line and only about 7 percent of the distribution is to the right of the dashed line. Thus, in this case, the probability of a Type II error has been reduced to about 0.07.

Comparing Samples of Unequal Size

Thus far, the discussion has centered on equal sample sizes. This section expands the *t* test for two groups to unequal sample sizes. In addition, the section introduces the notion of an experimental design.

A new resident physician has been asked by the senior physician with whom she is working to assist in a study. The study investigates the effect of physician interaction with patients on the degree of knowledge gained by the patients about breast cancer. When the patients come to the clinic, they will be given a brochure about breast cancer with information about its etiology, detection, treatment, and prognosis. They will all have waiting time adequate to read the brochure if they wish to do so. They will then be randomly divided into two groups. One group (the control group) receives no further information unless they ask for it. The second group (the experimental group) will have a 5- to 10-minute one-on-one discussion with the physician about breast cancer, providing the same information as was contained in the brochure. At the end of their visit, all patients will complete a short questionnaire that assesses their knowledge of breast cancer on a 20-point scale. The purpose of the study is to determine if the patients who have the one-on-one discussion with the physician score higher on the questionnaire than those who do not.

This is a classic experimental design (although not a double-blind randomized clinical trial). In this experiment we will introduce one modification in the classic design: The study will be carried out over a one-month period. During that time, the physicians expect to have about 65 women come to the clinic who are appropriate for the study. But because of the time that is involved in interacting with the experimental group, they do not feel that they can include more than 25 women in the experimental group. One decision, then, would be to say that only 25 women would be included in the control group. But this may not be the best decision. Because the control group costs no extra resources (the space required to take the brief test and its scoring is not a significant resource drain), it is a better strategy to include all women who are not in the experimental group as controls. Given that the physicians expect 65 women in total, the projected control group will consist of 40 women.

Conducting the *t* Test for the Unequal Sample Sizes: Using Pooled Variance

Let us now assume that the month has passed, the experiment has taken place, and post-intervention knowledge tests have been obtained for 65 women. How do we conduct the *t* test that will determine whether the two groups are different? Because the two group (or sample) sizes are different, we cannot use the *t* test as given in Equation 9.4. Instead, we need a formula for the *t* test that takes into account the fact that the two sample sizes are not the same. A pooled variance statistic adjusts for unequal sample sizes. The appropriate *t* test is as given in Equation 9.7.

$$t = \frac{\bar{x}_1 - \bar{x}_2}{\sqrt{s_p^2 \left(\frac{1}{n_1} + \frac{1}{n_2} \right)}} \tag{9.7}$$

where $s_p^2 = ((n_1 - 1)s_1^2 + (n_2 - 1)s_2^2)/((n_1 - 1) + (n_2 - 1))$, and s_1^2 is the sample variance for group 1, s_2^2 is the sample variance for group 2, n_1 is the sample size for group 1, and n_2 is the sample size for group 2.

The complete data set from this experiment (wholly fictional) is given in Chpt 9-1.xls. The results of the experiment, using those data, are shown in Figure 9.7. The figure shows, in columns A and B, some of the data from the study for both the Experimental group (the one that received

	E10	▼		=	=(E2-F2)/E9	
	A	B	C	D	E	F
1	Experimenta	Control		n	25	40
2	11	10		Xbar	10.04	7.525
3	12	3		s^2	7.123333	10.05064
4	13	5				
5	14	11		n-1	24	39
6	8	10		n-1*s^2	170.96	391.975
7	13	9				
8	11	4		s pooled	8.935476	
9	9	11		SE pooled	0.762106	
10	8	5		t	3.300065	
11	12	8		df	63	
12	12	4		Prob	0.001594	
13	7	8				

Figure 9.7 Results of a breast cancer experiment

the intervention) and the Control group (the one that did not). Columns E and F give the sample sizes, the mean, and the variance for each group, as well as the degrees of freedom for each group [$n - 1$] and [$n - 1 * s^2$]. Cells E8:E12 give the actual results of the *t* test. The value in cell E8 is the pooled variance following the formula for s_p^2 given in Equation 9.7. Cell E9 gives the pooled standard error, which is the denominator of the equation for *t* in Equation 9.7. The *t* value in cell E10 is calculated by using the formula in Equation 9.7. The degrees of freedom in cell E11 are the sum of cells E5 and F5 but are also $n1 + n2 - 2$. Cell E12 is the 95 percent confidence limit probability of finding a *t* value as large as 3.3 when there is actually no difference between the experimental group and the control group. This probability, at approximately 2 chances in 1,000, is very small. Therefore, the conclusion is drawn that there is a difference between the two groups. Furthermore, because the mean for the experimental group is larger than the mean for the control group, the conclusion is extended to say that the one-on-one discussion with the physician made a difference in the amount of knowledge that the women have. Table 9.1 contains the formulas for Figure 9.7.

The two *t* tests discussed thus far have different implications for what is actually known. The first *t* test, which compared discharges for men with discharges for women, was concerned only with whether there was a difference. The test does not and cannot say anything about the source of that difference. The difference might be due to differences in age between the men and women who were discharged, differences in their diagnoses or severity of illness, differences in length of stay, or other factors that have not been considered in the test. Other statistical procedures might shed light on the source of difference, but the *t* test cannot identify those possible differences. Conversely, if the assignment to the experimental and

Table 9.1   Formulas for Figure 9.7

Cell	Formula
E1	=COUNT(A2:A26)
F1	=COUNT(B2:A41)
E2	=AVERAGE(A2:A26)
F2	=AVERAGE(B2:A41)
E3	=VAR(A2:A26)
F3	=VAR(B2:A41)
E5	=E1-1
F5	=F1-1
E6	=E5*E3
F6	=F5*F3
E8	=(E6+F6)/(E5+F5)
E9	=(E8*((1/E1)+(1/F1)))^0.5
E10	=(E2-F2)/E9
E11	=E5+F5
E12	=TDIST(E10,E11,2)

the control groups for the second *t* test was adequately carried out, the *t* test does have the capability of indicating whether the experimental intervention has the ability to affect the knowledge women have about breast cancer. However, the ability of the *t* test to allow that conclusion to be drawn depends entirely on the adequacy of the random assignment process.

An Assumption of Equal Variance

The *t* tests discussed thus far carry with them an assumption that the variances of the two groups being compared are equal. With regard to the test for the difference between costs for men and women, the variances of the two groups (shown as the denominator in Equation 9.5) differ by only about 3 percent. With regard to the variances in the experimental setting, the values, shown as cells E3 and F3 in Figure 9.7, differ by about 41 percent. Is there a statistical test for the equivalence of variance between the two groups? In turn, if they are not equal, what can be done about that?

First, a test does exist for equivalence of variance in the *t* test setting. To examine this test, we will use the data from the experimental setting discussed in the second subsection of Section 9.2. The variances presented there differ by about 41 percent. The test of equivalence of variance is an *F* test. Whereas a *t* test is typically a test comparing mean values, an *F* test is typically a test comparing variances. The *F* test for the equivalence of variance for two groups in a *t* test setting is given in Equation 9.8. Chapter 10 contains detailed discussion on F tests and analysis of variance (ANOVA). The concept is introduced here for comparison to t tests.

$$F = \frac{s_1^2}{s_2^2} \tag{9.8}$$

where s_1^2 is the variance for one sample and s_2^2 is the variance for the other.

Testing for Equal Variance: The *F* Test

Refer to the example discussed in the second subsection of Section 9.2. The experimental group of 25 women has a variance of 7.12 (see Figure 9.7), whereas the control group has a variance of 10.05. So the F test for the difference between these two variances is that given in Equation 9.9 and has the value of 0.71. Whereas a t test has a single number representing degrees of freedom, an F test has two numbers representing degrees of freedom—one number for the numerator and one for the denominator. In this case, the degrees of freedom are 24 and 39 ($n_1 - 1$ for the experimental group and $n_2 - 1$ for the control group).

$$F = \frac{7.12}{10.05} = 0.71 \tag{9.9}$$

The F test is a test of equality of the variances, or $s_1^2 = s_2^2$. The F distribution is a nonsymmetrical distribution that generally looks like Figure 9.8. Figure 9.8 represents the F distribution for 24 and 39 degrees of freedom, but other F distributions are quite similar in appearance. The two dashed vertical lines indicate the lower and upper 95 percent limits. For 24 and 39 degrees of freedom, the F value must be approximately 0.5

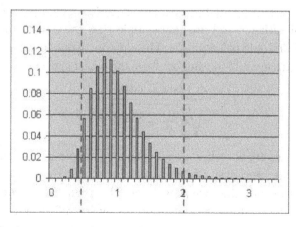

Figure 9.8 *F* distribution

or less (if the smaller variance is divided by the larger) or 2 or greater (if the larger variance is divided by the smaller) before the difference between the two variances is considered large enough to have come from populations in which the true variances are not equal. The actual value of the F test in Equation 9.9 (0.71) has a probability of occurrence of about 0.81. Because this probability is relatively high, the conclusion that we would reach is that the two variances are equal.

Unequal Variances: Now What?

In the case discussed earlier, the conclusion was drawn that the variances were equal. But what happens if the two variances prove not to be equal? In the case of unequal variances, the pooled variance formula in Equation 9.7 is no longer appropriate. Instead, the t test is conducted not by pooling the variance but by simply adding the variances divided by the sample sizes. In that case, the appropriate t test is given by Equation 9.10. It might be noted that when sample sizes are the same, the formula in Equation 9.10 will be exactly the same as the formula in Equation 9.4. The value of this is that if sample sizes are the same, the formula in Equation 9.4 can be used, regardless of whether variances are equal. But if the sample sizes are not the same, the formula given in Equation 9.7, or that given in Equation 9.10, will produce generally the same decision (although not the same numerical result for the t) most of the time. That is, if the decision to reject H0 was produced by Equation 9.7, it is highly likely that the same decision would be reached by using Equation 9.10.

$$t = \frac{\bar{x}_1 - \bar{x}_2}{\sqrt{\left(\frac{s_1^2}{n_1} + \frac{s_2^2}{n_2}\right)}} \tag{9.10}$$

To see the effect of the changes in the computation of the t test for unequal variance and unequal sample size, the t test as indicated in Equation 9.10 would be employed. The equation would produce the results shown in Equation 9.11 for the data from the breast cancer education study.

$$t = \frac{10.04 - 7.53}{\sqrt{\left(\frac{7.12}{25} + \frac{10.05}{40}\right)}} = 3.43 \tag{9.11}$$

If variances are known to be unequal and sample sizes are either equal or unequal, the appropriate degrees of freedom for the t test are reduced by the degree to which the variances differ. This reduction in the degrees of freedom for the t test may be carried out by several different formulas, all of which give approximately the same answer. But the most widely accepted method—the one most likely used by Excel—is given by the formula in Equation 9.12.

$$f = \frac{f_a f_b}{f_b c^2 + f_a (1 - c)^2}$$

(9.12)

where f is the adjusted degrees of freedom,

$$f_a = n_a - 1,$$
$$f_b = n_b - 1,$$

and

$$c = \frac{\left(\frac{s_a^2}{n_a}\right)}{\left(\frac{s_a^2}{n_a} + \frac{s_b^2}{n_b}\right)}$$

The formula in Equation 9.12 gives 57.48 as the degrees of freedom for the t test in Figure 9.7. We have already concluded that there is no difference in the variance of the two samples. However, a more conservative test would be to use 57 degrees of freedom (the nearest whole integer to the calculated value) to make the test. In that case, we would conclude that the probability of a t value as large as 3.43 would be 0.0011.

An important question with regard to the presumed unequal variance is the question of how much difference it makes if variances are unequal. First, it is useful to note that if sample sizes are equal, using the equal or unequal variance formulas will generally result in the same decision. In only rare situations, when the t test value was right around 2, calculated using either formula (and for equal sample size, the t from either formula is the same), would the unequal variance formula lead to a different decision. And in this situation, the unequal variance t test will always be less likely to reject H0. This is because the lower degrees of freedom for the unequal variance t test require a slightly larger value of t for *statistical significance*.

However, with both unequal variance and unequal sample sizes, it is essential to use the unequal variance t test. If the smaller sample also has the larger variance, the unequal variance t test is more likely to result in the acceptance of H0 than the equal variance t test. But if the smaller sample also has the smaller variance, the unequal variance t test is more likely than the equal variance t test to result in the rejection of H0. Thus, it is important, with the case of unequal sample sizes, to use the appropriate t test.

The Excel t Test Add-In

Excel provides two add-ins for a t test of two groups. To access the add-in within Excel, go to the Data ribbon, in the Analysis group, and click the Data Analysis option. In the Data Analysis menu the test is called t Test:

Figure 9.9 Dialog box for t test for equal variance

Two Sample Assuming Equal Variance and t Test: Two Sample Assuming Unequal Variance. Let us look at each of these with the data from the breast cancer education experiment as the example. After selecting Data Analysis, select t Test: Two Sample Assuming Equal Variance. The dialog box that appears is shown in Figure 9.9. In this dialog box, the data for the experimental group are included as variable 1 range, whereas the data for the control group are included as variable 2 range. Leaving the hypothesized mean difference blank is equivalent to putting in the value of zero. The labels box is checked because the first row contains the labels for the two data streams. The output will go on a new worksheet. Table 9.2 displays the steps for using Excel to calculate a t test.

Clicking OK will produce the result of this t test on a new worksheet. It can be seen, by comparing Figures 9.7 and 9.10, that the results computed by the formula in Equation 9.7 and the results of the add-in in Figure 9.10 are identical. The add-in also provides some additional information, particularly the level at which H0 would be rejected for one- and two-tail tests (t Critical one tail and t Critical two tail).

Differences in Results of Excel t Tests

Consider, now, the add-in for a t test assuming unequal variance. As stated before, to access the add-in within Excel, go to the Data ribbon, in the Analysis group, and click the Data Analysis option. Then select t Test: Two Sample Assuming Unequal Variance. When this option is selected, the dialog box that appears is nearly identical to the one shown in Figure 9.9. The difference is in the title. It is now t Test: Two Sample Assuming

	A	B	C	D
1	t-Test: Two-Sample Assuming Equal Variances			
2				
3		Experiment:	Control	
4	Mean	10.04	7.525	
5	Variance	7.12333	10.05064	
6	Observations	25	40	
7	Pooled Variance	8.93548		
8	Hypothesized Mean Difference	0		
9	df	63		
10	t Stat	3.30006		
11	P(T<=t) one-tail	0.0008		
12	t Critical one-tail	1.6694		
13	P(T<=t) two-tail	0.00159		
14	t Critical two-tail	1.99834		
15				
16				

Figure 9.10   Results of Excel *t* test for equal variance

	A	B	C
1	t-Test: Two-Sample Assuming Unequal Variances		
2			
3		Experiment:	Control
4	Mean	10.04	7.525
5	Variance	7.123333	10.05064
6	Observations	25	40
7	Hypothesized Mean Difference	0	
8	df	57	
9	t Stat	3.43459	
10	P(T<=t) one-tail	0.000556	
11	t Critical one-tail	1.672029	
12	P(T<=t) two-tail	0.001113	
13	t Critical two-tail	2.002466	
14			

Figure 9.11   Results of Excel *t* test for unequal variance

Unequal Variance. When the add-in is invoked, it produces a result—for the experimental data under consideration here—as shown in Figure 9.11.

There are three differences between the results shown in Figure 9.10 and those shown in Figure 9.11. The first is in the calculated value of the *t* test. It is 3.30 in Figure 9.10 and 3.43 in Figure 9.11. As noted previously, the value of 3.30 was calculated using Equation 9.7, whereas the value of 3.43 was calculated using Equation 9.10. A second is the absence of a pooled variance (s_p^2) value in Figure 9.11. This is because no pooled variance is calculated for the unequal variance *t* test. Finally, there is a difference in the degrees of freedom between the two figures. The equation for the equal variance degrees of freedom is simply $n_1 + n_2 - 2$, whereas the equation for the unequal variance degrees of freedom is found by using Equation 9.12.

Here are the steps for using the Excel t test add-in:

1. Go to the Data ribbon ➤ Analysis Group ➤ Data Analysis, and from the menu that appears select t Test: Two Sample Assuming Equal Variance.

2. In the Variable 1 Range input box type or highlight \$A\$1:\$A\$26.

3. In the Variable 2 Range input box type or highlight \$B\$1:\$B\$41.

4. Check the Labels checkbox (we included header labels when we inputted the Variable 1 Range and the Variable 2 Range).

5. Click the New Worksheet Ply radio button.

6. Click OK, and a table that resembles Figure 9.10 will appear.

Note: Do not change the Hypothesized Mean Difference—its default is blank, which translates into 0 for Excel—and do not change the Alpha value—the default is 0.05, and that is what we want.

EXERCISES FOR SECTION 9.2

1. Assume the following information for equal-sized samples, and make the appropriate t tests.

   a. Group 1: $\bar{x} = 25, s^2 = 27.8, n = 15$; Group 2: $\bar{x} = 23, s^2 = 27.8, n = 15$.

   b. Group 1: $\bar{x} = 25, s^2 = 27.8, n = 15$; Group 2: $\bar{x} = 29, s^2 = 27.8, n = 15$.

   c. Group 1: $\bar{x} = 125, s^2 = 92.6, n = 40$; Group 2: $\bar{x} = 121, s^2 = 92.6, n = 40$.

   d. Group 1: $\bar{x} = 125, s^2 = 92.6, n = 40$; Group 2: $\bar{x} = 131, s^2 = 92.6, n = 40$.

   e. Group 1: $\bar{x} = 11, s^2 = 15, n = 130$; Group 2: $\bar{x} = 11.5, s^2 = 15, n = 130$.

   f. Group 1: $\bar{x} = 11, s^2 = 15, n = 130$; Group 2: $\bar{x} = 12.5, s^2 = 15, n = 130$.

2. Determine the probability of the t test result in (a) through (f) of Exercise 1, and decide whether you would accept or reject the hypothesis of no difference between the two groups in each case.

3. Assume the following information for unequal size samples, and make the appropriate t tests.

   a. Group 1: $\bar{x} = 25, s^2 = 27.8, n = 30$; Group 2: $\bar{x} = 23, s^2 = 27.8, n = 15$.

   b. Group 1: $\bar{x} = 25, s^2 = 27.8, n = 30$; Group 2: $\bar{x} = 29, s^2 = 27.8, n = 15$.

   c. Group 1: $\bar{x} = 125, s^2 = 92.6, n = 40$; Group 2: $\bar{x} = 121, s^2 = 92.6, n = 25$.

   d. Group 1: $\bar{x} = 125, s^2 = 92.6, n = 40$; Group 2: $\bar{x} = 131, s^2 = 92.6, n = 25$.

    e. Group 1: $\bar{x} = 11, s^2 = 15, n = 130$; Group 2: $\bar{x} = 11.5, s^2 = 15, n = 90$.

    f. Group 1: $\bar{x} = 11, s^2 = 15, n = 130$; Group 2: $\bar{x} = 12.5, s^2 = 15, n = 90$.

4. Determine the probability of the *t* test result in (a) through (f) of Exercise 3, and decide whether you would accept or reject the hypothesis of no difference between the two groups in each case.

5. Use the data on the Cost worksheet of Chpt 9-1.xls that show the hospital cost for a randomly selected sample of 34 women and 34 men, and do the following:

    a. Calculate a *t* test of the hypothesis that cost for women is equal to cost for men against the alternative that they are not equal, assuming equal variance.

    b. Decide whether to accept or reject the hypothesis of equality.

6. Use the information given in the Breast C worksheet of Chpt 9-1.xls that show the data used for the analysis in Figure 9.7, and replicate the analysis shown in that figure.

7. Use the data on the Wait worksheet of Chpt 9-1.xls that represent the waiting time of a randomly selected group of people at an urgent-care clinic and a randomly selected group of people at an emergency clinic.

    a. Calculate a *t* test of the hypothesis that wait time in the urgent-care clinic is no different from wait time in the emergency clinic, assuming equal variance.

    b. Decide whether to accept or reject the hypothesis of equality.

8. Test the hypothesis of equality of variance for the following sets of data, and determine whether to accept or reject the hypothesis.

    a. For group 1: $s^2 = 9, n = 20$; for group 2: $s^2 = 5, n = 20$

    b. For group 1: $s^2 = 9, n = 50$; for group 2: $s^2 = 5, n = 50$

    c. For group 1: $s^2 = 9, n = 50$; for group 2: $s^2 = 5, n = 100$

    d. For group 1: $s^2 = 21, n = 20$; for group 2: $s^2 = 33, n = 20$

    e. For group 1: $s^2 = 21, n = 50$; for group 2: $s^2 = 33, n = 50$

    f. For group 1: $s^2 = 21, n = 50$; for group 2: $s^2 = 33, n = 100$

9. Test the hypothesis of equality of variance, and indicate the conclusion you reach.

    a. For the data on the Cost worksheet of Chpt 9-1.xls

    b. For the data on the Breast C worksheet of Chpt 9-1.xls

    c. For the data on the Wait worksheet of Chpt 9-1.xls

10. Use the unequal variance formula (Equation 9.10) for the *t* test to test the hypothesis of equality of wait time for the data on the Wait worksheet of Chpt 9-1.xls.

11. Use the Excel add-in for the equal variance *t* test, and conduct a *t* test for the data on the Cost worksheet of Chpt 9-1.xls. Do the results replicate those found in Exercise 5?

12. Use the Excel add-in for the equal variance *t* test, and conduct a *t* test for the data on the Breast C worksheet of Chpt 9-1.xls. Do the results replicate those found in Exercise 6?

13. Use the Excel add-in for the unequal variance *t* test, and conduct a *t* test for the data on the Wait worksheet of Chpt 9-1.xls. Do the results replicate those found in Exercise 10?

9.3   A *t* Test for Related Data

Thus far, the discussion of *t* tests has focused on two areas. These areas were on a population value determined a priori or on the question of whether two groups or samples are the same or different. This section addresses a *t* test that can be used when two sets of data are related. In particular, this is a test of whether two measurements for the same group of people (or organizations, or any other identifiable entities) are similar or different.

Calculation of the Test

To examine this *t* test, consider a group of persons with adult-onset diabetes who have come under care at a diabetes clinic. The clinic is confident that the symptoms of diabetes—especially high blood sugar—can be controlled through a combination of exercise, weight loss, and diet and lifestyle changes. To assess this belief, the clinic has enrolled a group of 40 volunteers, all with hemoglobin A1c (*HbA1c*) measures above 7.8 (in general, HbA1c levels above 7.8 indicate some difficulties in controlling blood sugar levels). The average HbA1c level for this group of 40 persons, at the time of enrollment in the study, was 8.49. The persons were counseled on diet, exercise, and lifestyle changes and had monthly meetings with their counselors to track progress toward agreed-upon goals. At the end of a six-month period, the HbA1c levels for these persons were again measured. The data for this study (entirely fabricated) are given in Chpt 9-2.xls. The mean HbA1c level for the entire group after the six-month study period was 8.25. The question is whether this reduction in HbA1c represents a statistically significant change.

The initial hypothesis for this study would typically be:

H0: The combination of exercise, weight loss, and diet and lifestyle changes has no effect on HbA1c levels

or

H0: $HbA1c_b = HbA1c_a$, where *b* refers to before and *a* to after.

Because there is some expectation that the HbA1c levels will be lowered by the combination of exercise, weight loss, and diet and lifestyle changes, the alternative hypothesis is:

H1: HbA1c levels will be lower after the intervention than before

or

H1: $HbA1c_b > HbA1c_a$

The test of the hypothesis, H0, just given, is carried out using the formula in Equation 9.13.

$$t = \frac{\overline{d}_{xb-xa}}{S.E._{\overline{d}}} \tag{9.13}$$

where $\overline{d}_{xb-xa}$ is the mean difference between the before and after measures, $S.E._{\overline{d}}$ is the standard error of the differences, and the degrees of freedom are $n - 1$ where n is the number of difference scores.

A partial file of the data for this before and after t test is given in Figure 9.12. The figure shows the before-data measure in column A, the after-data measure in column B, and the difference between the before- and after-data measures in column C. The mean difference value is given in cell F2 as 0.24, and the standard error of the difference is given in cell F5. The t test is shown in cell F6 (its calculation is shown in the formula line at the top). The probability of the occurrence of a t value as large as that shown in cell F6 is given in cell F7. The =TDIST() function is used with the t value of 2.4, 39 degrees of freedom and one tail (because the only result of interest is a result where after is less than before). The probability of getting a t value as large as 2.4 with a one-tail test is about 0.01. This means that we would reject the hypothesis that the HbA1c levels are equal before and

F6		= =F2/F5				
	A	B	C	D	E	F
1	Before	After	Difference			
2	7.97	8.10	-0.13		dbar	0.24
3	8.53	7.77	0.76		SD dbar	0.632652
4	8.27	8.20	0.07		n	40
5	8.40	8.67	-0.27		SE dbar	0.100031
6	8.23	7.72	0.51		t	2.406754
7	7.90	7.91	-0.01		Prob	0.010465
8	8.63	8.12	0.51			
9	8.56	7.48	1.08			
10	8.36	7.90	0.46			
11	7.92	8.84	-0.92			
12	8.96	8.46	0.40			

Figure 9.12 Calculation of before and after *t* test

Table 9.2   Formulas for Figure 9.12

Cell	Formula
F2	=AVERAGE(C2:C41)
F3	=STDEV(C2:C41)
F4	=COUNT(C2:C41)
F5	=F3/SQRT(F4)
F6	=F2/F5
F7	=TDIST(F6,F4,2)

after the intervention, and we would, in fact, accept the alternative, which is that HbA1c levels are lower after the intervention. Table 9.2 displays the formulas for Figure 9.12.

Excel Add-In for Related Data

Excel provides an add-in for a *t* test of the difference between related observations of this type. It is called *t* Test: Paired Two Sample for Means. The test is invoked precisely the same way as the *t* tests discussed in the fourth subsection of Section 9.2. When the test is invoked, you first see the dialog box shown in Figure 9.9. The *t* test that results from the data partially shown in Figure 9.12 is shown in Figure 9.13. That figure shows the mean before and the mean after, although these are not actually used in the calculation of the *t* test. It also shows the before and after variance, again not used in the *t* test. Also shown is a Pearson correlation. The *t* statistic and the probability of *t* are the same as those given in Figure 9.12.

	A	B	C	D
1	t-Test: Paired Two Sample for Means			
2				
3		Before	After	
4	Mean	8.49075	8.25	
5	Variance	0.271474	0.196487	
6	Observations	40	40	
7	Pearson Correlation	0.146592		
8	Hypothesized Mean Difference	0		
9	df	39		
10	t Stat	2.406754		
11	P(T<=t) one-tail	0.010465		
12	t Critical one-tail	1.684875		
13	P(T<=t) two-tail	0.020929		
14	t Critical two-tail	2.022689		
15				

Figure 9.13   Excel add-in for before and after *t* test

EXERCISES FOR SECTION 9.3

1. Use the data on the HbA1c worksheet in Chpt 9-2.xls.

   a. Replicate the results found in Figure 9.12.

   b. Replicate the results in Figure 9.13 with the Excel add-in for before and after measures.

2. The data on the Weight worksheet of Chpt 9-2.xls represent the weight of 25 people who went on a prescribed diet at the beginning of a one-year time period. The Before weights are their weights at the start of the program, and After are their weights one year later.

   a. Use the formula in Equation 9.13 to test the hypothesis that weight before equals weight after against the alternative that weight after is less than before, and indicate your conclusion.

   b. Use the Excel add-in for related data, and replicate the results found in (a).

3. A health payer organization is concerned about the time it takes a group of account assessors to process certain aspects of health care claims. They initiate a training program to reduce the time involved. Average processing time for a fixed set of claims is determined before and after the training program. The data are shown on the Time spreadsheet in Chpt 9-2.xls.

   a. Using the formula in Equation 9.13, test the hypothesis that processing time before and after training is the same against the alternative that processing time after is less than before, and indicate your conclusion.

   b. Use the Excel add-in for related data, and replicate the results found in (a).

KEY TERMS

=FREQUENCY()	*t* test
=TDIST()	Type I error
standard error	Type II error
statistical significance	

CHAPTER 10

ANALYSIS OF VARIANCE

There are three kinds of lies: lies, damned lies, and statistics.

—Benjamin Disraeli

Chapter 1 introduced several different questions that could be addressed using statistics. One of these was the question of whether eight hospitals in a hospital alliance differed from one another in length of stay, readmission rates, or cost per case. If we were interested in whether just two of the hospitals differed from one another, we could use a *t* test. As presented earlier, a *t* test is a test of whether a numerical variable is independent of a categorical variable that takes on only two values. But in this case, the question is whether a numerical variable is independent of a categorical variable that may take on more than two values—here, eight. One statistical test that can be used to determine if a numerical variable is independent of a multilevel categorical variable is *analysis of variance*, commonly referred to as ANOVA.

10.1 One-Way Analysis of Variance

A one-way analysis of variance is a technique used to compare means of two samples that can be used only for numerical data.

To simplify the example somewhat, we are going to assume that there are only four hospitals in the alliance. However, it should be noted that the principles would be the same for essentially any number of hospitals being observed. Now if we were to examine the question of whether the four hospitals in the hospital alliance differed on the measures of length of stay, readmission rates, or cost per case, we could use one-way analysis of variance. With length of stay, it is possible that we could obtain all the data for each hospital—for example, for the last month or the last year or the last 10 years. This would be an overwhelming amount of data for an example. For readmission rates, we might be able to get all the data for each hospital as long as the readmission was to the same hospital. Coordinating among hospitals in the alliance or with hospitals outside the alliance would be more difficult. So, in the case of length of stay, we might have too much information, and in the case of readmissions, we might have too little. But with regard to cost per case, we might be just right.

Recall that Chapter 7 discussed the likelihood that cost per case is not really known. But it might be possible for a hospital's chief financial officer, for example, to get a good idea of cost per case for a relatively small random sample of hospital discharges. Let us assume that the head of the hospital alliance has reached an agreement with the hospital CFOs. The hospital alliance will each select a random sample of 30 hospital discharges. In turn, using accounting procedures commonly agreed to, they will determine the cost of each of the 30 discharges for each hospital. When they have finished, they will have a cost figure assigned to each discharge. Before we discuss these specific hospital discharges, it will be useful to spend a little time discussing what analysis of variance means in relation to the t test. Let's discuss this with the average cost of hospital discharges as the subject.

Analysis of Variance: Relation to t Tests

If we were examining only the average cost of the discharges from two hospitals, what we would actually be examining with a t test could be characterized as shown in Figure 10.1, which shows two distributions: one around a mean discharge cost of $5,700 and one around a mean discharge cost of $9,400. For the sake of this discussion, each of these distributions is assumed to have a standard error of $800. The t test is a test of whether the two mean values, given their respective distributions, can be thought of as being different from each other. In the case of Figure 10.1, the t test would definitely indicate that these two means are different. More specifically, the mean discharge cost is not independent of the hospital of discharge because the two distributions overlap only slightly.

Analysis of variance examines essentially the same question, but for more than two levels of a categorical variable. Consider, for example, the graph shown in Figure 10.2, which shows the distribution around the average discharge cost for four hospitals, the lowest being $5,700 and

Figure 10.1 Average cost distribution for two hospitals

Figure 10.2 Average cost distribution for four hospitals

then rising to $6,300, $6,600, and finally $9,400. All of these hospitals are assumed to have equal standard errors of $800. Analysis of variance addresses the question of whether the average cost per discharge of any of the four hospitals can be seen as being different from any of the others. In the case of these four hospitals, it is quite likely that analysis of variance would show that their average costs per discharge are not all the same. This is apparent, as there is little overlap between the distribution of the hospital with the highest average costs and that of the other three hospitals.

Equations for One-Way Analysis of Variance

So how is analysis of variance carried out? Analysis of variance depends on two pieces of information. The first of these is the *between group variance*, sometimes referred to as the explained variance. The between group variance is associated with the differences between the groups—in this case, four different hospitals. The second is the *within group variance*, often referred to as the error variance. The within group variance is a measure of the difference between the observations within the groups—in this case, each individual hospital—and cannot be accounted for by any information available to the analysis.

Between Group Variance: SS_B

The between group variance (designated SS_B) is calculated as shown in Equation 10.1, which indicates that the between group variance requires that the grand mean for all observations—in this case, the 120 observations from all four hospitals—be subtracted from the mean for each group. In turn, this difference is then squared. The result for each hospital is then multiplied by the sample size from each hospital and summed across all *m* hospitals—here, four hospitals.

$$SS_B = \sum_{j=1}^{m} n_j(\bar{x}_j - \bar{\bar{x}})^2 \tag{10.1}$$

where *m* represents the number of separate groups, n_j designates the number of observations in each group, x_j designates the sample mean for group *j*, and $\bar{\bar{x}}$ designates the mean for all observations across all groups.

Within Group Variance: SS_W

The within group variance (designated SS_W) is calculated as shown in Equation 10.2, which says that the mean cost for the sample from each hospital is subtracted from each separate observation for a specific hospital and then squared. This result is summed over all observations for each group—hospital—and these results are then summed across all hospitals.

$$SS_W = \sum_{j=1}^{m} \sum_{i=1}^{n_j} (x_{ij} - \bar{x}_j)^2 \tag{10.2}$$

Although the between group variance SS_B and the within group variance SS_W are all that are required for the calculation of the analysis of variance, it is useful to know the formula for the total variance (SS_T). This is useful because $SS_T = SS_B + SS_W$. If there is ever any doubt about whether your calculations have been carried out correctly, it is possible to calculate all three values and be sure that, in fact, $SS_T = SS_B + SS_W$. The formula for SS_T is shown in Equation 10.3, which indicates that the grand mean for all observations is subtracted from each individual observation and that each of these results is squared. Then these are summed across all observations in each group and then across all groups.

$$SS_T = \sum_{j=1}^{m} \sum_{i=1}^{n_j} (x_{ij} - \bar{\bar{x}}_j)^2 \tag{10.3}$$

Calculation of One-Way Analysis of Variance for Four Hospitals

Now we'll look at an example of the analysis of variance calculation, using Microsoft Excel. Let's call the four hospitals in the alliance Albemarle Community, Beaufort Municipal, Catawba County, and Dare Regional. The CFOs of four hospitals in the alliance have agreed to select a random sample of 30 discharges and determine actual costs for these discharges. The data they generated are contained in the file Chpt 10–1.xls, and the first 14 observations are shown in Figure 10.3.

As should be clear from Figure 10.3, all of the first cost records (column C) are for a single hospital: Albemarle Community. The cost data for the other three hospitals are contained in rows 31 to 121. A discussion of the presentation in Figure 10.3 should begin with the *pivot table* in cells H2 : I8. This pivot table shows the average cost for each hospital (cells I4 : I7) and for all hospitals taken together (cell I8). The average cost per hospital and for all hospitals is obtained by changing Sum to Average in the Layout window for the pivot table (see Figure 4.25).

Computation of SS_T in Excel

The computation of SS_T is contained in column D, which is labeled (C-Xbarbar)^2. This indicates that the overall average (designated $\bar{\bar{x}}$ in Equations 10.1 and 10.3 and given as Xbarbar in the figure) is subtracted

	B	C	D	E	F	G	H	I	J	K	L
1	Hosp	Cost	(C-Xbarbar)^2	(C-Xbar)^2							
2	Albemarle	$5,342.61	2740146.38	1685779			Average of Cost				
3	Albemarle	$7,237.59	57427.93	355937			Hosp	Total	nj*(Xbar-Xbarbar)^2		
4	Albemarle	$11,801.95	23078428.01	26635553			Albemarle	6640.99	3822679.286		
5	Albemarle	$1,082.36	34994190.26	30898319			Beaufort	6253.90	16608449.72		
6	Albemarle	$2,379.59	21329237.54	18159493			Catawba	9380.71	170326344.6		
7	Albemarle	$8,469.39	2165139.35	3343062			Dare	5716.21	49286011.22		
8	Albemarle	$4,453.55	6473965.00	4784875			Grand Total	6997.95			
9	Albemarle	$4,745.26	5074606.60	3593776							
10	Albemarle	$11,963.80	24659678.64	28332352			SS	df	MS	F	p
11	Albemarle	$5,294.96	2900170.68	1811785		SST	2726170568	119			
12	Albemarle	$2,965.55	16260239.68	13508827		SSB	240043485	3	80014495	3.7334	0.01323
13	Albemarle	$3,896.16	9621093.45	7534068		SSW	2486127083	116	21432130		
14	Albemarle	$6,074.21	853293.28	321235			2726170568				
15	Albemarle	$7,217.18	48062.34	332000							

Figure 10.3 Analysis of variance for four hospitals

from the discharge cost figure in column C and then squared. The value of Xbarbar is taken from cell I8 in the pivot table. Each of the values in column D is summed in cell H11 and labeled SS_T in cell G11. The formula for cell H11 is =SUM(D2:D121). Although SS_T is not part of the test of whether the four hospitals differ from one another, it is an important check of MS_B, the mean square error between groups, and MS_W, the mean square error within groups.

The between group variance, SS_B, is calculated in cells J4:J7 and summed in cell H12. The values in cells J4:J7 are calculated by subtracting the grand total mean in cell I8 from each of the hospital means in cells I4:I7, squaring the result, and multiplying by the number of observations for each hospital—in this case, 30 for each. The result is then summed in cell H12, the formula for which is =SUM(J4:J7). Note that the 1.7E+08 in cell J6 is simply Excel's way of designating a number too large to display in the cell.

The within group variance, SS_W, is calculated in column E and summed in cell H13. The formulas used by Excel to calculate the values in column E are shown in the formula bar. The individual hospital averages, given in cells I4:I7, are subtracted from the cost of the discharges for each hospital and squared to get the values in column E. The first 30 values in column E use the average for Albemarle Community, given in cell I4; the next 30 use the average for Beaufort Municipal, given in cell I5; and so on for the other two hospitals. The results of all these operations are summed in cell H13, labeled SS_W. The formula for cell H13 is =SUM(E2:E121). The value shown in cell H14 is the sum of cells H12 and H13, to verify that, indeed, SS_B and SS_W actually sum to SS_T. Table 10.1 displays the associated formulas for the computation of SS_T in Excel.

The F Test for Differences in ANOVA

The test of whether hospital costs (a numerical variable) are independent of hospitals (a categorical variable that takes on four values) is an F test. The question raised is whether the variance of the numerical variable associated with a categorical variable that took on only two values was different for the two levels of the categorical variable.

You will recall that if it was, then the t test assuming equal variance was not strictly appropriate. Take note, though, that in the case of equal-sized groups for each level of the categorical variable, it was probably adequate.

The F test is a statistical test in which the test statistic has an F distribution if the null hypothesis is true.

Table 10.1 Formulas for Figure 10.3

Cell or Column	Formula	Action/Note
D Column	=(C2-$I$8)2	Copied to cell D121
E Column	=(C2-$I$4)2	For column B cells containing Albemarle
	=(C2-$I$5)2	For column B cells containing Beaufort
	=(C2-$I$6)2	For column B cells containing Catawba
	=(C2-$I$7)2	For column B cells containing Dare
H11	=SUM(D2:D121)	
J4	=30*(I4-$I$8)2	
J5	=30*(I5-$I$8)2	
J6	=30*(I6-$I$8)2	
J7	=30*(I7-$I$8)2	
H12	=SUM(J4:J7)	
H13	=SUM(E2:E121)	
H14	=SUM(H12:H13)	
I11	=COUNT(C2:C121)-1	
I12	=4-1	
I13	=I11-I12	
J12	=H12/I12	
J13	=H13/I13	
K12	=J12/J13	
L12	=FDIST(K112,I12,I13)	

The use of the F test to determine the independence of hospital costs and hospital categories is similarly a test of variances. But, in this case, it is a test of whether the between group variance—the variance that can be attributed to the differences between the hospitals—is large relative to the within group variance. The within group variance is the variance that cannot be explained by information about the different hospitals. It is considered error variance. But the F test of whether the between group variance is large relative to the within group variance is not directly a test of the relative size of SS_B and SS_W. If there are m different groups (in this case, four hospitals), then there are $m-1$ *degrees of freedom* in SS_B. If there are n_j separate observations in each group (in this case, 30 cost figures for each hospital, although the number could be different for each hospital), then there are $n_1-1+n_2-1+\ldots n_j-1$ degrees of freedom in SS_W. In Figure 10.3, the degrees of freedom for SS_B and SS_W are shown in cells I12 and I13, respectively. The degrees of freedom for SS_T are given in cell I11. It is the total number of observations minus one, and it should always equal the sum of the degrees of freedom for SS_B and SS_W.

Cells J12 and J13 in Figure 10.3 show what are known as the mean square between groups and the mean square within groups, respectively.

The mean square is found by dividing the between group variance and the within group variance by their respective degrees of freedom. The F test of whether the between group variance is large relative to the within group variance is actually calculated on the mean square values rather than on SS_B and SS_W. The formula for the F test is shown in Equation 10.4.

$$F = \frac{SS_B / df_{SS_B}}{SS_W / df_{SS_W}} = \frac{MS_B}{MS_W} \qquad (10.4)$$

The =FDIST() Function

As Equation 10.4 shows, the F test is the mean square between groups divided by the mean square within groups. The result of this operation is shown in cell K12 in Figure 10.3. The value of F is given as 3.7334. Now, of course, there arises the question of whether this F value is large or small. The probability of obtaining an F value as large as 3.7334 can be found with the =FDIST() function. The function takes three arguments: the F value itself and the degrees of freedom in the numerator and in the denominator. The actual probability of this F value is given in cell L12 as 0.01323. The Excel function statement for that value is =FDIST(3.7334,3,116) but in the figure is actually stated as cell references K12, I12, and I13. What the probability value of 0.01323 says is that there is a very low probability of getting an F value as large as 3.7334. Actually, there is only about one time in 100 sets of samples, if cost and hospital are actually independent of each other. In consequence, we would conclude that cost is not independent of the hospitals and that the hospitals do, in fact, differ in their costs.

The Excel Add-In for One-Way Analysis of Variance

Now we can turn to the calculation of analysis of variance by using the Excel ANOVA Single-Factor Data Analysis add-in. The data for the Excel single-factor ANOVA must be arranged differently from the data shown in Figure 10.3. The data must be arranged in columns, each column representing a single group—in this case, a single hospital. The first 14 discharge costs for each of the four hospitals are shown in Figure 10.4, arranged in four columns.

To access the ANOVA: Single-Factor option in the Data Analysis package within Excel, go to the Data ribbon, in the Analysis group, and click the Data Analysis option. From the Data Analysis menu choose ANOVA: Single-Factor. The dialog box shown in Figure 10.5 prompts you for the same type of information that most data analysis add-in dialogs require. The Input Range is the data to be used in the analysis and includes

	A	B	C	D
1	Albemarle	Beaufort	Catawba	Dare
2	$5,342.61	$6,844.89	$5,455.73	$1,035.75
3	$7,237.59	$6,283.80	$4,448.48	$6,130.58
4	$11,801.95	$5,206.09	$8,996.80	$2,584.28
5	$1,082.36	$22,030.51	$4,734.98	$2,635.85
6	$2,379.59	$5,372.86	$13,055.10	$5,371.03
7	$8,469.39	$2,197.14	$10,194.42	$14,433.99
8	$4,453.55	$13,472.69	$16,229.83	$2,283.88
9	$4,745.26	$8,486.18	$7,099.69	$3,630.39
10	$11,963.80	$2,447.01	$5,948.36	$4,775.36
11	$5,294.96	$19,182.24	$4,155.38	$6,084.66
12	$2,965.55	$10,021.34	$14,470.90	$1,414.80
13	$3,896.16	$1,594.57	$4,957.09	$6,630.33
14	$6,074.21	$4,412.80	$5,040.75	$5,139.11
15	$7,217.18	$7,000.21	$4,113.04	$16,346.71

Figure 10.4 Data arrangement for the Excel Single-Factor ANOVA add-in

Figure 10.5 ANOVA: Single-Factor dialog box

all cells A1:D31. This includes all 120 observations. Because the data are arranged in columns by hospital, the Grouped By Columns radio button is selected. The check box for the "Labels in the first row" is checked to indicate that the names of the hospitals are in cells A1, B1, C1, and D1. The Output Range radio button is selected to indicate that the output will be in the same spreadsheet, beginning in cell F2.

The Excel ANOVA Output

Figure 10.6 shows the output of the ANOVA: Single-Factor data analysis add-in. As indicated in the output range in Figure 10.5, the analysis output begins in cell F2. Cells F6 : F9 show the four hospitals. Cells G6 : G9 show the number of observations for each hospital. Cells G6 : G9 show the number of observations for each hospital, and cells I6 : I9 show the average cost for each. The variance in cells J6 : J9 is calculated by the standard variance formula given in Equation 6.3. An alternative way of calculating the within group variance would be to multiply each of the variance numbers by the degrees of freedom for each hospital (29) and sum them. Doing so would produce the same number as that shown in cell G15 as the within groups *sum of squares*. Cells G14, G15, and G17 show the between groups, within groups, and total sum of squares, respectively. You may note that these are the same values obtained in Figure 10.3 by our calculations. The mean square values in cells H14 and H15, which represent the sum of squares divided by the appropriate degrees of freedom, are also the same as those calculated in Figure 10.3, as are the *F* test value and the probability of the *F*.

The =FINV() Function

The additional information in Figure 10.6 is the number in cell L14 titled F crit, which stands for *F* critical. F crit is the value that must be reached by the *F* test (the division of MS_B by MS_W) in order to be at the 0.95 level of confidence. The value of F crit can be obtained with the =FINV() function. The =FINV() function takes three arguments: the level of significance (in this case, 0.05), and the degrees of freedom in MS_B

	F	G	H	I	J	K	L
1							
2	Anova: Single Factor						
3							
4	SUMMARY						
5	*Groups*	*Count*	*Sum*	*Average*	*Variance*		
6	Albemarle	30	199230	6640.985667	21757799.02		
7	Beaufort	30	187617	6253.895667	24442189.47		
8	Catawba	30	281421	9380.708667	23920882.37		
9	Dare	30	171486	5716.205	15607649.24		
10							
11							
12	ANOVA						
13	*Source of Variation*	*SS*	*df*	*MS*	*F*	*P-value*	*F crit*
14	Between Groups	240043484.8	3	80014494.95	3.733389769	0.01323	2.68281
15	Within Groups	2486127083	116	21432130.02			
16							
17	Total	2726170568	119				
18							

Figure 10.6 Output of the ANOVA: Single-Factor data analysis add-in

and MS_W. The F crit statement that produces the value in cell L14 L13 is =FINV(0.05,3,116).

The F test as discussed thus far provides a way to determine if a numerical variable treated as dependent is actually independent of a categorical variable that takes on more than two values. Why could the same F test not be used if the categorical variable takes on only two values, thus eliminating the need for the t test? The answer is that it could, but the t test has at least one advantage over the F test. The F test is always a two-tail test. There is no equivalent to the one-tail t test for the F test. In consequence, the t test remains useful if the categorical variable in question takes on only two values.

Where Do the Differences Lie in ANOVA?

The interpretation of the F test in either Figure 10.3 or Figure 10.6 is that at least one among the four hospitals under consideration is different from at least one other hospital in average cost. This is not a conclusion about the 30 sample observations from each hospital. Rather, it is a conclusion about all the discharges from the hospitals, assuming that the 30 discharges studied were drawn at random from all discharges. But determining that at least one hospital differs from at least one other is not the most satisfactory outcome. It might be pretty easy to decide that Catawba County hospital has higher costs (an average of $9,380.71 per discharge) than Dare Regional (an average of only $5,716.21). But what do we decide about Beaufort Municipal (at $6,253.90)? Does it have lower costs than Catawba, or higher costs than Dare? These questions cannot be answered directly by ANOVA, but they can be answered by several different statistical tests. Unfortunately for users of Excel, most of these tests rely on something called the studentized range statistic, which is often designated q_r. Excel does not provide probability distributions for the studentized range statistic, so this section will discuss a technique provided by Winer (1962). This technique can provide a direct comparison between each hospital and every other hospital, and the result can be interpreted using the F distribution, for which Excel does provide exact probabilities.

ANOVA: The Test of Differences

In our discussion of this statistical technique, it will be referred to as the test of differences between two means in ANOVA. It could equally be used to test one mean in comparison with all other means or two means in comparison with two others. However, this discussion will concentrate only on the test of two means at a time. The formula for this test is given in Equation 10.5.

$$F = \frac{(\bar{x}_1 - \bar{x}_2)^2 \left/ \left(\frac{1}{n_1} + \frac{1}{n_2} \right) \right.}{MS_w}$$

(10.5)

where $\bar{x}_1$ is the mean of the first group to be compared, $\bar{x}_2$ is the mean of the second, and n_1 and n_2 are the respective sizes of the two samples. MS_w is the mean square within groups taken from the original F test.

Equation 10.5 results in an F test with one degree of freedom in the numerator and degrees of freedom for MS_w (the mean square error) in the denominator. We can use this F test to determine which of the four hospitals is different from the others. If we do so, there will be six comparisons, as shown in Figure 10.7, which shows each hospital in cells F22 : F25. They have been reordered; the hospital with the lowest average cost is listed first. Cells G22 : G25 give the average cost per discharge for each hospital. The hospitals have been listed again in cells H20 : K20, with their average costs given in cells H21 : K21. Incidentally, the hospitals and their costs in cells H20 : K21 were generated by copying cells F22 : G25 and using the Paste Special ➤ Transpose command in cell H20. The six meaningful hospital cost comparisons are given in the cells above and to the right of the main diagonal of the resulting table. These six comparisons contrast each hospital with every other hospital.

The data in Table 10.2 represent the calculation of the formula given in Equation 10.5. The formula bar gives the calculation for cell I22. This is a comparison between Dare Regional and Beaufort Municipal. The dollar sign ($) convention as given in the formula bar allows the formula for cell I22 to be copied to the other five cells to produce the result for each comparison. The fact that the sample size is the same for each hospital

I22		=((I$21-$G22)^2/(1/30+1/30))/$I$15			
	F	G	H	I	J	K
20			Dare	Beaufort	Albemarle	Catawba
21			5716.21	6253.90	6640.99	9380.71
22	Dare	5716.21		0.202344	0.598554	9.3984502
23	Beaufort	6253.90			0.10487	6.8427353
24	Albemarle	6640.99				5.2533851
25	Catawba	9380.71				
26						
27			Dare	Beaufort	Albemarle	Catawba
28			5716.21	6253.90	6640.99	9380.71
29	Dare	5716.21		0.653675	0.440704	**0.002702**
30	Beaufort	6253.90			0.746645	0.0100837
31	Albemarle	6640.99				0.0237078
32	Catawba	9380.71				
33						
34		F Prob	0.008512			

Figure 10.7   Test of differences between two means in ANOVA

Table 10.2 Formulas for Figure 10.7

Cell or Column	Formula	Action/Note
I22	$=((I\$21-\$G22)^2/(1/30+1/30))/\$I\$15$	Copied to cells J22, K22, J23, K23, and K24
I29	$=FDIST(I22,1,116)$ Degrees of freedom in the numerator is 1 because we are comparing 2 events (i.e., $n=2$) and $DoF = n-1$ degrees of freedom in the denominator is equal to the DoF of MS_W, which is 116.	Copied to cells J29, K29, J30, K30, and K31
H34	$=1-(1-0.05)^\wedge(1/6)$	Alpha is chosen to be 0.05 and $c=6$ because six tests are being completed.

makes the term $(1/30 + 1/30)$ appropriate for each comparison. The last term, $\$I\$15$, refers to the mean square within groups (MS_W), given in cell I15 in Figure 10.6.

The second row in Table 10.2 contains the formula for the probabilities of the F values calculated in Figure 10.7. As you can see from Figure 10.7, the probability of an F as large as the 0.2023 in cell I22 is given as 0.6537 (cell I29). This means that if the average cost for Dare Regional and Beaufort Municipal were actually the same, an F value as large as 0.2023 would be obtained from the formula in Equation 10.5 about 65 percent of the time. Because our alpha level throughout this book is assumed to be 5 percent, we would clearly not reject the null hypothesis that costs per discharge for Dare and Beaufort are the same. But what do we conclude, for example, about Beaufort Municipal and Catawba County hospitals? In this case, the probability of the F value being as large as 6.843 is about 0.01. This number appears to be telling us that the costs per discharge for the Beaufort and Catawba hospitals are different. However, should we reject the null hypothesis that the two hospitals are no different in average costs per discharge? The answer is probably not, which needs a little explanation.

Rejecting/Accepting the Null Hypothesis When Using F Tests

In comparing each of the hospitals with every other hospital, six comparisons are made. And when a large number of comparisons are made following a significant overall F, the overall probability of alpha (α) increases. In other words, we run a higher risk of coming to the wrong conclusion. If we conduct six tests, the overall probability of alpha for all six tests will be $1 - (1 - \alpha)^6$. If the initial alpha is 0.05, this produces an overall probability for all six tests of about 0.26. Thus, if we conduct six tests, there is about one chance in four that a difference large enough to reject the null hypothesis at the 0.05 level will occur when we should not reject the null hypothesis. We run the risk of making the Type I error about one-fourth of the time. This risk is really too high.

Protecting against Alpha Inflation: Adjusting the F Probability

To protect against this inflation in the true value of alpha over six tests, we can reduce the actual probability level at which we will reject the null hypothesis by the result of the formula shown in Equation 10.6. In that equation, α_{Adj} is the adjusted value of alpha, and c represents the number of comparisons being made. Taking the cth root of $1 - \alpha$ would be a daunting task if it were being done with paper and pencil. Happily for us, Excel can take a cth root with very little difficulty. The F probability that provides an overall 0.05 level for alpha for all six tests taken together is given in cell H34 in Figure 10.7. This value is calculated using the Excel formula statement `=1-(1-0.05)^(1/6)`, which is the Excel equivalent of Equation 10.6 when alpha is 0.05 and c is 6. Based on this adjusted alpha for all six tests, we would conclude that only one comparison leads us to reject the null hypothesis of no difference. This is the comparison shown in bold in cell K29 of Figure 10.7—namely, that between Catawba County and Dare Regional. In other words, Catawba's costs are different from those of Dare, but no other average discharge costs are different. With this in mind, the significant F value obtained in both Figures 10.3 and 10.6 is a function of the difference between Catawba and Dare.

$$\alpha_{Adj} = 1 - (1 - \alpha)^{\left(\frac{1}{c}\right)} \tag{10.6}$$

It would not always be necessary to make all possible two-group or two-hospital comparisons following a significant overall F. In some cases, it may be sufficient simply to know that there is an overall difference. In turn, the test of differences between hospitals could be ignored. In other cases, it might be decided before the fact that if there are significant overall differences, it is because one group, such as Catawba County hospital, has greater costs than all the other three. In such a case, it would be reasonable to test Catawba against the other three only. This would result in only three comparisons, and the level of α_{Adj} would be, as expressed in Excel, `=1-(1-0.05)^(1/3)=0.017`.

Assumption of Equal Variances: The Bartlett Test

Like the first t test discussed in Chapter 9, the analysis of variance discussed here assumes equal variance across groups. There are several tests of the homogeneity of variance across groups, but the one discussed here is called the *Bartlett test*. The Bartlett test is a chi-square test and is carried out with the formula given in Equation 10.7. The formula in Equation 10.7 is

	F	G	H	I	J	K	L
1							
2	Anova: Single Factor						
3							
4	SUMMARY						
5	Groups	Count	Sum	Average	Variance	df*log(Var)	1/df
6	Albemarle	30	199230	6640.985667	21757799.02	212.7908339	0.03448
7	Beaufort	30	187617	6253.895667	24442189.47	214.2560631	0.03448
8	Catawba	30	281421	9380.708667	23920882.37	213.9845387	0.03448
9	Dare	30	171486	5716.205	15607649.24	208.6067874	0.03448
10						849.638223	0.13793
11							
12	ANOVA						
13	Source of Variation	SS	df	MS	F		
14	Between Groups	240043484.8	3	80014494.95	3.733389769		
15	Within Groups	2486127083	116	21432130.02		850.4035789	0.00862
16							0.11111
17	Total	2726170568	119			c	1.01437
18						Chi Square	1.73765
19						p	0.6286

Figure 10.8 Bartlett test for homogeneity of variance: Interpreting the Bartlett test

somewhat imposing, but, in practice, it is easily calculated using Excel. The result of the calculation is shown in Figure 10.8.

$$\chi^2 = \frac{2.303}{c} \left(df_{MS_W} \log MS_W - \sum_{j=1}^{m} df_{Gj} \log s_{Gj}^2 \right)$$

where

$$c = 1 + \frac{1}{3(m-1)} \left(\sum \frac{1}{df_{Gj}} - \frac{1}{df_{MS_W}} \right) \qquad (10.7)$$

Figure 10.8 replicates a part of the ANOVA output shown in Figure 10.6. The calculation of the Bartlett test is given in columns K and L. Cells K6 : K9 represent the degrees of freedom in each group (cells G6 : G9, respectively, minus 1, or 29) times the log of the variance (cells J6 : J9). These results are summed in K10, which represents the term in Equation 10.7. Cells L6 : L9 are 1 divided by the degrees of freedom in each group, and cell L10 is the sum of these, representing the term in the calculation of the term c. Cell K15 is cell H15 multiplied by the log of cell I15, and cell L15 is 1 divided by cell H15. Cell L16 is the result of the calculation of $1/(3 \times (m-1))$, where m is the number of groups being compared. The calculated value of c is shown in cell L17, and the calculated chi-square value is shown in L18. This chi-square statistic has $m - 1$, or three degrees of freedom. The probability value for a chi-square of 1.738 is given in cell L19 and was found using the =CHIDIST() function. The actual Excel statement is =CHIDIST(1.738,3). Table 10.3 contains the Excel formulas for completing the Bartlett test procedure.

Table 10.3   Formulas for Figure 10.8

Cell or Column	Formula	Action/Note
K6	=(G6-1)*LOG(J6)	Copied to cells K7, K8, and K9
K10	=SUM(K6:K9)	
L6	=1/G6	Copied to cells L7, L8, and L9
L10	=SUM(L6:L9)	
K15	=H15*LOG(I15)	
L15	=1/H15	
L16	=1/(3*(4-1))	Here the 4 represents m and is the number of groups being compared (i.e., Albemarle, Beaufort, Catawba, and Dare).
L17	=1+L16*(L10-(1/H15))	
L18	=(2.303/L17)*(H15*LOG(I15)-K10)	
L19	=CHIDIST(L18,3)	Here the 3 represents the degrees of freedom, which is $m - 1$ again with m being 4.

The interpretation of the Bartlett test is as follows. If the variances of the four hospitals are, in fact, the same—that is, the null hypothesis is true—we would expect to find a chi-square value as large as 1.738 about 60 percent of the times we drew samples of size 30 from each of the four hospitals. Because the likelihood of finding a chi-square value as large as 1.738 is so high, we will conclude that, in fact, the variances are the same.

The Bartlett test is one way of testing for the homogeneity of variance between the groups compared in ANOVA. However, it is not an essential part of the ANOVA process. When variances differ across the groups in the order of magnitude—for example, of 1 to 3 (i.e., the variance of one group is three times as large as the variance of another)—the results of ANOVA will not be greatly affected. Unless differences across the groups exceed the level of 1 to 3, ANOVA can be used with confidence.

Before we leave the one-way analysis of variance, it is important to comment on sample sizes. In the example given, all four hospitals contributed an equal number of observations—30—to the analysis. In many cases, it is not possible to obtain an equal number of observations for each group. In such a situation, everything that was discussed earlier in regard to ANOVA applies nonetheless. It is simply necessary to ensure that the appropriate number is used for n_j and for degrees of freedom for each group.

EXERCISES FOR SECTION 10.1

1. Use the data on the Costs worksheet of Chpt 10–1.xls, and replicate the calculations in Figure 10.3.

   a. Use a pivot table and the formula in Equation 10.1 to calculate the between group sum of squares (SS_B) for the costs in the four hospitals.

   b. Use the results of the pivot table from (a) and the formula in Equation 10.2 to calculate the within groups sum of squares (SS_W) for the costs in the four hospitals.

   c. Use the formula in Equation 10.3 to calculate the total sum of squares (SS_T) for the costs in the four hospitals.

   d. Determine the appropriate degrees of freedom, and use the formula in Equation 10.4 to calculate the F value for a test of the null hypothesis that the mean costs in the four hospitals are all the same.

   e. Use the =FDIST() function to obtain the probability of the F value, and draw the appropriate conclusion in regard to the null hypothesis.

2. The data on the Education worksheet of Chpt 10–1.xls represent the score received by three groups of women on a 20-point knowledge assessment of breast cancer risk following a visit to a breast cancer screening clinic. Persons 1 through 15 received no information, persons 16 through 30 received a pamphlet, and persons 31 through 45 received a brief face-to-face discourse on breast cancer risk from a physician. (The women were randomly selected—each to one of the three groups, and all received the face-to-face encounter with the physician following the experiment.)

   a. Use a pivot table and the formula in Equation 10.1 to calculate the between group sum of squares (SS_B) for the three groups of women.

   b. Use the results of the pivot table from (a) and the formula in Equation 10.2 to calculate the within groups sum of squares (SS_W) for the three groups of women.

   c. Use the formula in Equation 10.3 to calculate the total sum of squares (SS_T) for the three groups of women.

   d. Determine the appropriate degrees of freedom, and use the formula in Equation 10.4 to calculate the F value for a test of the null hypothesis that the mean knowledge scores of the three groups of women are all the same.

   e. Use the =FDIST() function to obtain the probability of the F value, and draw the appropriate conclusion in regard to the null hypothesis.

3. On a fresh spreadsheet, rearrange the data on the Costs worksheet of Chpt 10–1.xls into four columns, as shown in Figure 10.4.

   a. Use the ANOVA: Single-Factor data analysis add-in to carry out the analysis of variance.

   b. Confirm that the results are the same as those obtained in Exercise 1.

4. On a fresh spreadsheet, rearrange the data on the Education worksheet of Chpt 10–1.xls into three columns, each column representing one of each of the three groups of women in Exercise 2.

   a. Use the ANOVA: Single-Factor data analysis add-in to carry out the analysis of variance.

   b. Confirm that the results are the same as those obtained in Exercise 2.

5. Lay out a worksheet like the one shown in Figure 10.7, and replicate that figure for the data from the Costs worksheet of Chpt 10–1.xls.

   a. Use the formula in Equation 10.5 to calculate the F value for the difference between each hospital and every other.

   b. Use the formula in Equation 10.6 to calculate the adjusted value of alpha for the six comparisons.

6. Lay out a worksheet following the example in Figure 10.7, and make the comparison for the three groups from the Education worksheet of Chpt 10–1.xls.

   a. Use the formula in Equation 10.5 to calculate the F value for the difference between each education group.

   b. Use the formula in Equation 10.6 to calculate the adjusted value of alpha for the three comparisons.

7. Lay out a worksheet like the one shown in Figure 10.8, and replicate the Bartlett test for homogeneity of variance, as shown in that figure, using the formula in Equation 10.7.

8. Lay out a worksheet like the one in Figure 10.8, and conduct the Bartlett test for homogeneity of variance, using the formula in Equation 10.7, and decide whether the null hypothesis of equal variance should be accepted or rejected.

10.2   ANOVA for Repeated Measures

Two essentially different types of t test were discussed in Chapter 9. The first of these was a t test for differences between two unrelated groups. One-way analysis of variance is the multiple group extension of that t test. The second was the t test for a single group measured two times. The extension of that test is ANOVA for *repeated measures*. In this case, one group of people, or of organizations, is measured on some variable more than two times. The primary question: Is there is any difference between the several measurements?

> Repeated ANOVA tests the equality of means and is used when all components of a random sample are measured under a number of different conditions.

One of the questions that are of concern to the hospital alliance has to do with the cost of readmissions. In particular, it is suspected that the later admissions in a string of readmissions for the same person are likely to be more expensive than the earlier admissions. It is not always easy to track readmissions, particularly if they are at different hospitals. However, one of the hospitals in the alliance has been able to put together a list of several hundred people who were admitted to any one of the hospitals at least three times in the past three years. They have selected a random sample of 12 of these people and have determined the actual cost of each admission. The question then is, do these costs differ from admission to admission? If we were considering only a single readmission, it would be possible to use the t test for related data, comparing the mean for the first admission with the mean for the second. Because we are considering three admissions, it is more appropriate to use analysis of variance for repeated measures. It might also be pointed out that 12 people is a very small sample. Thirty people would be better. But 30 people would make an example that would take up too much spreadsheet space to be easily shown in this book. So we will stick with the smaller sample for illustrative purposes.

Variation within Repeated ANOVA: Effect versus Residual Variation

In considering analysis of variance for repeated measures, the total variation in the data (SS_T) can be divided into the variation between people—or between groups—(SS_B) and the variation within people or groups (SS_W). In general, differences that may exist between people or groups (SS_B) are not of interest to us. Rather, we are interested in the differences within people or groups (SS_W). In the example discussed here, differences within people are differences that may reflect different costs of hospital stays, depending on which admission is being considered. But SS_W can also be divided into two sources of variation. One source is the variation that is due to the differences in effect (i.e., costs of first, second, or third admissions) and is referred to as SS_A. The other is the variation that cannot be explained by whether the admission is first, second, or third. This last variation is generally referred to as residual variation (SS_R).

The formula for the variation within people (or groups) is given in Equation 10.8. Equation 10.8 says that the mean for each person or group i, $\bar{x}_i$, is subtracted from each observation for the person or group. The result is squared and summed over all people. In the example under discussion here, each person was admitted three times to the hospital. The average cost of all three admissions is subtracted from the cost of each and is then squared. And then each of these three values is summed over all 12 people.

$$SS_W = \sum_{j=1}^{m} \sum_{i=1}^{n} (x_{ij} - \bar{x}_i)^2 \tag{10.8}$$

where m is the number of different measurements.

Calculating Effect versus Residual Variation

The initial calculation of SS_W can be seen in column D in Figure 10.9, which shows an ID number for each person in the sample in column A and the number of the admission in column B. All admissions for the first seven people are shown in the figure. The data in the spreadsheet depicted in the figure actually occupy the first 37 rows of the spreadsheet. Column C is the cost of each admission for each person. Column D is the initial calculation of SS_W.

The Excel formula used for the calculation is shown in the formula bar in Figure 10.9. This formula indicates that the value in cell H4 was subtracted from the value in cell C2. The value in cell H4 is the mean cost for person 1, which was obtained using the pivot table function and the average option. The dollar sign ($) convention in cell D2 allows that formula to be copied to cells D3 and D4. Unfortunately, the calculation of SS_W is a little tedious, requiring that the $H$4 reference be changed to $H$5 for person 2, $H$6 for person 3, and so on. The result of the calculation of SS_W is shown in cell L4 in Figure 10.10. As the formula bar in that figure shows, SS_W is the sum of cells D2:D37 from Figure 10.9. Table 10.4 contains the formulas for calculating the ANOVA for repeated measures.

SS_A, which is the variation due to differences in admission costs or effect, is calculated from the formula in Equation 10.9, which indicates that SS_A is calculated by subtracting the grand mean from the mean for each admission. In this case, for example, as there are 12 people, there will be 12 first admissions averaged, and then 12 second and 12 third. Because this is a repeated measures ANOVA, n refers to the number of people or groups measured. There are n, or 12, people observed in this case, but mn,

	D2	▼	=	=(C2-$H$4)^2					
	A	B	C	D	E	F	G	H	I
1	Person	Admt	Cost	SSW	SST				
2	1	1	$2,319.69	1282669.50	4812620.72		Average of Cost		
3	1	2	$2,898.01	307170.89	2609674.22		Person ▼	Total	
4	1	3	$5,139.02	2845226.77	391327.05		1	3452.24	1126185
5	2	1	$4,193.34	19032.04	102475.93		2	4331.30	33182.97
6	2	2	$3,243.61	1183062.28	1612515.50		3	5036.12	273171.4
7	2	3	$5,556.94	1502201.58	1088853.41		4	5491.03	955645.8
8	3	1	$2,508.31	6389806.54	4020620.95		5	2814.97	2884864
9	3	2	$4,244.97	625913.05	72086.13		6	2673.46	3385607
10	3	3	$8,355.07	11015451.23	14757978.06		7	6388.47	3515668
11	4	1	$7,088.50	2551910.40	6630838.15		8	4504.25	84.85992
12	4	2	$4,932.22	312268.62	175361.10		9	7099.32	6686679
13	4	3	$4,452.37	1078814.60	3731.82		10	5705.89	1421885
14	5	1	$1,786.17	1058429.44	7438103.17		11	3348.01	1358278
15	5	2	$3,140.76	106139.12	1884301.48		12	3316.46	1432798
16	5	3	$3,517.98	494223.06	990977.67		Grand Total	4513.46	
17	6	1	$4,413.98	3029421.47	9895.99				
18	6	2	$1,599.82	1152695.69	8489289.96		Average of Cost		
19	6	3	$2,006.57	444737.83	6284490.51		Admt ▼	Total	
20	7	1	$6,767.15	143398.54	5079124.88		1	3898.89	377693.6
21	7	2	$2,713.24	13507315.55	3240787.05		2	3926.92	344022.7
22	7	3	$9,685.02	10867241.90	26745047.20		3	5714.56	1442647
23	8	1	$2,519.60	3938822.39	3975472.16		Grand Total	4513.46	
24	8	2	$7,210.54	7324023.61	7274248.02				

Figure 10.9 Data for ANOVA for repeated measures

	L4	▼	=	=SUM(D2:D37)			
	K	L	M	N	O	P	
1							
2		SS	df	MS	F	p	
3	SSB	69222144.55	11				
4	SSW	105175766.54	24				
5	SSA	25972353.07	2	12986177	3.607116	0.044168	
6	SSR	79203413.47	22	3600155			
7							
8	SST	174397911.09	35				
9							
10		174397911.09					

Figure 10.10 Results of ANOVA repeated measures

Table 10.4 Formulas for Figure 10.9

Cell or Column	Formula	Action/Note
D2	$=(C2-\$H\$4)^2$	Copied to cells D3 and D4
D5	$=(C2-\$H\$5)^2$ The logic for cells D2 and D5 continues for each group of three subsequent cells through cell D37.	Copied to cells D6 and D7 NOTE: Increment the row number, X, for the $\$H\$X$ command for each group of three.
E2	$=(C2-\$H\$16)^2$	Copied to cells E3 : E37
I4	$=(H4-\$H\$16)^2$	Copied to cells I5 : I15
I20	$=(H4-\$H\$23)^2$	Copied to cells I21 : I22

Table 10.5   Formulas for Figure 10.10

Cell or Column	Formula	Action/Note
L3	=3*(SUM(I4:I15))	
L4	=SUM(D2:D37)	
L5	=12*(SUM(I20:I22))	
L6	=L4-L5	
L8	=L3-L4	
M3	=12-1	Where 12 is m
M4	=12*(3-1)	Here the 12 represents m and the 3 represents n.
M5	=3-1	Where 3 is n
M6	=(3-1)*(12-1)	Where 3 is n and 12 is m
M8	=3*12-1	Where 3 is n and 12 is m
N5	=L5/M5	
N6	=L6/M6	
O5	=N5/N6	
P5	=FDIST(O5,M5,M6)	

or 36, total admissions. The squared value for the m, or three, admissions is then summed and multiplied by the number of people in the study, or 12. The result of this calculation is given in cell L5 in Figure 10.10. Table 10.5 contains the formulas for calculating the ANOVA repeated measures results in Figure 10.10.

$$SS_A = n \sum_{j=1}^{n} (\bar{x}_j - \bar{\bar{x}})^2 \qquad (10.9)$$

The residual variation, SS_R, is the difference between SS_W and SS_A. It is shown for this example in cell L6 in Figure 10.10. In cell L6, SS_R was actually calculated by $SS_W - SS_A$. The formula for SS_R is somewhat complicated but is as shown in Equation 10.10. In this case, there are 36 observations, $m \times n$ or 12 times 3. According to Equation 10.10, for each observation in the data set, the mean across all three admissions for each person $\bar{x}_i$ and the mean across all 12 people for each admission $\bar{x}_j$ are each subtracted from the individual observation corresponding to each of these means. The grand mean across all observations is added to this value, and the result is squared. Then this figure is added across all 36 admissions.

$$SS_R = \sum_{j=1}^{m} \sum_{i=1}^{n} (x_{ij} - \bar{x}_i - \bar{x}_j + \bar{\bar{x}})^2 \qquad (10.10)$$

The calculation of SS_R using the formula in Equation 10.10 is shown in Figure 10.11. The Excel statement for the term for SS_R corresponding

	A	B	C	D	E	F
F2			=(C2-D2-E2+$F$1)^2			
1	Person	Admt	Cost	Xbari	Xbarj	4513.46
2	1	1	$2,319.69	3452.24	3898.89	268305.58
3	1	2	$2,898.01	3452.24	3926.92	1043.58
4	1	3	$5,139.02	3452.24	5714.56	235882.90
5	2	1	$4,193.34	4331.30	3898.89	227158.15
6	2	2	$3,243.61	4331.30	3926.92	251153.55
7	2	3	$5,556.94	4331.30	5714.56	602.27
8	3	1	$2,508.31	5036.12	3898.89	3660483.05
9	3	2	$4,244.97	5036.12	3926.92	41866.16
10	3	3	$8,355.07	5036.12	5714.56	4485293.33

Figure 10.11 Calculation of SS_R

to the first admission for the first person is shown in the formula bar for cell F2. The value in cell D2 was taken from cell H4 in Figure 10.9, and the value in cell E2 was taken from cell H20, also from Figure 10.9. The grand mean, which is given in cell F1, was taken from cell H16 in Figure 10.9. As the formula bar shows, the value in cell D2 and the value in cell E2 are each subtracted from the value in cell C2. The grand mean in cell F1 is added to this total, and the result is squared. The sum of column F (excluding the mean in cell F1) is not shown, but it is exactly equal to the value shown for SS_R in cell L6 in Figure 10.10.

Although the between person variance SS_B and the total variance SS_T do not enter into the calculation of the F test, it is useful to know how they are derived. The formula for SS_T is exactly the same as the formula for SS_T for one-way ANOVA. That formula is shown in Equation 10.3. In this case, however, n_j will be only n because, with repeated measures on the same people or groups, the number of observations for each measurement will always be the same. The formula for SS_B is shown in Equation 10.11.

$$SS_B = m * \sum_{i=1}^{n}(\bar{x}_i - \bar{\bar{x}})^2 \qquad (10.11)$$

The initial steps in the calculation of both SS_T and SS_B are shown in Figure 10.9. SS_T is shown in column E and summed in cell L8 in Figure 10.10. The part within the parentheses for SS_B is calculated in cells I4:I15 in Figure 10.9, and the sum of those cells is multiplied by measurements (3) in cell L3 in Figure 10.10.

The degrees of freedom in repeated measures of ANOVA are given for this example in column M in Figure 10.10. The degrees of freedom for SS_B will always be $n - 1$. Degrees of freedom for SS_W will always be

	K	L
16	SSB	n-1
17	SSW	n(m-1)
18	SSA	m-1
19	SSR	(n-1)(m-1)
20	SST	nm-1

Figure 10.12 Degrees of freedom in repeated measures

$n(m-1)$. These, together, add to the degrees of freedom for SS_T, $nm-1$. The degrees of freedom for SS_A, $m-1$, and the degrees of freedom for SS_R, $(n-1)(m-1)$, add together to the degrees of freedom for SS_W. These respective degrees of freedom are shown in Figure 10.12.

The F test for the differences between the costs of admissions is the mean square, due to admissions, MS_A, divided by the mean square residual, MS_R. These are shown in cells N5 and N6, respectively, in Figure 10.10. The result of the division is shown in cell O5 in Figure 10.10. Cell P5 shows the probability of the F value, 0.044. This value says that if there were no difference in the cost of admissions across the three separate admissions considered, the probability of finding an F value as large as 3.6 would be about four chances out of 100 samples. Because the likelihood is so small under the null hypothesis of no difference, the conclusion is that the cost of admission is not independent of whether the admission is a first time, a first readmission (second admission), or a second readmission (third admission). In other words, the admission timing does matter in determining cost.

Where Do Observed Differences Lie?

As in one-way ANOVA, it is possible to consider, with the repeated measures design, where the differences between measures (in this case, admissions) might lie. The F test is again a test of the squared difference between two means—in this case, the mean cost of any admission. The formula for the F test is given in Equation 10.12, which is a modification of Equation 10.5. Equation 10.5 recognizes the fact that n is the same for each group and that the error mean square is designated mean square residual (MS_R). As with Equation 10.5, $\bar{x}_1$ refers to the mean of the first group in the comparison and $\bar{x}_2$ refers to the mean of the second. This F test has one degree of freedom in the numerator and degrees of freedom equal to that of MS_R in the denominator.

$$F = \frac{(\bar{x}_1 - \bar{x}_2)^2 / \frac{2}{n}}{MS_R} \tag{10.12}$$

In the case of the cost of the three admissions to the hospital, there could be three comparisons: that between admission 1 and admission 2, that between admission 1 and admission 3, and that between admission 2 and admission 3. The comparison across the three admissions is shown in Figure 10.13. The F test is shown as calculated in cells J29, K29, and K30. The formula for the F test as reproduced in Excel is shown in the formula bar for cell J29. Again, the use of the dollar sign ($) convention, as given in the formula bar, allows the contents of cell J29 to be copied to the other two cells directly. Cells J35, K35, and K36 show the probability of the F value given in the first three cells mentioned. Clearly there is no difference between admission 1 and admission 2, with a p value of 0.971. However, admission 3 appears to be different in cost from both admissions 1 and 2, with p values of 0.028 and 0.030 respectively. But because we have conducted three tests, the adjusted p value in cell H39 gives an overall level of 0.05 for all three tests, based on the formula in Equation 10.6. This says that for an overall level of 0.05 for all three tests, we must have a level of 0.017 for any individual test. This leaves us with the anomalous result that we have found a significant overall F, but with any of the three individual comparisons, we do not find significant F values. Although this is anomalous, it is not uncommon, especially if one is using the stringent criteria of the adjusted alpha level. From a practical standpoint, because there is a significant overall F value, and because the third admission is clearly more costly than the first two, it is appropriate in this case to consider the statistically significant difference to lie with the difference between the first two admissions and the third. Table 10.6 displays the Excel formulas for calculating the F tests in Figure 10.13.

J29		=	=((J$28-$H29)^2/(2/12))/$N$6	
	G	H	I	J	K
27	Admission			1	2	3
28				3898.89	3926.92	5714.56
29		1	3898.89	0	0.00131	5.494192
30		2	3926.92		0	5.325845
31		3	5714.56			0
32						
33	Admission			1	2	3
34				3898.89	3926.92	5714.56
35		1	3898.89		0.971457	0.028519
36		2	3926.92			0.030798
37		3	5714.56			
38						
39	p		0.017			

Figure 10.13 Comparison across three admissions

Table 10.6   Formulas for Figure 10.13

Cell or Column	Formula	Action/Note
J29	=((J$28-$H29)^2/(2/12))/$N$6	Copied to cells K29 and K30
J35	=FDIST(J29,1,22)	Copied to cells K35 and K36; the degrees of freedom are determined as 1 and 22 because two entities are being compared (i.e., $2 - 1 = 1$) in the numerator while the denominator has the same degrees of freedom as the MS_R (i.e., $(3 - 1)*(12 - 1)$).

Excel Add-In for Analysis of Variance with Repeated Measures

Excel does not provide a specific add-in for analysis of variance with repeated measures when only one group is under consideration (in this case, the one group is the 12 people, each of whom was admitted to the hospital three times). Excel does provide a repeated measures ANOVA when there is more than one group and more than one measure on each group. This is later discussed (in Section 10.3) as what is known as a *factorial design*.

EXERCISES FOR SECTION 10.2

1. Use the data given on the Readmit worksheet of Chpt 10-1.xls to replicate the analysis of cost of readmissions shown in Figures 10.9 and 10.10.

   a. Calculate SS_W—the variation within people—using the pivot table with person as the row variable (the pivot table should match that in cells G2:H16 in Figure 10.9) and the formula in Equation 10.8.

   b. Calculate SS_A—the variation due to differences in admission costs—using the pivot table with admission as the row variable (the pivot table should match that in cells G18:H23 in Figure 10.9) and the formula in Equation 10.9.

   c. Calculate SS_R—the residual variation—on a separate worksheet, using the formula in Equation 10.10, and confirm that it is equal to $SS_W - SS_A$.

   d. Calculate SS_B—the variation between people—using the pivot table in cells G2:H16 in Figure 10.9 and the formula in Equation 10.11.

   e. Calculate SS_T—the total variation—following the formula in Equation 10.3.

   f. Replicate the calculation of the F test statistic for the effect of readmission on cost, following the example in Figure 10.10.

   g. Use the formula in Equation 10.12 to replicate the results of the test of individual differences given in Figure 10.13.

2. The data on the HbA1c worksheet represent four measures of HbA1c readings for 10 people on an exercise and diet regimen. The measures were taken at equal intervals over the course of a year. Replicate the analysis of repeated measures for these data by doing the following:

   a. Calculate SS_W—the variation within people—using the pivot table with person as the row variable and the formula in Equation 10.8.

   b. Calculate SS_A—the variation due to differences across measurements—using the pivot table with measure as the row variable and the formula in Equation 10.9.

   c. Calculate SS_R—the residual variation—on a separate worksheet, using the formula in Equation 10.10, and confirm that it is equal to $SS_W - SS_A$.

   d. Calculate SS_B—the variation between people—using the formula in Equation 10.11.

   e. Calculate SS_T—the total variation—following the formula in Equation 10.3.

   f. Calculate the F test statistic for the effect of measure, following the example in Figure 10.10.

   g. Use the formula in Equation 10.12 to replicate the results of the test of individual differences given in Figure 10.13.

10.3   Factorial Analysis of Variance

Analysis of variance, like many special topics in statistics, is one to which entire books have been devoted. This chapter considers only one further application of analysis of variance, generally referred to as a factorial design. There are many different types of factorial designs. The one considered here is that in which there is a single numerical variable as the dependent variable and two categorical independent variables. For example, suppose the hospital alliance was interested not only in the differences among the four hospitals of the alliance but also in whether these differences were related to the sex of the patient. To simplify the calculations—and to present some variety in topics—instead of dealing with the cost of admission, this example will deal with the length of stay.

Factorial Example Applied to Hospital Admissions: Length of Stay and Gender

Consider that each hospital in the alliance has divided its admissions for the past year into those for males and those for females. In addition, each hospital randomly selects admissions for 10 males and for 10 females to include in the study. For each of these admissions, the length of stay is recorded and the data are submitted to analysis of variance. Figure 10.14

H12 | =(H3-$J12-H$16+$J$16)^2

	A	B	C	D	E	F	G	H	I	J	K	L
1	Hospital	Sex	LOS	SST	SSWC		Average of LOS	Sex ▾				
2	Albemarle	Male	4	4	0.16		Hospital ▾	Female	Male	Grand Total	SShosp	
3	Albemarle	Male	3	9	0.36		Albemarle	5.3	3.6	4.45	2.4025	
4	Albemarle	Male	5	1	1.96		Beaufort	6	4	5	1	
5	Albemarle	Male	4	4	0.16		Catawba	10.8	7.1	8.95	8.7025	
6	Albemarle	Male	8	4	19.36		Dare	6.2	5	5.6	0.16	
7	Albemarle	Male	6	0	5.76		Grand Total	7.075	4.925	6		
8	Albemarle	Male	3	9	0.36		SSsex	1.1556	1.1556			
9	Albemarle	Male	1	25	6.76							
10	Albemarle	Male	1	25	6.76		SShosp*sex	Sex				
11	Albemarle	Male	1	25	6.76		Hospital	Female	Male	Grand Total		
12	Beaufort	Male	3	9	1		Albemarle	0.0506	0.0506	4.45		
13	Beaufort	Male	1	25	9		Beaufort	0.0056	0.0056	5		
14	Beaufort	Male	3	9	1		Catawba	0.6006	0.6006	8.95		
15	Beaufort	Male	1	25	9		Dare	0.2256	0.2256	5.6		
16	Beaufort	Male	1	25	9		Grand Total	7.075	4.925	6		
17	Beaufort	Male	2	16	4							
18	Beaufort	Male	4	4	0			SS	df	MS	F	prob
19	Beaufort	Male	7	1	9		SShosp	245.3	3	81.77	4.53	0.0057
20	Beaufort	Male	13	49	81		SSsex	92.45	1	92.45	5.13	0.0266
21	Beaufort	Male	5	1	1		SShosp*sex	17.65	3	5.88	0.33	0.8064
22	Catawba	Male	2	16	26.01		SSWC	1298.6	72	18.04		
23	Catawba	Male	7	1	0.01		SST	1654	79			

Figure 10.14   ANOVA factorial analysis

shows the entire analysis of variance for the data derived from the sample of 10 males and 10 females, taken from each of the four hospitals. Column A shows the name of the hospital. Only the first 22 of 80 admissions are shown in the figure. All entries are males, and 10 are for Albemarle, 10 for Beaufort, and 2 for Catawba. Column B shows the sex of the person admitted. Column C shows the length of stay (LOS). Columns D and E are used in the calculations and are discussed later.

Table 10.7 contains the formulas for the calculations in Figure 10.14.

The first step in the analysis of variance is to obtain the mean LOS by hospital, by sex, and by sex for hospitals. These values are given in the pivot table, beginning in cell G1. The values in this pivot table were obtained using the average option, as was used in Figure 10.3 and Figure 10.9.

Calculation of SS_T: Total Sum of Squares Variation

Column D shows the initial calculations for SS_T, the total sums of squares. SS_T is one of the least important calculations. However, it is also one of the easiest and is therefore presented first. The formula for total sum of squares is given in Equation 10.13. Although the formula in Equation 10.13 appears complex with its triple summation signs, it is not. The symbols q and m in the formula refer to the number of levels of the first factor and the second factor, respectively. If we consider hospitals as the first factor, then there are four of these, so $q = 4$. Sex, then, is the second factor, and there are obviously two levels for sex and $m = 2$. The formula says to begin with the first person for the first hospital and sex group; following the

Table 10.7   Formulas for Figure 10.14

Cell or Column	Formula	Action/Note
		Create a pivot table for the data with Gender as the columns and Hospital as the rows.
D2	`=(C2-$J$7)^2`	Copied from cell D2 to cell D81
E	For Males	
	`=(C2-$I$3)^2`	Copied from cells E2 : E11
	`=(C2-$I$4)^2`	Copied from cells E12 : E21
	`=(C2-$I$5)^2`	Copied from cells E22 : E31
	`=(C2-$I$6)^2`	Copied from cells E32 : E41
	For Females	
	`=(C2-$H$3)^2`	Copied from cells E42 : E51
	`=(C2-$H$4)^2`	Copied from cells E52 : E61
	`=(C2-$H$5)^2`	Copied from cells E62 : E71
	`=(C2-$H$6)^2`	Copied from cells E72 : E81
K3	`=(J3-$J$7)^2`	Copied from cell K3 to cells K4, K5, and K6
H8	`=(H7-$J$7)^2`	Copied from cell H8 to I8
J12H16	`=J3=H7`	Copied from cell J12 to cell J16 Copied from cell H16 to cell I16
H12	`=(H3-$J$12-H$16-$J$16)^2`	Copied from cell H12 to cells H13, H14, H15, I12, I13, I14, and I15
H19	`=20*SUM(K3:K6)`	Where 20 is $m*n$, and $m=2, n=10$
H20	`=40*SUM(H8:I8)`	Where 40 is $q*n$, and $q=4, n=10$
H21	`=10*SUM(H12:H15)`	Where 10 is n
H22	`=SUM(E2:E81)`	
H23	`=SUM(D2:D81)`	
I19	`=3`	Where 3 is $q-1$ and $q=4$
I20	`=1`	Where 1 is $m-1$ and $m=2$
I21	`=3`	Where 3 is $(q-1)*(m-1)$ and $q=4, m=2$
I22	`=72`	Where 72 is $q*m*(n-1)$ and $q=4, m=2, n=10$
I23	`=79`	Where 79 is $q*m*n-1$ and $q=4, m=2, n=10$
J19	`=H19/I19`	
J20	`=H20/I20`	
J21	`=H21/I21`	
J22	`=H22/I22`	
K19	`=H19/J$22`	Copied to cells K20 and K21
L19	`=FDIST(K19,I19,I$22)`	Copied to cells L20 and L21

presentation in Figure 10.14, that would be Albemarle and a male. For that person, subtract the grand mean across all hospitals, sex groupings, and people (hence $\overline{\overline{x}}$), square the result; do this for every person in each sex group across all four hospitals, and sum it all up.

Column D contains the first part of the calculation. The calculation is the square of the difference between each observation and the grand mean.

The Excel formula for the first cell in the column that contains a number (cell D2) is $= (C2 - \$J\$7)\,\verb|^|2$. The dollar sign (\$) convention ensures that the grand mean is always used in the subtraction as the formula is copied to each cell in column D. The sum of all 80 calculations in column D is given as SS_T in cell H23.

$$SS_T = \sum_{k=1}^{q}\sum_{j=1}^{m}\sum_{i=1}^{n}(x_{ijk} - \overline{\overline{\overline{x}}})^2 \qquad (10.13)$$

Calculation of SS_{WC}: Sum of Squares within Cells Variation

The next sum of squares that may be discussed is SS_{WC}, which is the sum of squares within cells. The sum of squares within cells is that portion of the variation in the data that cannot be attributed either to the admitting hospital or to sex of the patient. Consequently, in this example, SS_{WC} is the error variance. It is calculated using the formula in Equation 10.14, which indicates that a mean value is subtracted from every observation, squared, and summed across all 80 patients. But in this case, the mean value that is subtracted is the mean for each hospital and sex grouping. These mean values are those in cells H3 : I6 in Figure 10.14. The initial calculation for SS_{WC} is carried out in column E. The Excel formula for cell E2 is $= (C2 - \$I\$3)\,\verb|^|2$. Cell I3, however, is in the terms given in Equation 10.14 or in this case only the term $\overline{x}_{11}$. It is the appropriate term to be subtracted only from the first 10 observations (males in Albemarle). For males in Beaufort, the appropriate term changes to cell I4, and so on. This can be a little tedious, but it is necessary for the calculation. The sum of all the calculations in column E is given in cell H22 as 1298.6.

$$SS_{WC} = \sum_{k=1}^{q}\sum_{j=1}^{m}\sum_{i=1}^{n}(x_{ijk} - \overline{x}_{jk})^2 \qquad (10.14)$$

Calculation of SS_{rows}: Sum of Squares between Rows Variation

The sum of squares due to the differences between hospitals are given in Equation 10.15. The equation is given as SS_{rows}, because hospitals are the rows in the pivot table in Figure 10.14. It should be clear that this is a general formula that applies to any two-factor factorial design, not just to this specific one. The formula for SS_{rows} says that the overall average for all 80 observations is subtracted from the average for each hospital. This average is calculated across all people in a given hospital and both sex groups, hence the designation $\overline{\overline{x}}_q$. That result is then squared and added across all four hospitals. Because there are m times n, or 20 observations for each hospital, the resulting sum is multiplied by 20. The first step in the calculation of SS_{rows}, or, in this case, SS_{hosp}, is given in cells K3:K6. The Excel formula for cell K3 is $= (J3-\$J\$7)\wedge2$. The formula in cell K3 can then be copied to the other three cells. The sum of the cells K3:K6 is then multiplied by m times n in cell H19. The Excel formula for H19 is $=20*sum(K3:K6)$.

$$SS_{rows} = mn \sum_{k=1}^{q}(\bar{\bar{x}}_q - \bar{\bar{x}})^2 \tag{10.15}$$

Calculation of SS_{cols}: Sum of Squares between Columns Variation

The sum of squares due to differences by sex are calculated in essentially the same way as the sum of squares due to hospitals. Because sex is the column designation in the pivot table in Figure 10.14, the formula for the sum of squares due to sex is given as SS_{cols} in Equation 10.16. It can be seen that Equations 10.15 and 10.16 are quite similar. The initial computation of SS_{cols}—in this case SS_{sex}—is given in cells H8 and I8 in Figure 10.14. The Excel formula for cell H8 is $= (H7-\$G\$7)\wedge2$. The sum of cell H8 and cell I8 is multiplied by q times n ($q*n=40$) in cell H20.

$$SS_{cols} = qn \sum_{j=1}^{m}(\bar{\bar{x}}_m - \bar{\bar{x}})^2 \tag{10.16}$$

Calculation of $SS_{rows \cdot cols}$: Sum of Squares Due to Interaction Variation

The only sum of squares left to calculate is what is known as the sum of squares due to interaction. In a factorial design, SS_{rows} and SS_{cols} (or the sum of squares due to the hospitals and the sum of squares due to sex) are known as *main effects*. But there may also be an effect that is due to what is called interaction. The computation of the sum of squares due to interaction is given in Equation 10.17. This equation says to take the mean for each sex and hospital ($\bar{x}_{jk}$), subtract the appropriate mean for sex ($\bar{\bar{x}}_j$) and the appropriate mean for hospital ($\bar{\bar{x}}_k$), add the grand mean ($\bar{\bar{x}}$), square the result, and add it across all sex and hospital groups. The initial calculation of $SS_{rows \cdot cols}$—in this case, $SS_{hosp \cdot sex}$—is carried out in cells H12:I15. The Excel formula for cell H12, following Equation 10.17, is given in the formula bar in Figure 10.14. The result of the calculations is found in cell H21. It sums cells H12:I15 and multiplies that result by n

(which is 3 in this case). As an overall check of the variation calculations, you can confirm that the sum of cells H19 : H22 is equal to SS_T in cell H23.

$$SS_{rows \cdot cols} = n \sum_{k=1}^{q} \sum_{j=1}^{m} \left(\bar{x}_{jk} - \bar{\bar{x}}_j - \bar{\bar{x}}_k + \bar{\bar{\bar{x}}} \right)^2 \qquad (10.17)$$

The degrees of freedom for this analysis are given in cells I19 : I23. These degrees of freedom are calculated according to the equations shown in Figure 10.15. It should also be noted that the degrees of freedom shown in cells I19 : I22 add to the total degrees of freedom in cell I23.

    There are three F tests of interest in this analysis. There is an F test for the main effect of hospitals, an F test for the main effect of sex, and an F test for the interaction between the two. The divisor in each of these F tests is the within cell variation SS_{WC}. The mean square values for each of these four elements are given in cells J19 : J22, and are the SS values divided by degrees of freedom. The F tests are given in cells K19 : K21, and the probabilities of these F values, based on =FDIST(), are given in cells L19 : L21. The conclusion from these F tests and their probabilities is that there is a main effect due to hospitals (length of stay is not independent of hospital) and a main effect due to sex (length of stay is not independent of sex), but there is no effect due to interaction.

Excel Add-In for Factorial ANOVA

Excel provides two add-ins in the Data Analysis package for factorial analysis of variance. Only one of those, ANOVA: Two-Factor with Replication, is discussed here. This is the analysis that will produce the results given in Figure 10.14. To carry out the analysis using ANOVA: Two-Factor with Replication, it is necessary first to rearrange the data in Figure 10.14 as they are shown in Figure 10.16. Only the observations for Albemarle and the first five observations for males and females, respectively, are shown for Beaufort in Figure 10.16. The remaining observations continue to row 41

	N	O
1		
2	rows	q-1
3	cols	m-1
4	rows*cols	(q-1)(m-1)
5	within cells	qm(n-1)
6	total	qmn-1
7		

Figure 10.15   Degrees of freedom in two-factor factorial ANOVA

Figure 10.16 Data arrangement for ANOVA: Two-Factor with Replication

of the spreadsheet. It should be clear that the observations for males are shown in column B and those for females are shown in column C. Also shown in Figure 10.16 is the ANOVA: Two-Factor with Replication dialog box for carrying out the analysis. In that dialog, the input range is given as $A$1:$C$41. This indicates that Excel recognizes that there will be a row of labels at the top of the data and a row of labels in the left column. Rows per sample is given as 10, which means Excel will appropriately treat each 10 rows as a different set of observations. The output range is given as $E$2, which means the output will begin in that cell.

ANOVA in Excel Using the Data Analysis Package: Step-by-Step Instructions

Follow these step-by-step instructions to invoke the Data Analysis package in Excel and complete the required inputs for ANOVA output.

1. Go to the Data ribbon, in the Analysis group, and click the Data Analysis option.

2. After you click the Data Analysis option, a screen resembling Figure 10.16 will appear. In that screen choose the ANOVA: Two-Factor with Replication option. A dialog box, as shown in Figure 10.16, will appear.

3. In the Input Range box, enter $A$1:$C$41 or highlight cells A1 through C41.

4. In the Rows per sample field, enter 10.

5. Click the Output Range radio button, and enter $E$2 in the field.

6. Click OK, and the ANOVA output will be created.

	E	F	G	H	I	J	K
36	ANOVA						
37	Source of Variation	SS	df	MS	F	P-value	F crit
38	Sample	245.3	3	81.77	4.53	0.0057	2.73
39	Columns	92.45	1	92.45	5.13	0.0266	3.97
40	Interaction	17.65	3	5.88	0.33	0.8064	2.73
41	Within	1298.6	72	18.04			
42							
43	Total	1654	79				
44							

Figure 10.17   Results of ANOVA: Two-Factor with Replication

Partial results of the ANOVA: Two-Factor with Replication are shown in Figure 10.17. Only the ANOVA table is shown in the figure, but several tables of averages precede the ANOVA results; they occupy rows 2 to 35 but are not shown in the figure. As the figure shows, the results of the Excel ANOVA add-in are the same as those calculated in Figure 10.16. The only difference is the value of F_{crit}, given in column K. Again, these are the levels that the F values would have to reach to be significant at the 0.05 level.

When one-way analysis of variance was discussed, we indicated that both the formulas and the Excel add-in allowed for different sample sizes across the different groups. Neither the formulas given in this section (for a two-factor ANOVA) nor the Excel add-in permits unequal group sample sizes. It is possible to carry out two- or multifactor analysis of variance with unequal sample sizes in groups. However, the analysis becomes much more complicated and is often more easily performed using dummy variables in multiple regression, which is discussed in Chapter 13.

Repeated Measures in a Factorial Design

The title of the Excel add-in ANOVA: Two-Factor with Replication suggests that at least one of the factors is being measured more than one time. However, using the ANOVA: Two-Factor with Replication add-in for a repeated measure design is not as straightforward as one might wish. As indicated in Figure 10.17, the results are not appropriate to repeated measures on the same set of persons or organizations. The results seen in Figure 10.17 are appropriate, as used in the figure, to a single measure on any included observation.

If the Excel add-in for ANOVA: Two-Factor with Replication is actually used to carry out analysis of variance in a factorial design wherein one variable is measured more than one time, some additional work must be done to get to the appropriate answers. To see that, let us consider a simple example. The data in Figure 10.18 show the length of stay for

	A	B	C
1		Male	Female
2	Admit 1	4	4
3		3	6
4		5	2
5		4	2
6		8	4
7	Admit 2	3	7
8		1	13
9		3	3
10		1	5
11		1	2
12	Admit 3	2	10
13		7	7
14		3	16
15		14	4
16		3	11

Figure 10.18 Simple data for repeated measures in a factorial design

five men and five women for three different hospital admissions. This represents a factorial design with repeated measures on one variable: hospital admissions. The observation in cell B2, 4, represents a four-day stay for the first man on the spreadsheet. Cell B7 represents the same person's length of stay for his second admission, and cell B12 represents his length of stay for his third admission. Similarly, the 4 in cell C2 represents the length of stay for the first woman on the spreadsheet. Her second stay is represented by cell C7, and her third stay is represented by cell C12. If we use the ANOVA: Two-Factor with Replication add-in to analyze these data, the result is as shown in Figure 10.19. The conclusion that one would draw from this analysis is that there is a difference among the three admissions, but not between the two sexes, in length of stay. This would be based on the fact that the probability for the F related to the samples (the three admissions) is less than 0.05, whereas the probability related to the columns (male and female) is not less than 0.05. We would also conclude no *interaction effects*.

	E	F	G	H	I	J	K
29							
30	ANOVA						
31	Source of Variation	SS	df	MS	F	P-value	F crit
32	Sample	89.26667	2	44.63333	3.735007	0.038705	3.402832
33	Columns	38.53333	1	38.53333	3.224547	0.085144	4.259675
34	Interaction	45.26667	2	22.63333	1.894003	0.172285	3.402832
35	Within	286.8	24	11.95			
36							
37	Total	459.8667	29				
38							

Figure 10.19 ANOVA results for repeated measures in a factorial design

Dividing within Cell Variation in Repeated Measures ANOVA

But this conclusion would not take into account the fact that the three admissions were for the same group of people. In comparing what is given in the ANOVA printout (Figure 10.19) with what is appropriate for a repeated measures design, Figure 10.20 (adapted from Winer 1962) is useful. As the figure shows, the between cell variation is the same for both repeated and nonrepeated measures. It can be divided into variation due to the columns, variation due to the rows, and the interaction between columns and rows. Where the nonrepeated measure design has only one error term, however—that being the within cell variation—the repeated measures design has two error terms. The within cell variation can be divided into variation due to subjects within groups (one source of error) and variation due to rows (the repeated measure) times subjects within groups (the second source of error). It turns out that the appropriate error term to construct the F test for differences between columns is subjects within groups, whereas the appropriate error term for differences between rows and for the column and row interaction is rows times subjects within groups. Thus, the F test for nonrepeated measures is not appropriate for the repeated measures case.

Using Excel to Calculate within Cell Variation

To find the values for subjects within groups and for rows times subjects within groups, it is necessary to have the mean value for each person across all measures, something not produced by the Excel add-in. Figure 10.21 shows the analysis for two factors when one is a repeated measure. The average for each person across all measures is obtained in cells E2 : F6.

	N	O	P	Q	R	S	T
1	Two variable factorial design				Two variable factorial design		
2	No repeated measures				Repeated meaures on rows		
3	Variation		df		Variation		df
4	Total		qmn-1		Total		qmn-1
5	Between Cells		qm-1		Between Cells		qm-1
6	Columns		m-1		Columns		m-1
7	Rows		q-1		Rows		q-1
8	Columns*Rows		(m-1)(q-1)		Columns*Rows		(m-1)(q-1)
9							
10	Within Cells		qm(n-1)		Within Cells		qm(n-1)
11						Subjects within		m(n-1)
12						Groups		
13						Rows * Subjects		m(n-1)(q-1)
14						within Groups		
15							

Figure 10.20   Sources of variation and degrees of freedom in factorial designs

E2		▼		=	=AVERAGE(B2,B7,B12)	
	A	**B**	**C**	**D**	**E**	**F**	**G**

	A	B	C	D	E	F	G
1		Male	Female				
2	Admit 1	4	4		3	7	
3		3	6		3.667	8.667	
4		5	2		3.667	7	
5		4	2		6.333	3.667	
6		8	4		4	5.667	
7	Admit 2	3	7				
8		1	13		1.284	0.360	
9		3	3		0.218	5.138	
10		1	5		0.218	0.360	
11		1	2		4.840	7.471	
12	Admit 3	2	10		0.018	0.538	
13		7	7				
14		3	16		4.133333	6.4	
15		14	4				
16		3	11				
17							
18	Source		SS	df	MS	F	p
19	Between Subj		99.8667	9			
20	Sex		**38.5333**	1	38.53333	5.026087	0.055262
21	Subj w G		61.3333	8	7.666667		
22							
23	Within Subjects		360	20			
24	Admissions		**89.2667**	2	44.63333	3.167357	0.069361
25	Admissions * Sex		**45.2667**	2	22.63333	1.60615	0.23138
26	Admissions*subj w G		225.467	16	14.09167		
27							
28	Total		459.867	29			
29							

Figure 10.21 Appropriate analysis for repeated measures, two-factor design

As there are 10 people, there are 10 averages. The way in which the average is produced is shown in the formula bar. This can be copied directly to all the cells in E2:F6 to obtain the appropriate average values. Cells E14 and F14 contain the overall average for men and the overall average for women. The formula for the sum of squares for subjects within groups is given in Equation 10.18. This equation says to take the average for each person across all three measures. The designation $\bar{x}_{k(ij)}$ means that the ij observations are nested within the k measures. From the average the overall mean is subtracted for each level of j. The result is then squared, summed, and multiplied by the number of repeated measures.

$$SS_{subjwG} = q \sum_{j=1}^{m} \sum_{k=1}^{n} (\bar{x}_{k(ij)} - \bar{\bar{x}}_j)^2 \tag{10.18}$$

The initial steps in this operation can be seen in cells E8:F12. Cells E14 and F14 contain the mean for each sex group ($\bar{\bar{x}}_j$). The Excel formula for cell E8 is $= (E2 - E\$14)^{\wedge}2$. The dollar sign (\$) convention allows this formula to be copied to every cell in E8:F12 to produce the terms to be summed for subjects within groups. The formula is completed in cell C21 by multiplying the sum of E8:F12 by 3, the number of repeated measures.

The appropriate analysis of variance table is shown in cells A18 : G28. The sources of variation are divided into those that are between subjects and those that are within subjects. The three quantities in bold are those that came from the Excel analysis shown in Figure 10.19. Subjects within groups, plus the column variable—sex—adds to the total between subjects variation of 99.87. Subtracting the between subjects variation from the total variation (cell C28) provides the total for within subjects variation. Subtracting the two values given in Figure 10.19 for admissions and the interaction term produces the term admissions times subjects within groups. The degrees of freedom appropriate to each of these sources of variation are given in column D. The appropriate F test for the difference between the sexes is the mean square for sex divided by the mean square for subjects within groups. The appropriate F test for both admissions and the interaction term requires the mean square for admissions times subjects within groups as the divisor. When these appropriate tests are carried out, we would no longer conclude that there is a difference across admissions, as we incorrectly concluded in Figure 10.19. Table 10.8 contains the formulas for the ANOVA Factorial Analysis in Figure 10.21.

ANOVA and Lean/Six Sigma Practices within the Health Care Industry

It must be noted that ANOVA does not stand alone when applied out in the field. The vast majority of the time it is employed under the auspices of Lean and Six Sigma. Lean and Six Sigma are approaches to improving processes. Manufacturing has applied Lean/Six Sigma to production systems very successfully over the past 30 years in one shape or form (e.g., statistical process control, Toyota Production System, just-in-time inventory). Although health care professionals do not like to think of health care as a production system, health care does have a production system. However, health care workers are not production workers but knowledge workers. In turn, the principles of Lean and Six Sigma can be applied to health care.

The goal of Lean is to reduce waste and cut lead times, while the goal of Six Sigma is to reduce variation and improve quality. ANOVA is employed in the Six Sigma arena to analyze data and ferret out where process variation

Table 10.8   Formulas for Figure 10.21

Cell or Column	Formula	Action/Note
E2	=AVERAGE(B2,B7,B12)	Copied from cells E2:F6
E8	=(E2-E$14)^2	Copied from cells E8:F12
E14	=AVERAGE(B2:B16)	Copied from cells E14:F14
C21	=3*SUM(E8:E12)	Where 3 is q
C20	=38.53333	Given in previous ANOVA, Figure 10.19
C19	=C20+C21	This creates the between subjects source variation.
C23	=C28-C19	This creates the total within subjects variation.
C26	=C23-C24-C25	This creates the within subjects interaction variation for admissions and subjects within groups.
D19	=9	Where 9 is $m*n-1$, $m=2$, $n=5$
D20	=1	Where 1 is $m-1$, $m=2$
D21	=8	Where 8 is $m*(n-1)$, $m=2$, $n=5$
D23	=20	Where 20 is $m*n*(q-1)$, $m=2$, $n=5$, $q=3$
D24	=2	Where 2 is $q-1$, $q=3$
D25	=2	Where 2 is $(m-1)*(q-1)$, $m=2$, $q=3$
D26	=16	Where 16 is $m*(n-1)*(q-1)$, $m=2$, $n=5$, $q=3$
E20	=C20/D20	Copied to cell E21
E24	=C24/D24	Copied to cells E25 and E26
F20	=E20/E21	Copied to cells F24 and F25
G20	=FDIST(F20,D20,D21)	
G24	=FDIST(F24,D24,D$26)	Copied to cell G25

occurs. Most health care professionals understand hypothesis testing and its use in areas such as medical/drug testing. However, simply put, hypothesis testing and in turn ANOVA are employed to find out "what depends on what." For example, "Does lab testing lateness depend on day of the week?" By employing ANOVA to analyze changes made to a process (e.g., alter the lab testing schedules), the source of variation can be identified and i process changes can then be implemented that reduce the identified variation. All this leads to the goal of Six Sigma, reduced variation, while pushing to meet the goal of Lean, which is waste reduction and reduced lead times. In all, ANOVA is a very powerful tool within the Lean Six Sigma arena to identify variation and begin the improvement process. It should be noted that entire textbooks and courses are dedicated to Lean Six Sigma. The authors encourage readers to seek out material in these topics as this is only a very brief statement on the area of Lean Six Sigma.

EXERCISES FOR SECTION 10.3

1. Use the data on the LOS worksheet in Chpt 10–1.xls, and replicate the analysis given in Figure 10.14.

    a. Replicate the pivot table given in cells G1 : J7 in Figure 10.14.

    b. Use the formula in Equation 10.13 to calculate SS_T as shown in column D in Figure 10.14.

    c. Use the formula in Equation 10.14 to calculate SS_{WC} as shown in column E in Figure 10.14.

    d. Use the formula in Equation 10.15 to calculate SS_{rows} (difference between hospitals) as shown in column K and cell H19 in Figure 10.14.

    e. Use the formula in Equation 10.16 to calculate SS_{cols} (difference between sexes) as shown in cells H8 : I8 and H20 in Figure 10.14.

    f. Use the formula in Equation 10.17 to calculate $SS_{rows \cdot cols}$ (interaction between hospital and sex) as shown in cells H12 : I15 and cell H21 in Figure 10.14.

    g. Determine the appropriate degrees of freedom, calculate the mean square values, and carry out the F tests as shown in cells I18 : K23 in Figure 10.14.

2. The data on the Wait worksheet of Chpt 10–1.xls represent the waiting time in minutes for 72 emergency room visits. The visits were randomly selected with 12 taken from among true emergencies and 12 taken from among nonemergencies for each of three shifts. Use the factorial analysis of variance to determine whether there is a difference between shifts and between emergencies and nonemergencies in waiting time in the emergency room.

    a. Replicate the pivot table given in cells G1 : J7 in Figure 10.14 for the Wait data.

    b. Use the formula in Equation 10.13 to calculate SS_T as shown in column D in Figure 10.14 for the Wait data.

    c. Use the formula in Equation 10.14 to calculate SS_{WC} as shown in column E in Figure 10.14 for the Wait data.

    d. Use the formula in Equation 10.15 to calculate SS_{rows} (difference by emergency status) as shown in column K and cell H19 in Figure 10.14 for the Wait data.

    e. Use the formula in Equation 10.16 to calculate SS_{cols} (difference between shifts) as shown in cells H8 : I8 and H20 in Figure 10.14 for the Wait data.

    f. Use the formula in Equation 10.17 to calculate $SS_{rows \cdot cols}$ (interaction between shift and emergency) as shown in cells H12 : I15 and cell H21 in Figure 10.14 for the Wait data.

g. Determine the appropriate degrees of freedom, calculate the mean square values, and carry out the *F* tests as shown in cells I18 : K23 in Figure 10.14 to determine if there is a main effect of emergency status, a main effect of shift, or an interaction.

3. Rearrange the data for hospital LOS as given in Figure 10.16, and carry out the analysis of variance using the ANOVA: Two-Factor with Replication add-in. Confirm that the results are the same as those found in Exercise 1.

4. Rearrange the data for waiting time in the emergency room with shift as the column variable (three columns) and emergency or other as the row variable (first 12 rows emergency, last 12 rows other), and carry out the analysis of variance using the ANOVA: Two-Factor with Replication add-in. Confirm that the results are the same as those found in Exercise 2.

5. Use the data on the worksheet Readmit2 in Chpt 10–1.xls, and replicate the analysis given in Figure 10.21.

   a. Generate the ANOVA: Two-Factor with Replication results for the data on the Readmit2 worksheet as the first step.

   b. Generate the appropriate sum of squares for subjects within groups, using the formula in Equation 10.18.

   c. Complete the analysis as shown in cells A18 : H28 in Figure 10.21.

6. The data on the Test-Retest worksheet of Chpt 10–1.xls represent 18 women who were randomly assigned to three educational formats at a breast cancer screening clinic. Six women received no educational intervention, six women received a pamphlet, and six received face-to-face information from a physician. The women were measured on a 20-point scale of knowledge at the beginning and at the end of the visit. Replicate the analysis in Figure 10.21 for these women.

   a. Generate the ANOVA: Two-Factor with Replication results for the data on the Test-Retest worksheet as the first step.

   b. Generate the appropriate sum of squares for subjects within groups, using the formula in Equation 10.18.

   c. Complete the analysis as shown in the cells in Figure 10.21, using Figure 10.20 for the appropriate degrees of freedom.

KEY TERMS

=CHIDIST()	factorial design
=FDIST()	interaction effect
=FINV()	main effect
analysis of variance	pivot table
Bartlett test	repeated measures
between group variance	sum of squares
degrees of freedom	within group variance

CHAPTER 11

SIMPLE LINEAR REGRESSION

I can prove anything by statistics except the truth.

—George Canning

Linear regression is a statistical method for determining the relationship between one or more *independent variables* and a single *dependent variable*. In this chapter we look at what is called simple linear regression. Simple linear regression is the relationship between a single independent variable and a single dependent variable.

11.1 Meaning and Calculation of Linear Regression

> Linear regression is a method of organizing data that uses the least squares method to determine which line best fits the data.

To examine what is meant by the relationship between an independent variable and a dependent variable, consider the four graphs shown in Figure 11.1. The figure shows examples of four different possible relationships between two variables. The black points in each graph represent individual observations (50 in all but difficult to count). The horizontal axis (from 0 to 20) represents the value of any individual observation on the independent variable. This variable is commonly designated x. The vertical axis (from 0 to 20) represents the value of each individual observation on the dependent variable. The dependent

Figure 11.1 Examples of relationships

variable is commonly designated y. So if one looks at the point farthest to the right in chart (a), that individual observation has a value of approximately 15 on the variable x (the horizontal axis) and 15 on the variable y (the vertical axis). If we look at the point farthest to the right in chart (b), that observation has a value of approximately 15 on the variable x, but about 5 on the variable y.

Analyzing Relationships between Dependent and Independent Variables

Each of the charts in Figure 11.1 demonstrates a possible relationship, briefly described in the chart title, between the variable x and the variable y. Chart (a) shows a positive relationship between x and y. This means that observations with larger values of x tend also to have larger values of y. Chart (b) shows a negative relationship between x and y. In this case, observations with larger values of x tend to have smaller values of y. In general, knowing something about x in either chart (a) or chart (b) will allow you to predict something about y even if you have no other knowledge of y.

Chart (c) shows another type of relationship between x and y—in this case, no relationship at all. In chart (c), observations with small values of x tend to have both large and small values of y, and observations with large values of x also appear to have both large and small values of y. In general, knowing something about the value of x is no better than knowing nothing about x in predicting values of y for data that conform to chart (c). Chart (d) shows yet a different type of relationship between x and y, one that is called a nonlinear relationship. In chart (d), knowledge of x will provide a better prediction of y than no knowledge of x, but because the relationship is not linear, simple linear regression, as discussed in this chapter, will not be adequate to describe the relationship. Simple linear regression will provide us with no useful information about chart (d).

Chapter 13 discusses ways to adapt *regression analysis* to deal with chart (d), but, for now, only linear relationships will be discussed. Producing charts with Microsoft Excel is important and fairly easy (see Chapter 2). Charts give us the ability to determine whether linear regression can adequately describe a relationship.

Linear Regression: Fitting a Line to Data

Linear regression can describe the data in chart (a) and chart (b) in Figure 11.1, but what does that mean? What it means is that the regression process will assign a *best-fitting straight line* to the data. What does best-fitting mean? We will soon provide a formal definition of best-fitting, but for now, think of it as a line through the data that goes through the means of both x and y and comes as close as possible to all the points in the data set. Consider specifically chart (a) in Figure 11.1. This chart is reproduced as Figure 11.2. In addition to the data points shown in Figure 11.1, Figure 11.2 shows the best-fitting straight line. This is the line that comes closest to all points in the data set while at the same time going through the true mean of both x and y.

A straight line in a two-dimensional space (the space defined by the values of x on the horizontal axis and y on the vertical axis) can be described with an equation, as shown in Equation 11.1. Any point on the line is the joint graphing of a selected value of x and the value of y defined by Equation 11.1. If we know that b_1 is 0.5 and b_0 is 2, then if x is 5, y will be 4.5. If x is 10, y will be 7. If x is 0, y will be 2.

$$y = b_1 x + b_0 \tag{11.1}$$

Figure 11.2 Positive relationship with the best-fitting straight line

The Equation of a Line: Slope Intercept Form

In Equation 11.1, the two coefficients b_1 and b_0 have particular meanings. The coefficient b_1 is frequently referred to as the slope of the line. In concrete terms, b_1 is the distance the line rises in a vertical direction as x increases by one unit. So if x increases from 2 to 3, y increases by one half unit. The coefficient b_0 is frequently referred to as the intercept of the line. It represents specifically the point at which the line crosses the y-axis, or the value of y when x is equal to 0.

If we are representing the points in Figure 11.2 with the best-fitting straight line, we must recognize that most of the points do not fall on the straight line. Actually, almost none of them do. To account for this, the equation shown in Equation 11.1 is likely to be modified in one of two ways, both shown in Equation 11.2. The representation in Equation 11.2a indicates that the straight-line equation is only an estimate of the true value of y. The $\hat{y}$ designation (pronounced y hat by statisticians) indicates that the value produced by the straight-line equation is an estimate of the true value of y. The representation in Equation 11.2b is the actual value of y rather than an estimate. The e at the end of the equation indicates that some value e (termed the error) must be added to the formula in order to produce the true value of y.

$$\hat{y} = b_1 x + b_0 \tag{11.2a}$$

$$y = b_1 x + b_0 + e \tag{11.2b}$$

What Does Regression Mean in Practical Terms?

To get a better understanding of what a straight-line prediction of y by x means in practical terms, let us consider 20 hospital admissions, the length of stay of each admission, and the charges for the stay. Figure 11.3 shows data on 20 hospital admissions that were randomly selected from a file of 2,000 admissions. First, regression is a statistical test of the independence of the two variables—the length of stay and the total charges. The implicit null hypothesis is that the two variables are independent. If we reject that null hypothesis, we are left with the conclusion that the two variables are dependent on each other. But the nature of this dependence is very explicit. If we look back at Equations 11.2a or 11.2b, either indicates explicitly that the value of y is dependent on the value of x but not the other way around. In terms of the data shown for the 20 hospital stays in Figure 11.3, it is quite likely that total charges are dependent on the length of stay. However, it would make little logical sense to suggest that the length of hospital stay was dependent on what was charged for the stay.

	A	B	C
1	Stay	LOS	Charges
2	1	3	$2,614
3	2	5	$4,307
4	3	2	$2,449
5	4	3	$2,569
6	5	3	$1,936
7	6	5	$7,231
8	7	5	$5,343
9	8	3	$4,108
10	9	1	$1,597
11	10	2	$4,061
12	11	2	$1,762
13	12	5	$4,779
14	13	1	$2,078
15	14	3	$4,714
16	15	4	$3,947
17	16	2	$2,903
18	17	1	$1,439
19	18	1	$820
20	19	1	$3,309
21	20	6	$5,476
22			

Figure 11.3 Twenty hospital stays

Furthermore, what does it mean to reject the null hypothesis of independence? Because regression deals with linear relationships, rejecting the null hypothesis of independence would mean finding a linear relationship between, for example, the length of stay and the charges for which the slope of the line could be determined to be different from zero. To see if it is likely that we will be able to find such a straight line, consider the graph of the length of stay and the charges as shown in Figure 11.4. In Figure 11.4 it is possible to see that the data from the 20 hospitals suggest that as the

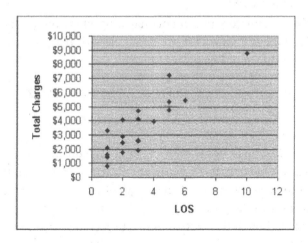

Figure 11.4 Length of stay and charges

length of stay increases, total charges also increase. The short lengths of stay have the lowest costs, and the longer lengths of stay have the highest costs. The single 10-day stay has the highest cost of all.

The Linear Relationship: How Is it Determined?

The data also appear to show a linear relationship. It is relatively easy to imagine a straight line that begins at about $2,000 when LOS is 1 day and then goes up to about $9,000 when LOS is 10 days. Imagining such a straight line, we could say that its slope—that is, the change in the dollar value of total charges as LOS changes by one day—is the difference between $2,000 and $9,000, divided by the difference between 1 day of stay and 10 days of stay. If we accept this logic, the slope of the straight line through the data in Figure 11.4 could be tentatively calculated as given in Equation 11.3. From a practical standpoint, then, we could conclude that for these hospitals (and the hospitals from which the sample of 20 was taken), as the length of stay increases by one day, the total charges increase by $777.78.

$$\text{Slope} = b_1 = (\$9,000 - \$2,000)/(10 - 1) = \$777.78 \tag{11.3}$$

Furthermore, by finding the dollar value of the straight line at any point along its path, we can predict what the actual dollar value of any number of days of stay will be. Typically, the dollar value that is used as the reference point for setting the position of the line for all points is the dollar value of 0 on the *x-axis*. Although a hospital stay of zero days may not actually exist, the straight line through the data will cross the *y*, or vertical, *axis* at some point. That point, known as the intercept, could be calculated as $2,000 (the cost of a one-day stay) minus $777.78 (the slope of the line) or, as given in Equation 11.4, $1,222.22.

Based on the simple expedient of imagining where the straight line runs through the data in Figure 11.4, we come up with the predictor equation for charges, as shown in Equation 11.5.

$$\text{Intercept} = b_0 = \$2,000 - \$777.78 = \$1,222.22 \tag{11.4}$$

$$\text{Charges} = \$777.78 \text{ LOS} + \$1,222.22 \tag{11.5}$$

Equation 11.5 matches the format of a straight line, as it is given in Equation 11.1. What does this mean in practical terms? It means that if a hospital wishes to project the cost of any length of stay in the hospital, it can do so by multiplying the length of stay by $777.78 and adding a constant amount of $1,222.22. Although this will not indicate precisely what the charges for any individual stay will be, it can be a good guideline on the average.

But before we can accept this result as a good guideline for anticipating the total charges, we must be able to reject the null hypothesis of independence between the charges and the length of stay. We have so far done nothing that would allow us to reject that null hypothesis, although we would feel, just by looking at the data in Figure 11.4, that we should reject that hypothesis in favor of the explicit hypothesis given in Equation 11.5. Equation 11.5 states that charges are dependent on the length of stay. Furthermore, though we have found a line that may seem to fit the data, we may not necessarily have found the best-fitting straight line. Both of these issues are taken up in the next section.

Calculating Regression Coefficients

In the previous section we considered how we might estimate *regression coefficients* based on a simple examination of the plot of the data in a two-dimensional space. In this section we actually calculate the coefficients, using formulas that produce the exact coefficients b_1 and b_0. These coefficients are then used to create the best-fitting straight line through the data. At this point, it is probably useful to define the best-fitting straight line formally. The best-fitting straight line is the line that minimizes the sum of squared differences between each individual data point and the line predicted by the coefficients. The formal definition of a best-fitting straight line can be seen in Equation 11.6.

$$\sum (y - \hat{y})^2 = min \tag{11.6}$$

Given the formal definition of a best-fitting straight line, as shown in Equation 11.6, the two formulas for the coefficients b_1 and b_0 are as given in Equations 11.7 and 11.8. The formulas in Equations 11.7 and 11.8 are derived using calculus.

The regression coefficient is the ratio of the covariation between both variables to the variation of the independent variable.

Some discussion of the derivation is developed in Chapter 12, but there is no assumption that you need to understand calculus in order to proceed.

$$b_1 = \frac{\sum (x - \bar{x}) * (y - \bar{y})}{\sum (x - \bar{x})^2} \tag{11.7}$$

$$b_0 = \bar{y} - b_1 \bar{x} \tag{11.8}$$

	G2		▾		≡ =E22/D22		
	A	B	C	D	E	F	G
1	Stay	LOS (x)	TC (y)	x-xbar	y-ybar		
2	1	3	$2,614	-0.15	-981.236	b1	$ 803.99
3	2	10	$8,769	6.85	5173.884	b0	$1,062.59
4	3	2	$2,449	-1.15	-1146.55		
5	4	3	$2,569	-0.15	-1026.45		
6	5	3	$1,936	-0.15	-1658.96		
7	6	5	$7,231	1.85	3635.564		
8	7	5	$5,343	1.85	1747.464		
9	8	3	$4,108	-0.15	512.984		
10	9	1	$1,597	-2.15	-1998.24		
11	10	2	$4,061	-1.15	466.134		
12	11	2	$1,762	-1.15	-1833.62		
13	12	5	$4,779	1.85	1184.044		
14	13	1	$2,078	-2.15	-1516.85		
15	14	3	$4,714	-0.15	1118.464		
16	15	4	$3,947	0.85	351.534		
17	16	2	$2,903	-1.15	-692.406		
18	17	1	$1,439	-2.15	-2156.3		
19	18	1	$820	-2.15	-2774.94		
20	19	1	$3,309	-2.15	-285.736		
21	20	6	$5,476	2.85	1881.184		
22		3.15	$3,595.15	94.55	76016.95		

Figure 11.5 Calculation of coefficients

Given the formulas in Equations 11.7 and 11.8, it is possible to proceed to find the coefficients for the best-fitting straight line mathematically rather than rely on the eyeball method. The calculations for finding the coefficients are developed in Figure 11.5.

Using Excel to Calculate the Regression Coefficients

In Figure 11.5, the means of the length of stay and the total charges are shown in cells B22 and C22, respectively. Each value of x minus the mean of x is shown in column D, and each value of y minus the mean of y is shown in column E. Cell D22, which is the denominator in the formula in Equation 11.7, takes advantage of the Excel =SUMSQ() function, which finds the sum of the squares of a stream of numbers. In this case, the function was invoked as =SUMSQ(D2:D21). Cell E22, which is the numerator in the formula in Equation 11.7, takes advantage of the Excel =SUMPRODUCT() function, which finds the sum of the product of two streams of numbers. In this case, the function was invoked as =SUMPRODUCT(D2:D21,E2:E21). The value of b_1, shown in cell G2, was calculated, as the formula bar shows, by dividing the value in cell E22 by that in cell D22. The value of b_0, shown in cell G3, was calculated by subtracting cells B22*G2 from cell C22.

Table 11.1 Formulas for Figure 11.5

Cell or Column	Formula	Action/Note
B22	=AVERAGE(B2:B21)	
C22	=AVERAGE(C2:C21)	
	=B2−B$22	Copied from cells D2:D21
E2	=C2−C$22	Copied from cells E2:E21
D22	=SUMSQ(D2:D21)	
E22	=SUMPRODUCT(D2:D21,E2:E21)	
G2	=E22/D22	
G3	=C22−G2*B22	

The result of this calculation is the set of coefficients b_1 and b_0 for a best-fitting straight line through the data, as defined by Equation 11.6. Although the coefficients are not exactly the same as those estimated by the eyeball method in the first subsection of Section 11.1, they are certainly of the same order of magnitude. Table 11.1 displays the formulas for the calculation of the linear regression coefficients in Figure 11.5.

EXERCISES FOR SECTION 11.1

1. Use the data on the Hospital charges worksheet of Chpt 4-1.xls, and generate the following *xy* charts. (The first variable in each case should be considered the independent variable.)

    a. Age with LOS

    b. Age with Charges

    c. Charges with Medicare

2. Which, if any, of the charts in (a), (b), or (c) (preceding) appear to be the best to fit a linear model and why? Which appear to be the worst?

3. Use the data on the HDI worksheet of Chpt 6-1.xls, and generate the following *xy* charts. (The first variable in each case should be considered the independent variable.)

    a. AdLit99 with LifeEx99

    b. GrossEnrol99 with LifeEx99

    c. GDP/c (PPP99) with LifeEx99

4. Which, if any, of the charts in (a), (b), or (c) (preceding) appear to be the best to fit a linear model and why? Which appear to be the worst?

5. Use the following values of b_1 and b_0 and the values of the independent variable x to determine the values of y, and graph the resulting numbers.

    a. $b_1 = .5, b_0 = 3, x = 2, 5, 9, 14$

    b. $b_1 = 1.2, b_0 = 2120, x = 225, 321, 452, 511$

    c. $b_1 = 2.73, b_0 = 534, x = 150, 231, 344, 427$

    d. $b_1 = .0002, b_0 = 60, x = 40, 60, 80, 100$

6. Use the data on the Charges worksheet of Chpt 11-1.xls to replicate the calculation of b_1 and b_0, shown in Figure 11.5.

7. The data on the U5Mort worksheet of Chpt 11-1.xls represent female literacy (FemLit) and under-five mortality (U5Mort) for 114 countries of the world, each having more than 1 million inhabitants. The data were taken from the *State of the World's Children 2001* (2000). Use these data to calculate b_1 and b_0 for FemLit as a predictor of U5Mort, following the example in Figure 11.5.

11.2   Testing the Hypothesis of Independence

We have determined the coefficients for the straight-line equation that best fits the data in Figures 11.4 and 11.5. The question now is, can we use this information to determine whether we will accept or reject the implicit null hypothesis of independence between the charges and the length of stay? In looking at the data, it appears clear that we should reject the null hypothesis, because the points so clearly show that as the length of stay increases, the charges increase. But we can calculate both a measure of the degree of this relationship and a statistical test for the null hypothesis.

Calculation of Total Variance

Both the calculation of the degree of the relationship and the statistical test (an F test) for the null hypothesis depend on calculating variances. In this case, the variances are all with respect to the dependent variable, y. The total variance in y is as shown in Equation 11.9, which is the mean of y subtracted from each value of y and the result squared and then summed across all values of y (thus SS_T, which stands for sum of squares—total).

$$SS_T = \sum (y - \bar{y})^2 \tag{11.9}$$

Dividing the Total Variance: Regression Variance and Error Variance

The total variance in y can be considered as being divided into two portions. One portion is that which can be accounted for with the knowledge of the regression coefficients. This portion is termed sum of squares due to regression, or SS_R, and shown in Equation 11.10. The second portion is that which cannot be accounted for with the knowledge of the regression coefficients. This portion is termed sum of squares due to error, or SS_E, shown in Equation 11.11. In both Equations 11.10 and 11.11, the representation is as given in Equation 11.2. Also, $SS_T = SS_R + SS_E$.

$$SS_R = \sum (\hat{y} - \bar{y})^2 \qquad (11.10)$$

$$SS_E = \sum (y - \hat{y})^2 \qquad (11.11)$$

Calculating the Degree of Relationship: R^2 or Coefficient of Determination

The calculation of the degree of the relationship between the length of stay and the charges is the calculation of a ratio of the amount of variation that can be accounted for by the regression line and the total variation. This ratio is sometimes called the coefficient of determination but is almost universally referred to as R^2. The formula for R^2 is given in Equation 11.12.

$$R^2 = SS_R/SS_T \qquad (11.12)$$

The calculation of the degree of the relationship between the length of stay and the charges is the calculation of a ratio of the amount of variation that can be accounted for by the regression line and the total variation.

The calculation of R^2 is given in Figure 11.6, in which several of the calculations deserve explanation. The values in cells H2:H21 are calculated using the formula in Equation 11.2a. These are the predicted values of y ($\hat{y}$), based on the regression coefficients in cells G2 and G3. It should be noted that the average of the predicted values is exactly the same as the average of the actual values of y. This will always be true and is a way to check the accuracy of calculations. The values in cells I2:I21 represent the difference between the predicted values of y and the mean of y ($\hat{y} - \bar{y}$). The mean of this column, shown in cell I22, should always be 0. The values in cells J2:J21 represent the difference between each value of y and the predicted values of y ($y2\hat{y}$). Again, the mean of these data, shown in cell J22, will always be 0.

The total sum of squares (SS_T), shown in cell G5, were calculated using the =SUMSQ() function on cells E2:E21. The sum of squares that can be accounted for by the regression equation (SS_R)—typically called the sums of

	A	B	C	D	E	F	G	H	I	J
1	Stay	LOS (x)	TC (y)	x-xbar	y-ybar			yhat	yhat-ybar	y-yhat
2	1	3	$2,613.91	-0.15	-981.236	b1	$ 803.99	$3,474.55	-$120.60	-$860.64
3	2	10	$8,769.03	6.85	5173.884	b0	$ 1,062.59	$9,102.46	$5,507.31	-$333.43
4	3	2	$2,448.60	-1.15	-1146.55			$2,670.56	-$924.58	-$221.96
5	4	3	$2,568.70	-0.15	-1026.45	SST	78485804.6	$3,474.55	-$120.60	-$905.85
6	5	3	$1,936.19	-0.15	-1658.96	SSR	61116626.0	$3,474.55	-$120.60	-$1,538.36
7	6	5	$7,230.71	1.85	3635.564	SSE	17369178.6	$5,082.52	$1,487.38	$2,148.19
8	7	5	$5,342.61	1.85	1747.464			$5,082.52	$1,487.38	$260.09
9	8	3	$4,108.13	-0.15	512.984	R^2	0.7787	$3,474.55	-$120.60	$633.58
10	9	1	$1,596.91	-2.15	-1998.24			$1,866.57	-$1,728.57	-$269.66
11	10	2	$4,061.28	-1.15	466.134	MSR	61116626.0	$2,670.56	-$924.58	$1,390.72
12	11	2	$1,761.53	-1.15	-1833.62	MSE	964954.4	$2,670.56	-$924.58	-$909.03
13	12	5	$4,779.19	1.85	1184.044			$5,082.52	$1,487.38	-$303.33
14	13	1	$2,078.30	-2.15	-1516.85	F	63.3363	$1,866.57	-$1,728.57	$211.73
15	14	3	$4,713.61	-0.15	1118.464	p	2.64E-07	$3,474.55	-$120.60	$1,239.06
16	15	4	$3,946.68	0.85	351.534			$4,278.53	$683.39	-$331.85
17	16	2	$2,902.74	-1.15	-692.406	S.E.	982.3209	$2,670.56	-$924.58	$232.18
18	17	1	$1,438.85	-2.15	-2156.3	S.E.b1	101.0235	$1,866.57	-$1,728.57	-$427.72
19	18	1	$820.21	-2.15	-2774.94			$1,866.57	-$1,728.57	-$1,046.36
20	19	1	$3,309.41	-2.15	-285.736	t	7.96	$1,866.57	-$1,728.57	$1,442.84
21	20	6	$5,476.33	2.85	1881.184	p	2.64E-07	$5,886.51	$2,291.36	-$410.18
22		3.15	$3,595.15	94.55	76016.95			$3,595.15	$ 0.00	$ 0.00

Figure 11.6   Calculation of R^2 and F

squares due to regression—were calculated using the =SUMSQ() function on cells I2:I21. R^2, shown in cell G9, was calculated by Equation 11.12. The value of R^2 can range from 0.00 to 1.00 and literally means the proportion of variation in the dependent variable y that can be predicted, knowing the values of the independent variable x and the coefficients for the best-fitting straight line through the data. In this case, 78 percent of the variation in charges can be accounted for by knowledge of the length of stay. Table 11.2 displays the formulas for the calculation of R^2 and F for Figure 11.6.

Understanding Explained versus Unexplained Variance

The sum of squares due to error (SS_E)—that proportion of the variation in y that cannot be accounted for by knowledge of x, shown in G7—are calculated using the =SUMSQ() function on cells J2:J21. The unexplained portion of the variation, SS_E, accounts for the 22 percent of the variation in charges that cannot be accounted for by knowing the length of stay. The portion of the variation that can be accounted for by regression is known also as the explained variance, and the portion that cannot be accounted for is known as the unexplained variance.

It might be useful to consider again what explained variance and unexplained variance mean in terms of the chart first shown in Figure 11.4. That chart is reproduced in Figure 11.7, with several additions. The solid line sloping from the lower left to the upper right is the best-fitting straight line through the points, as defined by the regression coefficients calculated in Figure 11.6. The dashed horizontal line represents the mean of the

Table 11.2 Formulas for Figure 11.6

Cell or Column	Formula	Action/Note
H2	=G$2*B2+G$3	Copied from cells H2:H21
H22	=AVERAGE(H2:H21)	
I2	=H2−C$22	Copied from cells I2:I21
J2	=C2−H2	Copied from cells J2:J21
I22	=SUM(I2:I21)	
J22	=SUM(J2:J21)	
G5	=SUMSQ(E2:E21)	
G6	=SUMSQ(I2:I21)	
G7	=SUMSQ(J2:J21)	
G9	=G6/G5	
G11	=G6/1	G6 is divided by 1 because the degrees of freedom is 1.
G12	=G7/18	G6 is divided by 18 because the degrees of freedom is 20 minus 2.
G14	=G11/G12	
G15	=FDIST(G14,1,18)	Degrees of freedom are 1 and 18 for the =FDIST() function.
G17	=SQRT(G7/18)	Eighteen is the degrees of freedom or $n − 2$, $n = 20$.
G18	=G17/SQRT(D22)	
G20	=G2/G18	
G21	=TDIST(G20,18,2)	=TDIST() contains three arguments: the first is the calculated t value, the second the degrees of freedom, and the third a 1 or a 2, indicating a one-tailed or two-tailed test. Here we choose 2 as we are conducting a two-tailed test.

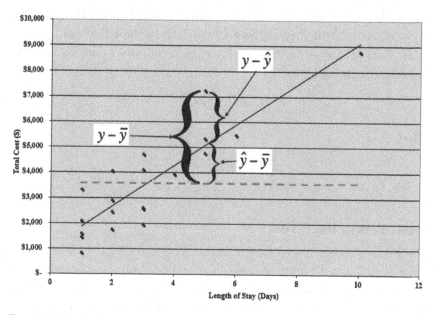

Figure 11.7 Total variance, regression variance, and error variance

points shown in cell C22 in Figure 11.6. There are three labeled brackets. The bracket labeled $y - \bar{y}$ represents the total variation for the length of stay of five days, shown in cell B7 in Figure 11.6. That bracket represents the value of charges for that stay—$7,230.71—minus the mean charges for all stays—$3,595.15, or $3,635.56. The bracket labeled $\hat{y} - \bar{y}$ represents the difference between the predicted value for that stay—$5,082.52—and the mean of all stays—$3,595.15, or $1,487.38. This is the portion of the variation in the charges for this stay that can be predicted using the regression equation. The bracket labeled $y - \bar{y}$ represents the difference between the actual charges for this particular stay—$7,230.71—and the predicted value of $5,082.52, or $2,148.19. This is the portion of the variation in the charges for this stay that cannot be predicted with the regression equation. When all these differences for each point are squared and summed, the values of SS_T, SS_R, and SS_E are generated.

Testing the Null Hypothesis: Is the Model Predicting Well?

The R^2 value tells us the degree of relationship between the length of stay and charges. In this case, the length of stay accounts for 78 percent of the variance in the charges. This would generally be considered a very high degree of relationship. But still not yet discussed explicitly is the resolution of the question of whether we can reject the null hypothesis of independence between the two variables. The resolution of that question is given formally by the F test shown in cell G14 in Figure 11.6. This F test is calculated by the formula given in Equation 11.13, the formula in which is usually described as the division of the mean square due to regression by the mean square error. The mean square values are found by dividing SS_R and SS_E by their respective degrees of freedom.

$$F = MS_R/MS_E \tag{11.13}$$

where

$$MS_R = SS_R/1$$
$$MS_E = SS_E/(n - 2)$$

Interpreting the F Test

The F value shown in cell G14 of Figure 11.6 is 63.33, a relatively large value of F. The probability of this F is given in cell G14 as 2.64E-07. This indicates that the F value calculated would have been found approximately three times out of 10 million different samples of 20 observations if charges were independent of the length of stay. Because this is an extremely small probability, we reject the null hypothesis of independence and conclude that the two variables are, in fact, not independent. In other words, charges and length of stay are related.

There are several additional values in Figure 11.6. These include the overall *standard error* of estimate (*S.E.*) in cell G17, the standard error of b_1 (*S.E. b_1*) in cell G18, a *t test* in cell G20, and the probability of the *t* in cell G21. Each of these deserves some discussion.

Calculating Standard Error and *t* Tests

The standard error shown in cell G17 is the average error of the actual observations around the regression line shown in Figure 11.7. It is calculated using the formula given in Equation 11.14.

$$S.E._{reg} = \sqrt{\frac{SS_E}{(n-2)}}$$ (11.14)

The standard error of b_1 (*S.E. b_1* in cell G18) is the average variation of the coefficient, b_1. The coefficient b_1 in any regression analysis is a sample-based estimate of the true population coefficient b_1. As a sample mean value $\bar{x}$, an estimate of the true population mean m has a range within which there is a probability of the true mean being found; so, too, the coefficient, b_1, has a similar range. That range is determined by the *S.E. b_1*. But the *S.E. b_1* also serves another function. Just as a *t* test can be conducted by dividing appropriate mean values by their standard errors, a *t* test can be conducted to determine whether the coefficient b_1 is different from 0. If the *t* test does not produce a *t* value large enough to reject the implied null hypothesis that b_1 is 0, the conclusion would have to be that the null hypothesis of independence of the variables x and y would be rejected. The standard error of b_1 is calculated using the formula in Equation 11.15.

$$S.E.\ b_1 = \frac{S.E._{reg}}{\sqrt{\sum (x - \bar{x})^2}}$$ (11.15)

t Test versus *F* Test: Why Calculate Both?

The *t* test to determine if b_1 is different from 0 is shown in Equation 11.16, and the value of the *t* test for the length of stay and the charges is shown in cell G20 in Figure 11.6. The probability of the *t* test is shown in cell G21. You will note that it is exactly the same as the probability of the *F* test in cell G15. This is no accident. In simple linear regression with a single *predictor variable*, the probability of the *F* test will always be the same as the probability of the t test. This is because the F test of the general hypothesis of independence is exactly the same as the t test of the null hypothesis that the coefficient b_1 is zero. In multiple regression, which we will take up in Chapter 12, the F test and the individual t tests for regression coefficients will not have the same probabilities. Therefore, we must calculate both the F statistic and the associated t statistics.

$$t = \frac{b_1}{S.E.\ b_1} \tag{11.16}$$

What to Do about the Intercept, b_0?

It is useful to note that there is no comparable test in this analysis to determine whether the coefficient b_0 is different from zero. In this analysis no standard error for b_0 has been determined, but the primary reason no test for b_0 is conducted is that whether b_0 is different from 0 has no bearing on the rejection or nonrejection of the null hypothesis of independence. The coefficient b_0 is simply an anchor for the left side of the regression line. Whether it is 0 or different from 0 is usually not central to the analysis. In the analysis discussed here, no value for b_0 has even been found. We will see when we move to multiple regression, however, that a value for the standard error of b_0 will be produced by the analysis.

EXERCISES FOR SECTION 11.2

1. Use the data from the Charges worksheet of Chpt 11-1.xls and the calculations of b_1 and b_0 carried out in Exercise 6 of Section 11.1 to replicate the calculations shown in Figure 11.6.

   a. Calculate the total sum of squares (SS_T) as given in Equation 11.9 and shown in cell G5 in Figure 11.6. (Use the =SUMSQ() function on the data in column E.)

   b. Calculate the predicted values of TC in column H by using the formula in Equation 11.1.

   c. Calculate the difference between $\hat{y}$ and $\bar{y}$ in column I and the value of SS_R (sum of squares due to regression) by using Equation 11.10 and the =SUMSQ() function on the data in column I.

   d. Calculate the values of $\bar{y}$ in column J and the value of SS_E (sums of squares due to error) by using Equation 11.11 and the =SUMSQ() function on the data in column J.

   e. Calculate the value of R^2 by using Equation 11.12.

   f. Calculate the degrees of freedom for SS_R and SS_E as shown in Equation 11.13 and the values of MS_R and MS_E, using the same formula. Calculate the value of F from the same formula.

      g. Determine the probability of F with the $=\texttt{FDIST()}$ function and the appropriate degrees of freedom.

      h. Determine the standard error of regression by using the formula in Equation 11.14.

      i. Determine the standard error of b_1 by using the formula in Equation 11.15.

      j. Calculate the t value for b_1 by using the formula in Equation 11.16, and determine its probability with the $=\texttt{TDIST()}$ function.

2. Use data on the U5Mort worksheet in Chpt 11-1.xls and the results of the calculation of b_1 and b_0 for FemLit as a predictor of U5Mort from Exercise 7 of Section 11.1, and replicate the complete analysis in Figure 11.6.

      a. Calculate the total sum of squares (SS_T) as given in Equation 11.9. (Use the $=\texttt{SUMSQ()}$ function.)

      b. Calculate the predicted values of $\texttt{U5Mort()}$ in column H by using the formula in Equation 11.1.

      c. Calculate the difference between and $\bar{y}$ in column I and the value of SS_R (sum of squares due to regression) by using Equation 11.10 and the $=\texttt{SUMSQ()}$ function on the data in column I.

      d. Calculate the values of $y - \hat{y}$ in column J and the value of SS_E (sum of squares due to error) by using Equation 11.11 and the $=\texttt{SUMSQ()}$ function on the data in column J.

      e. Calculate the value of R^2 by using Equation 11.12.

      f. Calculate the degrees of freedom for SS_R and SS_E as shown in Equation 11.13 and the values of MS_R and MS_E, using the same formula. Calculate the value of F from the same formula.

      g. Determine the probability of F with the $=\texttt{FDIST()}$ function and the appropriate degrees of freedom.

      h. Determine the standard error of regression by using the formula in Equation 11.14.

      i. Determine the standard error of b_1 by using the formula in Equation 11.15.

      j. Calculate the t value for b_1 using the formula in Equation 11.16, and determine its probability with the $=\texttt{TDIST()}$ function.

11.3   The Excel Regression Add-In

Now that we have worked through the steps of regression analysis, we can look at the capabilities of the Excel regression add-in. When Data Analysis is invoked, the dialog box shown again in Figure 11.8 will appear. When Regression is selected, as it is in the figure, the Regression dialog box,

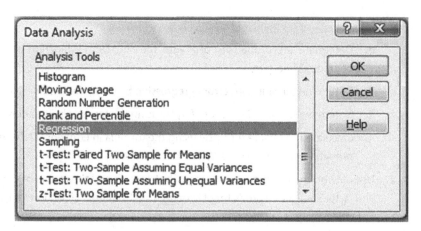

Figure 11.8 Excel Data Analysis add-in dialog box

Figure 11.9 Regression dialog box

shown in Figure 11.9, appears. In Figure 11.9, several things should be noted. First, the field labeled Input Y Range contains the cell reference to the y *variable*, total charges, which is in cells C1:C21. The field labeled Input X Range contains the cell references for length of stay, which is in cells B1:B21. The box named Labels is checked, indicating that the first row in each column is a label. If cells B1 and C1 were not included in the input range fields and the Labels box were checked, Excel would treat the values 3 for the length of stay and $2,613.91 as labels and would not include that observation in the analysis.

The box labeled "Constant is Zero" should never be checked. There is an analysis known as weighted least squares that involves the assumption that the constant is 0, but, in general, that box should be left unchecked. The confidence level is given as 95 percent by default. It is possible to change this to another level by checking the Confidence Level box. The final item in the Regression dialog box that must be indicated is where the output is to go. It can go on the same sheet, on a new worksheet, or in a new workbook. If we check the Output Range radio button and then enter E1 in the corresponding field, the output will be placed on the same sheet in cell E1. Several other options in this dialog box produce additional results, but in general we will not use those in this book.

Linear Regression in Excel Using the Data Analysis Package: Step-by-Step Instructions

Follow these step-by-step instructions to invoke the Data Analysis package in Excel and complete the required inputs for linear regression analysis.

1. Go to the Data ribbon, in the Analysis group, and click the Data Analysis option.

2. A dialog box (Figure 11.8) will appear. Here, choose the Regression option. Another dialog box (Figure 11.9) will appear.

3. In the Input Y Range field, enter $C$1:$C$21 or highlight cells C1 through C21.

4. In the Input X Range field, enter $B$1:$B$21 or highlight cells B1 through B21.

5. Click the Output Range radio button, and enter $E$1.

6. Click OK, and the Regression output will be created.

Analyzing the Excel Regression Output

Clicking OK in the Regression dialog box (Figure 11.9) will produce the results shown in Figure 11.10. The table shown here is exactly as it appears in the regression output for any set of data. The labels cannot be completely seen because the column is not wide enough—for example, Adjusted R in cell E6 is actually Adjusted R square. Similarly, andard Err in cell G16 is really Standard Error, but the cell is too narrow for the entire title to show. It is possible to see the entire titles by putting the cursor between, for

	E	F	G	H	I	J	K	L	M
1	SUMMARY OUTPUT								
2									
3	*Regression Statistics*								
4	Multiple R	0.88244							
5	R Square	0.7787							
6	Adjusted R Square	0.7664							
7	Standard Error	982.321							
8	Observations	20							
9									
10	ANOVA								
11		*df*	*SS*	*MS*	*F*	*Significance F*			
12	Regression	1	61116626	61116626	63.3363	2.63936E-07			
13	Residual	18	17369179	964954.365					
14	Total	19	78485805						
15									
16		*Coefficients*	*Standard Erro*	*t Stat*	*P-value*	*Lower 95%*	*Upper 95%*	*Lower 95.0%*	*Upper 95.0%*
17	Intercept	1062.59	386.67085	2.74804159	0.01323	250.2222667	1874.95289	250.222267	1874.95289
18	LOS(x)	803.987	101.02355	7.95840979	2.6E-07	591.7442002	1016.2294	591.7442	1016.2294
19									

Figure 11.10 Results of using the regression add-in

example, columns E and F at the top of the sheet and double-clicking. But after a little use, the absence of complete labels will not be a problem.

But let us look at the various different numbers that are produced by the regression analysis add-in. The first number in the table is labeled Multiple R. This value, which is often called the *correlation coefficient*, represents the correlation between the two variables, x and y. The correlation coefficient can be calculated by the formula shown in Equation 11.17. It can also be found by taking the square root of R^2 in cell G9 in Figure 11.6. One caveat to taking the square root of R^2 to find r, however, is that r may be negative or positive. If the value of b_1 is negative, the actual value of r in two-variable linear regression will be negative. However, the Multiple R shown in the Excel regression result will always be positive.

$$r = \frac{\sum (x - \bar{x})(y - \bar{y})}{\sqrt{\sum (x - \bar{x})^2 \sum (y - \bar{y})^2}} \qquad (11.17)$$

Multiple R

Multiple R represents the strength of the linear relationship between the actual and the estimated values for the dependent variables. The scale ranges from -1.0 to 1.0, where 1.0 indicates a good direct relationship and -1 indicates a good inverse relationship.

R Square

R^2 is a symbol for a coefficient of multiple determination between a dependent variable and the independent variables. It tells how much of the variability in the dependent variable is explained by the independent variables. R^2 is a goodness-of-fit measure, and the scale ranges from 0.0 to 1.0.

Adjusted R Square

In the adjusted R square, R^2 is adjusted to give a trucr estimate of how much the independent variables in a regression analysis explain the dependent variable. Taking into account the number of independent variables makes the adjustment.

Standard Error of Estimates

The standard error of estimates is a regression line. The error is how much the research is off when the regression line is used to predict particular scores. The standard error is the standard deviation of those errors from the regression line. The standard error of estimate is thus a measure of the variability of the errors. It measures the average error over the entire scatter plot.

The lower the standard error of estimate, the higher the degree of linear relationship between the two variables in the regression. The larger the standard error, the less confidence can be put in the estimate.

t Statistic

The rule of thumb says the absolute value of t should be greater than 2. To be more accurate, the t table has been used.

The critical values can be found in the back of most statistical textbooks. The critical value is the value that determines the critical regions in a sampling distribution. The critical values separate the obtained values that will and will not result in rejecting the null hypothesis.

F Statistic

The F statistic is a broad picture statistic that intends to test the efficacy of the entire regression model presented.

A hypothesis is tested that looks at H0: $B_1 = B_2 = 0$. If this hypothesis is rejected, this implies that the explanatory variables in the regression equation being proposed are doing a good job of explaining the variation in the dependent variable Y.

The R^2 value shown in cell F5 is exactly the same value as that calculated for R^2 by using the formula shown in Equation 11.12 and as given in cell G9 in Figure 11.6.

The adjusted R square (cell E6) represents the reduction of the actual R^2 to reflect the number of independent variables in the prediction equation (as shown in Equation 11.2). The terms "independent variables," "regressors," and "predictor variables" are all considered synonymous. In the case of two-variable regression, there is always only one independent variable. In turn, the adjusted R^2 is very close to the R^2 value. However, the more independent variables, regressors, or predictor variables that are included in the regression equation, the larger will be the R^2. This is because every additional independent variable reduces the size of SS_E. To counter this, the adjusted R^2 reduces the value of R^2 to reflect this decrease in SS_E. The formula for the adjusted R^2 is shown in Equation 11.18. More is said about the adjusted R^2 in Chapter 12.

$$R^2_{adj} = 1 - (1 - R^2)\frac{n-1}{n-2} \tag{11.18}$$

The standard error, what we labeled *S.E.* in Figure 11.6 (cell G17), is shown in cell F7 of the Excel regression output (Figure 11.10). The number of observations—20—is confirmed in cell F8 in Figure 11.10. The ANOVA section of the Excel regression output also matches our previous calculations. SS Regression in Figure 11.10, cell G12 at 61,116,626, matches the value of SS_R in cell G6 in Figure 11.6. A brief examination of the two figures will show that all the *SS* values and *MS* values in Figure 11.10 match their corresponding values in Figure 11.6. The *F* test value of 63.336 is the same in both figures, as is the probability of *F*, 2.64E-07.

Similar results are found with regard to the coefficients themselves. The coefficients b_1 and b_0, shown as LOS(x) and Intercept, respectively, in Figure 11.10, are the same in both figures, as is the standard error of b_1. The standard error of b_0 was not calculated in Figure 11.6. In general, whether b_0, the intercept term, can be shown to be different from 0 is irrelevant to the decision to reject the null hypothesis of independence between the two variables in the analysis. The intercept represents no more than an anchor to establish the position of the regression line. But because the standard error of b_0 is given in the Excel regression output, it is useful to know how it can be calculated. The formula for the standard error of b_0 is given in Equation 11.19. Although Σx^2 is not calculated in Figure 11.6, it is easy to confirm with =SUMSQ(C2:C21) that it is 293, and the term in the denominator in Equation 11.19 is $\sqrt{6.4539}$, which gives a value for *S.E.* b_0 of 386.67.

$$S.E.\ b_0 = \frac{S.E._{\cdot reg}}{\sqrt{\dfrac{n\sum(x - \bar{x})^2}{\sum x^2}}} \tag{11.19}$$

The *t* statistic for the coefficient b_1 as shown in Figure 11.10 was calculated in cell G20 in Figure 11.6. These both match, as do their probabilities. The *t* statistic for b_0 was not calculated in Figure 11.6, but if it had been, it would have equaled that found in the Excel regression output. The last four columns in rows 16 to 18 in Figure 11.10 give upper and lower 95 percent limits for the coefficients b_1 and b_0. If the user requests a level of confidence other than 95 percent, the upper and lower limits will then be given as the last two sets of cells. These values, though not found in Figure 11.6, can be found in exactly the same way that upper and lower 95 percent limits are found for a mean value. The lower value of 591.744, for example, which is shown in cell J18 (and L18) in Figure 11.10, is calculated exactly as shown in Equation 11.20. The other limits can be found in the same way.

$$\text{Lower} = b_1 - t_{18}\ \text{S.E.}\ b_1 = 803.987 - 2.101 \times 101.024 = 591.744 \quad (11.20)$$

EXERCISES FOR SECTION 11.3

1. Use the data from the Charges worksheet of Chpt 11-1.xls, and do the following:

   a. Generate the regression analysis by using the Tools ➤ Data Analysis Regression add-in, and replicate the analysis shown in Figure 11.10.

   b. Make sure that all the values in this result equal those found in Exercise 1 of Section 11.2.

2. Use the data from the U5Mort worksheet of Chpt 11-1.xls, and do the following:

   a. Generate the regression analysis by using the Tools ➤ Data Analysis Regression add-in, and replicate the analysis in Exercise 2 of Section 11.2.

   b. Make sure that all the values in this result equal those found in Exercise 2 of Section 11.2.

11.4   The Importance of Examining the Scatterplot

The scatterplots shown in Figure 11.1 provide one example of data not appropriate for two-variable regression: chart (d). This relationship is curvilinear and, consequently, is not best described by using a straight line. This section looks at some other cases in which regression analysis must be used very carefully. The presentation in this section is inspired by a similar presentation in *Statistics for Managers Using Microsoft Excel* (Levine, Stephan, and Szabat 2007; Levine, Stephan, and Szabat 2013) and *Spreadsheet Modeling for Business Decisions* (Kros 2014).

A scatterplot is a way to graphically display a collection of points, each having the value of one variable determining the position on the horizontal axis and the value of the other variable determining the position on the vertical axis.

Four different data sets are shown in Figure 11.11. For each of these data sets, the best-fitting straight line is defined by the equation $y = 0.50x + 1.55$. (The best-fitting straight line for data set 4 is actually $y = 0.51x + 1.55$.) If you calculate the regression coefficients b_1 and b_0 for each of these data

	A	B	C	D	E	F	G	H	I	J	K	L
1	Data set one			Data set two			Data set three			Data set four		
2	X	Y		X	Y		X	Y		X	Y	
3	5	5		5	4		5	7		5	3	
4	6	4		7	6		7	6		5	4	
5	6	6		9	5		9	6		5	5	
6	7	4		11	8		11	6		14	5	
7	7	5		13	7		13	6		14	9	
8	7	6		15	10		15	7		14	13	
9	8	4		17	9		17	8		22	5	
10	8	6		19	12		19	10		22	16	
11	9	5		21	11		21	13		22	20	
12	20	12		23	14		23	17		22	10	

Figure 11.11 Four data sets

sets, they will be essentially equal for each data set. But only one of these data sets could be considered appropriate for simple linear regression with one predictor variable, x.

Visual Inspection of the Scatterplots: Attempting to Identify Relationships

The xy scatterplots of these four data sets, along with the best-fitting straight lines, are shown in Figure 11.12. When looking at this figure, it should be possible to see why only one of these data sets—data set 2—is appropriate for simple linear regression analysis. Although the equation for the best-fitting straight line for data set 1 is exactly the same as that for

Figure 11.12 Scatterplots of four data sets where $y = .5x + 1.55$

data set 2, that line depends entirely on the value at $x = 20$ and $y = 12$. If that value were not included, the coefficient of b_1 would have been 0 and there would be no relation between x and y at all. In essence, the entire relationship found between x and y in this case depends on a single data point. The single data point in this case is often called an outlier. When outliers are present, it is important to decide whether they are unduly affecting the regression results.

Data set 3 is inappropriate for simple linear regression because the data actually show a curved relationship between x and y. Regression can be used to describe the data in data set 3, but it must be curvilinear regression, which is taken up in Chapter 13. In essence, a straight-line relationship between x and y is not the correct model for describing the way the x variable affects the y variable in data set 3.

Examining the Variance of the Data: The Constant Variance Assumption

Data set 4 may be a little more difficult to see as being inappropriate for simple linear regression. The points do tend to lie along the straight line defined by the regression equation. However, they do not seem to depict a nonlinear relationship as in data set 3, and the line is not defined by a single outlier as in data set 1. The problem with the use of simple linear regression to analyze data set 4 is that the variance in the data is not the same at each point where a value of x is recorded. When x is 5, the three values taken on by y have an average variance (the difference between each value of y at $x = 5$ and the mean of the values of y at $x = 5$ divided by the number of values of y at $x = 5$) of 0.33. The three values taken on by y when $x = 14$ have an average variance of 5.33. The four values taken on by y when $x = 22$ have an average variance of 10.89.

One of the basic assumptions of simple linear regression is that the variance of y across all values of x is constant. In the case of the data in data set 4, this is clearly not the case. As the value of x increases, the variance in y increases. Most authors of statistics texts agree that the results of regression analysis are not greatly affected by violating this assumption of equal variance. More important, the more appropriate analysis of the data in data set 4 would be an analysis called weighted least squares. Weighted least squares are discussed in Chapter 14, but in a different context. For those interested in a general treatment of weighted least squares, any good introductory text in econometrics will provide a discussion of its calculation and use.

11.5 The Relationship between Regression and the *t* Test

This section considers the relationship between regression and the *t* test. Remember that *t* tests were discussed in Chapter 9. The one that is particularly examined here is the *t* test for two different groups. Consider the example given in Chapter 9 of the two groups of women, one of which received information from a physician about breast cancer and the other of which received only written information. In turn, the question that was asked was, "Between the two groups, did this result in different knowledge about breast cancer?" The results of the *t* test, with both equal and unequal variance assumptions, were shown in Figures 9.10 and 9.11. The mean knowledge assessment scores for the two groups were 10.040 for the women who received information from a physician and 7.525 for the women who received only a pamphlet. For the equal variance assumption, the pooled variance was 0.762 and the value of the *t* statistic ((10.040 − 7.525)/0.762) was 3.3.

Using Excel's Regression Function to Perform a *t* Test

Figure 11.13 shows the data for the comparison between the two groups redone using regression analysis. The dependent variable in the regression

	D	E	F	G	H	I
1	SUMMARY OUTPUT					
2						
3	*Regression Statistics*					
4	Multiple R	0.383909				
5	R Square	0.147386				
6	Adjusted R Sq	0.133853				
7	Standard Error	2.989227				
8	Observations	65				
9						
10	ANOVA					
11		df	SS	MS	F	ignificance F
12	Regression	1	97.31115	97.31115	10.89043	0.001594
13	Residual	63	562.935	8.935476		
14	Total	64	660.2462			
15						
16		Coefficient	andard Err	t Stat	P-value	Lower 95% Up
17	Intercept	7.525	0.472638	15.92127	9.23E-24	6.580507	8.
18	Group	2.515	0.762106	3.300065	0.001594	0.992051	4.|
19						

Figure 11.13 Regression as a *t* test

is the score received by each woman, whether in the experimental or control group, on the knowledge test. The independent variable is a variable that is coded 1 if the woman is in the experimental group and 0 if she is not. Such a variable is called a dummy variable, probably because it does not actually represent a numerical variable but, rather, serves as a categorical variable that can be treated as a numerical variable.

In examining Figure 11.13, it is possible to see that the Intercept term in cell E17 (7.525) is the mean of the control group. The coefficient indicated as Group is the coefficient on the dummy variable that takes on only the values 1 and 0. As such, the value of 2.515 is not a slope but is, rather, the value that is added to the intercept to get the mean of the experimental group. It is easy to see that $7.525 + 2.515 = 10.040$. Furthermore, it is possible to see that the t test on the coefficient for group, which is precisely the difference between the control group and the experimental group divided by the pooled variance (0.762), is exactly the same as the t test for two groups assuming equal variance. This will always be the case. Whenever a dummy variable is employed in regression, the coefficient will be the difference between the mean of the group coded 0 and the mean of the group coded 1. The t test for the coefficient will be exactly the same as the t test for the difference in means.

It is important to note that when a variable is employed in a regression context, a dummy actually defines two different regression equations. In this simple case of a single dummy variable, the original regression equation, shown in Equation 11.21, actually becomes two equations as shown in Equation 11.22. It should be clear that these values are just the mean of the group designated 0 and the group designated 1 by the dummy variable, respectively.

$$y - \text{hat} = b_1 x + b_0 \qquad (11.21)$$

$$(y - \text{hat}|x = 0) = b_0,$$

$$\text{and } (y - \text{hat}|x = 1) = b_1 + b_0 \qquad (11.22)$$

EXERCISES FOR SECTION 11.5

1. Use the data on the Cost worksheet of Chpt 9-1.xls that show the hospital cost for a randomly selected sample of 34 women and 34 men.

   a. Rearrange the data so that they can be analyzed using regression, and add an independent variable that is 1 for women and 0 for men.

b. Test the hypothesis that the cost for women is equal to the cost for men (against the alternative that they are not equal) using regression.

2. Use the data on the Breast C worksheet of Chpt 9-1.xls to complete the following. Figure 11.13 displays the simple regression analysis output for these data.

   a. Rearrange the data so that they can be analyzed using regression, and add an independent variable that is 1 for the women in the experimental group and 0 for the women in the control group.

   b. Replicate the analysis shown in Figure 11.13.

3. Use the data on the Wait worksheet of Chpt 9-1.xls that represent the waiting time of a randomly selected group of people at an urgent-care clinic and a randomly selected group of people at an emergency clinic.

   a. Rearrange the data so that they can be analyzed using regression, and add an independent variable that is 1 for Emergency and 0 Urgent care.

   b. Test the hypothesis that waiting time is equal for both groups (against the alternative that they are not equal) using regression.

KEY TERMS

=FDIST()	predictor variable
=SUMPRODUCT()	regression analysis
=SUMSQ()	regression coefficient
=TDIST()	standard error
best-fitting straight line	*t* test
correlation	*x*-axis
dependent variable	*x* variable
independent variable	*y*-axis
linear regression	*y* variable

CHAPTER 12

MULTIPLE REGRESSION: CONCEPTS AND CALCULATION

Smoking is one of the leading causes of all statistics.

—Liza Minnelli

LEARNING OBJECTIVES

- Understand the nature of multiple regression and the calculation of basic multiple regression results

- Understand the relationship between multiple regression and matrices

Chapter 11 considered simple linear regression, its calculation, and its interpretation. This chapter extends the simple linear regression model to include more than one *predictor variable*. This is what is known as *multiple regression*. This chapter will consider the nature of multiple regression and the calculation of the basic multiple regression results.

Appendix A, "Multiple Regression and Matrices," discussing the multiple regression and matrix algebra, can be found at the end of the book.

12.1 Introduction

Health care professionals are often faced with the need to describe and analyze relationships between outcomes and predictors. They seek to identify and explain trends, test hypotheses, and/or develop forecasting models. Linear regression models are able to incorporate complex mathematical functions to describe the associations between sets of variables. Given the availability of data in health care administration databases, the application of linear regression can result in improved health care decision making.

In introducing the multiple regression model, we will contrast it to simple linear regression. In this contrast, the Microsoft Excel regression add-in, considered in Chapter 11, will be extended to multiple regression.

Multiple regression analysis is a way for us to understand more about the relationship between several independent or predictor variables and a dependent or criterion variable.

The Extension of Simple Linear Regression

The simple linear regression model is shown in Equation 12.1. In the simple linear regression model, the coefficient b_1 represents the slope of the regression line in an xy graph. The coefficient b_0 represents the intercept of the regression line, or the value of the *dependent variable y* when the *independent variable x* is equal to 0. The symbol e represents the error—the difference between the actual values of y and the predicted values of y.

$$y = b_1 x + b_0 + e \tag{12.1}$$

The multiple regression model extends the simple linear regression model to include more than one independent variable. In the context of the presentation in Equation 12.1, the multiple regression model could be presented as shown in Equation 12.2. In Equation 12.2, the subscript m represents any number of independent variables, and the three dots in a row represent the b coefficients and x variables from 2 to m that are included in the equation but not shown.

$$y = b_1 x_1 + b_2 x_2 + \cdots + b_m x_m + b_0 + e \tag{12.2}$$

The relationship in the simple linear regression model can be envisioned as a line (the regression line) in a two-dimensional graph where, by convention, the horizontal axis is the x variable and the vertical axis is the y variable. This was illustrated in Chapter 11. In simple terms, the relationship of a single independent variable to a dependent variable can be pictured in a two-dimensional space. If there were two independent variables (x variables), it would be possible to picture this relationship as a plane in a three-dimensional space—although this is not easily shown on a two-dimensional medium, such as paper.

If there are more than two independent variables, it becomes impossible to picture this on paper as well. If there are m independent variables, the logical extension is that we should be able to construct a model of all the variables at the same time by producing an m dimensional figure in an $m + 1$ dimensional space. Although human beings can easily deal with the notion of only three dimensions at a time, it becomes virtually impossible to picture graphically the simultaneous relationship of all x variables to the y variable in $m + 1$ dimensions. For the purposes of understanding multiple regression, it is not necessary to form this mental picture. We simply need to understand that each independent x variable may have some effect on y that is assessed simultaneously with the effect of all other x variables.

Purpose of Multiple Regression: Dependent and Independent Variable Relationships

The purpose of *multiple regression analysis* is essentially the same as that of linear regression. We are trying to understand whether there is any relationship between each of the independent variables x and the dependent variable y and in turn what that relationship may be. To do this for simple regression, we learned that two algebraic formulas can be used to find directly the values of b_1 and b_0.

Similarly, there is a direct algebraic strategy for finding all the coefficients b_m and b_0 in the multiple regression model. However, the use of this strategy is mathematically complex enough that, until the advent of modern computers, the solution of multiple regression relationships beyond a very few independent variables x was rarely attempted. Fortunately, the Excel add-in that allows us to do simple linear regression easily also allows us to do multiple regression with up to 16 independent variables x. In general, few practical applications of multiple regression require that many independent variables.

To examine the way in which Excel can be used for multiple regression, let us consider the data shown in Figure 12.1. In the figure, the variable y is cost per hospital case for 10 hospitals. The variable $X1$ is the size of the hospital in number of beds. The variable $X2$ is a measure of the extent to which the administrator of the hospital can accurately compare his hospital with other hospitals, in terms of costs. An administrator who has a more accurate view of the competition receives a higher score on the visibility scale.

The data shown in Figure 12.1 are wholly fabricated. However, they were fabricated with the recognition that larger hospitals are frequently

	B	C	D
1	Y	X1	X2
2	Cost	Size	Visibility
3	2750	225	6
4	2400	200	37
5	2920	300	14
6	1800	350	33
7	3520	200	11
8	2270	250	21
9	3100	175	21
10	1980	400	22
11	2680	350	20
12	2720	275	16
13			

Figure 12.1 Cost data for 10 hospitals

thought to have lower case costs than smaller hospitals, and hospitals whose administrators are knowledgeable about the competition are also likely to have lower case costs. Even though these data are for only 10 hypothetical hospitals, they can be used to demonstrate both the regression capability of Excel and the calculation of the *regression coefficients.*

Multiple Regression Using Excel's Data Analysis Add-In

The first step in the description of the use of Excel for multiple regression is a discussion of how the Data Analysis Regression add-in can be used to carry out multiple regression. Recall the initial Regression dialog box, shown in Figure 12.2. This figure also shows the entries needed to produce the regression results. As with simple linear regression, the dependent variable, which is cost, is shown in the Input Y Range field as $B$2:$B$12. The independent variable, however, shown in the Input X Range field, is now different from the simple linear regression model. For multiple regression, the entry for the *x* variable is given as $C$2:$D$12. Excel has been instructed to select not a single column but two contiguous columns to be included as the independent variable data.

Figure 12.2   Initial Regression dialog box

As was the case with single variable regression, the Labels box has been checked to indicate that the first cell in each row of data is to be treated as a data label. The last important component in the regression window is the output range, which, in this case, is given as cell F1 in the spreadsheet in which the data appear. Clicking OK in this dialog box carries out the multiple regression operation and shows the results beginning in cell F1.

Multiple Linear Regression Using Excel's Data Analysis Package: Step-by-Step Instructions

Follow these step-by-step instructions to invoke the Data Analysis package in Excel and complete the required inputs for linear regression analysis.

1. Go to the Data ribbon, in the Analysis group, and click the Data Analysis option.

2. A dialog box (Figure 11.8) will appear. Here, choose the Regression option. Another dialog box (Figure 12.2) will appear.

3. In the Input Y Range field, enter $B$2:$B$12 or highlight cells B2:B12.

4. In the Input X Range field, enter $C$2:$C$12 or highlight cells C2:C12.

5. Click the Output Range radio button, and enter $F$1.

6. Click OK, and the Regression output will be created (see Figure 12.3).

	F	G	H	I	J	K	L
1	SUMMARY OUTPUT						
2							
3	Regression Statistics						
4	Multiple R	0.8340336					
5	R Square	0.6956121					
6	Adjusted R Sq	0.6086441					
7	Standard Error	323.9537					
8	Observations	10					
9							
10	ANOVA						
11		df	SS	MS	F	Significance F	
12	Regression	2	1678818.023	839409	7.998485	0.015559511	
13	Residual	7	734621.9772	104946			
14	Total	9	2413440				
15							
16		Coefficients	Standard Error	t Stat	P-value	Lower 95%	Upper 95%
17	Intercept	4240.131	435.6084415	9.733813	2.56E-05	3210.081442	5270.18054
18	Size	-3.7623152	1.442783962	-2.60768	0.035032	-7.17395474	-0.3506757
19	Visibility	-29.895527	11.66297571	-2.56328	0.037372	-57.4740623	-2.3169913

Figure 12.3 Multiple regression output

Interpreting the Output from Excel's Multiple Regression Package

The results of the multiple regression are shown in Figure 12.3. This figure is quite similar to that for simple linear regression. However, instead of having one named variable (other than the intercept), there are two: Size and Visibility. The interpretation of the multiple regression output given in Figure 12.3 is essentially the same as the interpretation for simple linear regression. The interpretation of the Regression Statistics section is essentially the same as that of simple linear regression, except that now the adjusted R square takes into account the two independent variables. The analysis of variance (ANOVA) is interpreted just as it was in simple linear regression, but it should be noted that there are now two degrees of freedom in the regression and $n - 3$ in the residual. The regression coefficients are also interpreted exactly as in simple linear regression except that there are now two slope coefficients rather than one.

There is an important point to consider when interpreting the slope coefficients: In simple linear regression we saw that the regression line could be graphed quite clearly as a straight line in a two-dimensional space. In other words, the graph is two-dimensional with the x or independent variable on the horizontal axis and the y or dependent variable on the vertical axis. With two independent variables, a graph of the predicted values would have to be a plane (a two-dimensional figure) in a three-dimensional space.

By extension, if we were to hope to graph the results of, for example, five independent variables, a five-dimensional figure in a six-dimensional space would have to be created. Because the average human being cannot generate a mental image of any space with more than three dimensions, it should be apparent that it would be impossible to produce a visual image of the results of most multiple regression analyses. In short, the useful visual aids are pretty much limited to simple linear regression.

There is another point to clarify when looking at the coefficients from multiple regression: These coefficients are computed simultaneously. If either coefficient were calculated independently (i.e., in a simple linear regression), it would not be equal to the coefficients calculated in multiple regression. This point is true except in that unusual situation in which there is absolutely no relationship between the two independent variables. Furthermore, the *R square* obtained from multiple regression is not the sum of the *R square* that would be obtained from two simple linear regressions with the same two variables. In fact, either of the two independent variables may produce nearly as large an R square as the two variables taken together.

Multiple R

Multiple R represents the strength of the linear relationship between the actual and the estimated values for the dependent variables. The scale ranges from -1.0 to 1.0, where 1.0 indicates a good direct relationship and -1 indicates a good inverse relationship.

R Square

R^2 is a symbol for a coefficient of multiple determination between a dependent variable and the independent variables. It tells how much of the variability in the dependent variable is explained by the independent variables. R^2 is a goodness-of-fit measure, and the scale ranges from 0.0 to 1.0.

Adjusted R Square

In the adjusted R square, R^2 is adjusted to give a truer estimate of how much the independent variables in a regression analysis explain the dependent variable. Taking into account the number of independent variables makes the adjustment.

Standard Error of Estimates

The standard error of estimates is a regression line. The error is how much the research is off when the regression line is used to predict particular scores. The standard error is the standard deviation of those errors from the regression line. The standard error of estimate is thus a measure of the variability of the errors. It measures the average error over the entire scatter plot.

The lower the standard error of estimate, the higher the degree of linear relationship between the two variables in the regression. The larger the standard error, the less confidence can be put in the estimate.

t Statistic

The rule of thumb says the absolute value of t should be greater than 2. To be more accurate, the t table has been used.

The critical values can be found in the back of most statistical textbooks. The critical value is the value that determines the critical regions in a sampling distribution. The critical values separate the obtained values that will and will not result in rejecting the null hypothesis.

F Statistic

The F statistic is a broad picture statistic that intends to test the efficacy of the entire regression model presented.

A hypothesis is tested that looks at H0: $B_1 = B_2 = 0$. If this hypothesis is rejected, this implies that the explanatory variables in the regression equation being proposed are doing a good job of explaining the variation in the dependent variable Y.

The Solution to the Multiple Regression Problem

In Chapter 11, we learned how to calculate the regression coefficients from original data and found that the results we obtained were exactly the same as those obtained by the Excel Data Analysis Regression package. In this chapter we are going to look at how the results of multiple regression can be found. In general, because the multiple regression coefficients are found simultaneously, the formula for the solution of the multiple regression problem is not as easily expressed as the solution for the simple linear regression.

This section examines the case of two independent variables as the simplest multiple regression case. Also, this section introduces the use of some relatively elementary calculus. You do not need to understand the calculus involved to use the results or do anything else in this book. However, those who do understand calculus should be able to see how it is possible to arrive at the equations necessary to solve the multiple regression problems. Recall that the criterion for a best-fitting regression result is as that shown in Equation 12.3. If there are two independent variables, as discussed earlier in Section 12.1, then Equation 12.3 can be defined as shown in Equation 12.4, where b_0 represents the coefficient for the intercept.

$$\Sigma(y - \hat{y})^2 = minimum \tag{12.3}$$

$$\hat{y} = b_1 x_1 + b_2 x_2 + b_0 x_0 \tag{12.4}$$

If $\hat{y}$ is as given in Equation 12.4, then the problem of multiple regression is to find the coefficients b_j that minimize the expression in Equation 12.5.

$$\Sigma(y - b_1 x_1 + b_2 x_2 + b_0 x_0)^2 = minimum \tag{12.5}$$

The Calculus behind the Formulas

Calculus provides a direct solution to the problem of finding the formulas that provide the coefficients b_j that minimize the expression in Equation 12.5. The solution is to take the partial derivative of Equation 12.5, with respect to each of the three b_j coefficients. Although how this is done may not be clear to you if you don't understand calculus, don't despair. It is important to know only that it *can* be done; you will never have to know how to do it in order to understand anything else in this section of the book—or in the book in general.

Using calculus, the partial derivative of Equation 12.5 is found, with respect to each of the three b_j coefficients. The result will be three new equations, as shown in Equation 12.6.

$$\frac{\partial}{\partial b_1} = -2\sum x_1(y - b_1 x_1 - b_2 x_2 - b_0 x_0)$$

$$\frac{\partial}{\partial b_2} = -2\sum x_2(y - b_1 x_1 - b_2 x_2 - b_0 x_0)$$

$$\frac{\partial}{\partial b_0} = -2\sum x_0(y - b_1 x_1 - b_2 x_2 - b_0 x_0) \qquad (12.6)$$

It is the case that if we set the equations in Equation 12.6 equal to 0, we can solve for the regression coefficients that will best fit the original dependent variable data. After setting the three equations equal to 0, we can drop the partial derivative signs in the equations (the symbols in front of the equal signs). After a little algebra, we end up with the three formulations in Equation 12.7.

$$\sum x_1 y - b_1 \sum x_1^2 - b_2 \sum x_1 x_2 - b_0 \sum x_1 x_0 = 0$$

$$\sum x_2 y - b_1 \sum x_1 x_2 - b_2 \sum x_2^2 - b_0 \sum x_2 x_0 = 0$$

$$\sum x_0 y - b_1 \sum x_1 x_0 - b_2 \sum x_2 x_0 - b_0 \sum x_0^2 = 0 \qquad (12.7)$$

or

$$b_1 \sum x_1^2 + b_2 \sum x_1 x_2 + b_0 \sum x_1 x_0 = \sum x_1 y$$

$$b_1 \sum x_1 x_2 + b_2 \sum x_2^2 + b_0 \sum x_2 x_0 = \sum x_2 y$$

$$b_1 \sum x_1 x_0 + b_2 \sum x_2 x_0 + b_0 \sum x_0^2 = \sum x_0 y$$

Solving the Simultaneous Equations Using Excel

Equation 12.7 represents a set of simultaneous equations. Because both the independent variables denoted by x and the dependent variable y are known values, all of the terms in Equation 12.7 that involve summations of x or y can be calculated. Hence, they are known values. But the coefficients b_j are what we are interested in discovering. They are the unknown values. With that in mind, you might recognize the second three expressions in Equation 12.7 as being three equations with three unknowns. In general, a set of equations with an equal number of unknowns can be solved simultaneously for the unknown values. Thus, we should be able to solve this set of three equations for the coefficients b_j that we wish to find. If you remember high school algebra, you know that you can solve this problem with *successive elimination*.

Calculating the X and Y Summations

The first step in the successive elimination process is to find the various summations involving x and y. Figure 12.4 shows the calculation of the various known values required by the simultaneous equations in Equation 12.7 for our data. The data were originally given in Figure 12.1 and are repeated here. The values in cells G6:G11 were found by using the =SUMPRODUCT () function, which multiplies two separate strings of data together and sums the result of all the multiplication operations. The construction of the =SUMPRODUCT () statement can be seen in the formula line in Figure 12.4 for the variables *X1* (Size) and *X2* (Visibility).

You can also see in the formula line that the =SUMPRODUCT () function takes two arguments: the data range for the first variable and the data range for the second variable. The values in cells G3:G5 could also have been produced by using the =SUMPRODUCT () function, with the same range entered for each argument. But they were actually produced by using the =SUMSQ () function, which takes one argument and acts by squaring each subsequent value and putting the sum of those operations into the appropriate cell. Table 12.1 displays the formulas for the calculation of sums in Figure 12.4.

Solving for the Coefficients: Successive Elimination

With the various sums calculated that are called for in the three simultaneous equations given in Equation 12.7, it is possible to undertake the solution

G6		= =SUMPRODUCT(B3:B12,C3:C12)				
A	B	C	D	E	F	G
1 Y	X1	X2	X0			
2 Cost	Size	Visibility	Intercept			
3 2750	225	6	1		X1^2	794375
4 2400	200	37	1		X2^2	4833
5 2920	300	14	1		X0^2	10
6 1800	350	33	1		X1X2	55825
7 3520	200	11	1		X1X0	2725
8 2270	250	21	1		X2X0	201
9 3100	175	21	1		X1Y	6896750
10 1980	400	22	1		X2Y	497750
11 2680	350	20	1		X0Y	26140
12 2720	275	16	1			

Figure 12.4 Calculation of sums

Table 12.1 Formulas for Figure 12.4

Cell or Column	Formula
G3	=SUMSQ(B3:B12)
G4	=SUMSQ(C3:C12)
G5	=SUMSQ(D3:D12)
G6	=SUMPRODUCT(B3:B12,C3:C12)
G7	=SUMPRODUCT(B3:B12,D3:D12)
G8	=SUMPRODUCT(C3:C12,D3:D12)
G9	=SUMPRODUCT(A3:A12,B3:B12)
G10	=SUMPRODUCT(A3:A12,C3:C12)
G11	=SUMPRODUCT(A3:A12,D3:D12)

A20		■	=D15/D16		
	A	**B**	**C**	**D**	**E**
14		b1	b2	b0	
15		794375	55825	2725	6896750
16		55825	4833	201	497750
17		2725	201	10	26140
18					
19		794375	55825	2725	6896750
20	13.55721	756831.5	65522.01	2725	6748103
21		37543.53	-9697.01	0	148646.8
22					
23		794375	55825	2725	6896750
24	272.5	742562.5	54772.5	2725	7123150
25		51812.5	1052.5	0	-226400
26					
27		37543.53	-9697.01		148646.8
28	-9.21332	-477365	-9697.01		2085895
29		514908.5	0		-1937248
30		-3.76232			
31					

Figure 12.5 Successive elimination for b_j

to the equations. The solution for coefficient b_j is shown in Figure 12.5. Rows 15 to 17 in Figure 12.5 represent the three simultaneous equations. The b0, b1, and b2 designations in row 14 represent the coefficient by which each of the numbers in the corresponding row must be multiplied to produce the values in column E, which represent the sums of X1Y, X2Y, and X0Y, respectively.

Successive elimination for the solution of b_j proceeds by eliminating, successively, each of the other two coefficients. This is equivalent to finding the value of the equations when the values by which the other coefficients are multiplied are equal to 0. Rows 19, 20, and 21 show the result of finding an equation with two variables and two unknowns with b_0 eliminated. Row 15 is replicated in row 19. To produce row 20, row 16 is multiplied by the value in cell A20, which is found by dividing cell D15's value by cell D16's value.

You will note that the result in cell D20 is exactly the value in cell D19. Row 20 is then subtracted from row 19 to produce row 21, which is essentially one equation with two rather than three unknown values, b_1 and b_2. The same process is repeated in rows 23 to 25. Row 15 is again copied to row 23, but now, to produce row 24, row 17 is multiplied by the value in cell A24, which is cell D15 divided by cell D17. Again, the result in cell D23 is the same as that in D24. Subtracting row 24 from row 23 produces a second equation with two unknowns in row 25.

The final step of this successive elimination is shown in rows 27 to 29. Row 21, the first of the two equations in two unknowns that were found, is copied to row 27. Row 28 is the result of multiplying row 25 by the value in cell A28, which is cell C21 divided by cell C25. Again, note that the values in cells C27 and C28 are equal. Now, subtraction of row 28 from row 27 leaves a single variable (b_1) with a nonzero value. The solution to the equation in row 29 is shown in cell B30. You can confirm that that is the same value that was found for the coefficient of Size in Figure 12.3, the Excel Data Analysis ➤ Regression–produced result.

The other two coefficients can be found in much the same way. It should be clear that successive elimination is a tedious process involving a lot of division, multiplication, and subtraction. Because it is also what is known as an iterative process, it can be very difficult to set up in a systematic way on a spreadsheet. Moreover, as the number of coefficients gets larger, the amount of work involved in the successive elimination approach to solving simultaneous equations grows geometrically. Basically, it is not a very efficient way to do multiple regression. Fortunately, there is a much more efficient way to solve simultaneous equations—essentially to solve the multiple regression problem—and Excel can deal with it quite effectively. But to understand that strategy for finding multiple regression coefficients, it is necessary to understand a little about matrix math, which is the topic of Appendix A that accompanies Chapter 12 (see p. 481).

EXERCISES FOR SECTION 12.1

1. Use the data shown in Figure 12.1 (also given on the Hospitals worksheet in Chpt 12-1.xls).

   a. Replicate the analysis given in Figure 12.3 by using the Tools ➤ Data Analysis ➤ Regression add-in.

   b. Replicate the analysis given in Figure 12.5, and find the coefficient for b_1 by using successive elimination.

    c. Find the other two coefficients by the same method, and make sure they match those given in Figure 12.3.

2. The data on the SWC worksheet of Chpt 12-1.xls is taken from the *State of the World's Children 2001* (2000). It shows rates of under-five mortality (U5Mort), female literacy (FemLit), and access to safe water (SafeW) for 113 countries of the world, each with more than 1 million inhabitants. Use the data to do the following:

    a. Carry out an analysis such as that given in Figure 12.3 by using Excel's regression add-in. To access the regression add-in, go to the Data ribbon, in the Analysis group, click the Data Analysis option, and then choose the Regression option.

    b. Carry out an analysis such as that given in Figure 12.5, and find the coefficient for b_1 by using successive elimination to find the coefficient for FemLit.

    c. Find the other two coefficients by the same method.

KEY TERMS

#NUM!	independent variable
=MDETERM()	inverse
=MINVERSE()	matrix
=MMULT()	multiple regression
=SUMPRODUCT()	predictor variable
=SUMSQ()	*R square*
=TDIST()	regression analysis
=TRANSPOSE()	regression coefficient
array	scalar
dependent variable	transpose
determinant	vector

CHAPTER 13

EXTENSIONS OF MULTIPLE REGRESSION

Statistics: the mathematical theory of ignorance.

—Morris Kline

Chapter 12 provided an introduction to *multiple regression*, and this chapter continues that discussion. In particular, we consider the use and effect of dummy variables in multiple regression, the selection of best models in multiple regression, correlation among independent variables and the effect of this correlation, and the assessment of nonlinear relationships.

13.1 Dummy Variables in Multiple Regression

Chapter 11 discussed the correspondence between regression and the *t* test. That chapter also showed that the results of both analyses were essentially the same when a *dummy variable* alone was employed as the predictor variable in regression. This section examines the inclusion of a dummy variable, along with other continuous variables in multiple regression analysis, to produce what is sometimes called analysis of covariance (ANCOVA).

A Dummy Variable with No Interaction

Suppose we examine again the data shown in Figure 11.3. Those data show 20 hospital stays and the total charge for each. But this time we will include a second variable: sex of the patient. The length of stay and charges data were taken from actual hospital discharge records. However, the included sex variable was made up to fit

	A	B	C	D
1	Stay	LOS (x1)	Sex (x2)	TC (y)
2	1	3	0	$2,613.91
3	2	10	0	$8,769.03
4	3	2	1	$2,448.60
5	4	3	0	$2,568.70
6	5	3	0	$1,936.19
7	6	5	1	$7,230.71
8	7	5	1	$5,342.61
9	8	3	1	$4,108.13
10	9	1	0	$1,596.91
11	10	2	1	$4,061.28
12	11	2	0	$1,761.53
13	12	5	0	$4,779.19
14	13	1	1	$2,078.30
15	14	3	1	$4,713.61
16	15	4	0	$3,946.68
17	16	2	1	$2,902.74
18	17	1	0	$1,438.85
19	18	1	0	$820.21
20	19	1	1	$3,309.41
21	20	6	0	$5,476.33

Figure 13.1 Data for 20 hospital days with sex as a dummy variable

	H	I	J	K	L
16		Coefficients	Standard Error	t Stat	P-value	Low
17	Intercept	143.6974749	285.4721068	0.503368	0.621165	-4
18	LOS (x1)	875.0476353	62.5665606	13.98587	9.35E-11	74
19	Sex (x2)	1544.552164	273.445291	5.648487	2.89E-05	96
20						

Figure 13.2 Results of regression for 20 hospitals

the example we will discuss. The new data set for the 20 discharges is shown in Figure 13.1, and it shows the length of stay as $x1$ and sex as $x2$. It should be clear that sex is a categorical variable that has been labeled 1 and 0 (1 = female; 0 = male). This allows the categorical variable *sex* to be treated as a numeric variable in regression (as shown in Chapter 11).

Now, if the *regression coefficients* for the two *independent variables* and the intercept are calculated for these data, the results are as shown in Figure 13.2. It can be seen in the figure that the coefficients for both length of stay and sex are different from 0, according to the t tests and probabilities of t (cells K18 and 19 and L18 and 19, respectively).

The Equation for Predicted Values of Total Costs

With the results shown in Figure 13.2, the equation for the predicted values of total charges (TC), given the length of stay and the sex of the patient, is as shown in Equation 13.1. But because sex takes on only the two values 1 and 0, the predicted values of total charges actually form two lines—one when the categorical variable *sex* is coded 0 (male) and one when sex is coded

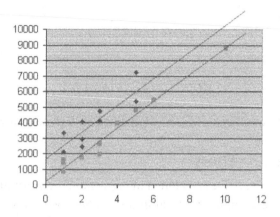

Figure 13.3 Graph of cost data by length of stay

1 (female). The equation of these two lines is as shown in Equation 13.2. The parts within the parentheses in Equation 13.2 are read TC_{pred}, given that *sex* equals 0 (male), and TC_{pred}, given that *sex* equals 1 (female).

$$TC_{pred} = 875.05 \text{ LOS} + 1544.55 \, sex + 143.70 \quad (13.1)$$

$$(TC_{pred}|sex = 0) = 875.05 \text{ LOS} + 143.70, \text{and}$$

$$(TC_{pred}|sex = 1) = 875.05 \text{ LOS} + 1{,}688.25 \quad (13.2)$$

It should be clear that these two lines are exactly parallel to each other (they have the same slope of $875.05) and are exactly $1,544.55 apart ($1688.25 − $143.70). The predicted lines for male and female patients among the 20 in the data set are shown in Figure 13.3. Also shown in the figure are the actual observations. The observations for women are shown as black diamonds and for men as gray squares. As the two parallel predictor lines show, the cost goes up by $875.05 per day, but for every day, the cost is higher for women than for men by $1,544.55. It might also be noted that the two regression lines defined by the equations in Equation 13.1 and Equation 13.2 account for 92 percent of the variance in total charges ($R^2 = 0.92$).

General Formula for Multiple Regression Analysis Using a Dummy Variable

Having looked at the effect of a single dummy variable added to a *regression analysis*, it is useful to provide a general formula for the effect of a dummy variable alone in a multiple regression model. This is shown in Equation 13.3.

$$\text{if } \hat{y} = b_1 x + b_D D + b_0,$$

then

$$(\hat{y}|D = 0) = b_1 x + b_0, \qquad\qquad (13.3)$$

and

$$(\hat{y}|D = 1) = b_1 x + (b_D + b_0)$$

where D is the dummy, and b_D is the coefficient of the dummy.

The Interaction Effect

When a dummy variable is included in regression, the effect of the dummy could be more complex than simply to define two parallel regression lines. It is possible that the two lines (or planes, or hyperspaces) defined by the dummy variable may not be parallel. But for this to occur, the regression analysis would have to include not only the dummy variable but also an interaction term between the dummy variable and at least one continuous variable.

Consider again the data for hospital charges shown in Figure 13.1. Now include an interaction between the continuous variable length of stay and the dummy variable sex, as shown in Figure 13.4. In that figure, it can be seen that the interaction is simply the multiplication of the continuous variable

	A	B	C	D	E
1	Stay	LOS (x1)	Sex (x2)	x1*x2	TC (y)
2	1	3	0	0	$2,613.91
3	2	10	0	0	$8,769.03
4	3	2	1	2	$2,448.60
5	4	3	0	0	$2,568.70
6	5	3	0	0	$1,936.19
7	6	5	1	5	$7,230.71
8	7	5	1	5	$5,342.61
9	8	3	1	3	$4,108.13
10	9	1	0	0	$1,596.91
11	10	2	1	2	$4,061.28
12	11	2	0	0	$1,761.53
13	12	5	0	0	$4,779.19
14	13	1	1	1	$2,078.30
15	14	3	1	3	$4,713.61
16	15	4	0	0	$3,946.68
17	16	2	1	2	$2,902.74
18	17	1	0	0	$1,438.85
19	18	1	0	0	$820.21
20	19	1	1	1	$3,309.41
21	20	6	0	0	$5,476.33
22					

Figure 13.4 Hospital charges with dummy and interaction

		Coefficients	Standard Error	t Stat	P-value	Low
36		Coefficients	Standard Error	t Stat	P-value	Low
37	Intercept	205.7500125	312.5326393	0.658331	0.519687	-4!
38	LOS (x1)	857.5456375	71.35928576	12.0173	2.01E-09	70(
39	Sex (x2)	1293.925913	533.9772408	2.423186	0.027613	1(
40	x1*x2	88.21714028	160.2076205	0.550643	0.589485	-2!

Figure 13.5 Regression coefficients with dummy and interactions

by the dummy variable. When the dummy variable is 0, the interaction term ($x1*x2$) is 0. When the dummy variable is 1, the interaction term is equal to the continuous variable.

We now carry out regression analysis with charges as the *dependent variable* and the three independent variables as shown in Figure 13.4. The resulting regression coefficients, their standard errors, and the appropriate t tests are shown in Figure 13.5. These regression coefficients also account for 92 percent of variance. The fact that the interaction term adds nothing to the regression equation in terms of the variance accounted for is confirmed by the t statistic for the interaction term, shown in cell L40. The t statistic is 0.55, which has a 59 percent probability of occurrence under the null hypothesis that charges are independent of the interaction between the length of stay and sex. In essence, we conclude that the coefficient on the interaction term is 0.

A Dummy Variable with an Interaction

We now consider an example in which the interaction term is statistically significant. In other words, can we conclude that the coefficient on the interaction term is different from 0? Such an example is shown in Figure 13.6. This figure shows the same charges and the same length of stay as those shown in Figures 13.1 and 13.4. However, the sex designations have changed to present a different picture of the data. If regression is carried out using only the dummy variable with no interaction term, the results are as shown in Figure 13.7.

Of the regression coefficients shown in Figure 13.7, only the coefficients for length of stay and the intercept are different from 0. Sex is no longer a statistically significant predictor of charges. In this case, it would be a reasonable practice to simply drop sex from the analysis and predict charges with the length of stay only, except for one thing. It may be that the interaction between the length of stay and sex could have a statistically significant relationship to charges. To determine if it does, it would be necessary to analyze all three variables—the length of stay, sex, and the length of stay/sex interaction—simultaneously. The coefficients that result

	A	B	C	D	E
1	Stay	LOS (x1)	Sex (x2)	x1*x2	TC (y)
2	1	3	0	0	$2,613.91
3	2	10	0	0	$8,769.03
4	3	2	1	2	$2,448.60
5	4	3	1	3	$2,568.70
6	5	3	1	3	$1,936.19
7	6	5	1	5	$7,230.71
8	7	5	0	0	$5,342.61
9	8	3	1	3	$4,108.13
10	9	1	1	1	$1,596.91
11	10	2	0	0	$4,061.28
12	11	2	1	2	$1,761.53
13	12	5	0	0	$4,779.19
14	13	1	0	0	$2,078.30
15	14	3	0	0	$4,713.61
16	15	4	0	0	$3,946.68
17	16	2	1	2	$2,902.74
18	17	1	1	1	$1,438.85
19	18	1	1	1	$820.21
20	19	1	0	0	$3,309.41
21	20	6	0	0	$5,476.33
22					

Figure 13.6 Hospital charges with dummy and interaction: Modified example

	I	J	K	L	M
37		Coefficients	Standard Error	t Stat	P-value	Low
38	Intercept	1488.76838	533.051131	2.792919	0.01249	3€
39	LOS (x1)	755.066654	108.7859451	6.940847	2.38E-06	5₂
40	Sex (x2)	-544.16469	473.0625337	-1.1503	0.265944	-1
41						

Figure 13.7 Regression coefficients with dummy only: Modified example

	I	J	K	L	M
16		Coefficients	Standard Error	t Stat	P-value	Low
17	Intercept	1959.00894	483.7201956	4.04988	0.000929	93
18	LOS (x1)	637.506515	101.7513079	6.26534	1.13E-05	42
19	Sex (x2)	-2280.0527	747.4511603	-3.05044	0.007632	-3
20	x1*x2	667.841641	242.5195211	2.753764	0.014124	15

Figure 13.8 Regression coefficients with dummy and interaction: Modified example

from this analysis are shown in Figure 13.8. In that figure it is possible to see that not only is the coefficient for sex statistically different from 0, but so, too, is the interaction coefficient.

In addition, the coefficient on the length of stay remains statistically significant. What does this mean in terms of the prediction of charges?

It means not only will charges be predicted by two lines with different intercepts for males and females, but also the slopes of those lines will be different. This can be seen in the equations for the two lines, as shown in Equation 13.4. For men (*sex* = 0), the charge increases by $637.51 for each additional day of stay, with a fixed cost of $1,959.01 for a stay of zero days. For women, the cost increases by $1,305.35 per day of stay from a fixed cost of −$321.04 for a stay of zero days. Of course, because no hospital admission will be a zero-day stay, the intercept terms represent only the *y*-axis anchor for the respective lines.

$$(TC_{pred}) = 637.51 \text{ LOS} + 22,280.05 \text{ } sex + 667.84 \text{ LOS} \cdot sex + 1,959.01,$$

or

$$(TC_{pred}|sex = 0) = 637.51 \text{ LOS} + 1,959.01,$$

and

$$(TC_{pred}|sex = 1) = 1,305.35 \text{ LOS} - 321.04 \tag{13.4}$$

Now that we have seen that the regression lines are different, it may be useful to see how these are pictured in a two-dimensional graphic presentation. Figure 13.9 shows the graph of the charges data with the two regression lines as defined by Equation 13.4, included in the graph. The more steeply sloped graph with the intercept below 0 is the line for women. The actual observations for women are shown as diamonds. The less steeply sloped graph with the regression line crossing the *y*-axis at about $2,000 is the slope for men. The actual observations for men are shown as squares.

It should be remembered that these examples, although based on actual charge and length of stay data, have fabricated data for sex. The sex variable

Figure 13.9 Hospital charges with dummy and iteration graphed

has been manipulated in each case just presented to produce the outcomes that have been found. It is highly unlikely that over a large sample of data any difference would be found for men and women in hospital charges. In addition, the result of an *interaction effect* would be even more unlikely. Nevertheless, there are many situations in which dummy variables and interaction terms could have realistic meaning. With that in mind, it is useful to present a general formula for determining the slope and intercept of lines when dummy variables and interactions are present. Such a formula is given in Equation 13.5.

$$\text{if } \hat{y} = b_1 x + b_D D + b_2 xD + b_0,$$

then

$$(\hat{y}|D = 0) = b_1 x + b_0,$$

and

$$(\hat{y}|D = 1) = (b_1 + b_2)x + (b_D + b_0) \tag{13.5}$$

where D is the dummy, and b_D is the coefficient of the dummy.

If there is more than one continuous independent variable, the slope of the line defined by the continuous variable will change only for those variables for which there are dummy continuous variable interaction terms.

General Comments on Dummy and Interaction Terms

Let's assume that an interaction is expected and an interaction term is included in an analysis with a continuous variable and a 1/0 dummy. In turn, the full regression model, including the interaction term, should be run. If the interaction term is not different from 0 (i.e., if the absolute t value is less than 2), the interaction term can be dropped. Then the analysis can be rerun with only the continuous variable and the dummy variable included. This simpler model will describe the data as adequately as the more complex model, including the interaction. If, in this further analysis, the coefficient for the dummy is not different from 0, it is possible to drop the dummy as well and simply predict the dependent variable on the basis of the continuous variable (or continuous variables).

Let's now assume that an interaction term is included in an analysis and the coefficient for the interaction term is different from 0 but the coefficients for the continuous variable and the dummy variables are not different from 0. A similar decision as previously mentioned may be made. It is sometimes possible to drop the continuous variable and the dummy variable and predict the dependent variable solely on the strength of the interaction variable itself. The results of the analysis may produce slightly different coefficients, but the predicted values of the dependent variable will be very much the same.

Example of Using Only the Interaction Term as the Predictor

To see an example of this, consider the imaginary hospital charge data shown in Figure 13.10. In this data set, *Inpatient*=1 means that the patient was actually in the hospital during the length of stay indicated, whereas *Inpatient*=0 means that the patient was being treated during the time period indicated as *LOS* (length of stay) on an outpatient basis. The question is whether there is an interaction effect of *LOS* and *Inpatient*.

Using the Data Analysis ➤ Regression add-in produces the coefficients shown in Figure 13.11. In that figure it can be seen by the *t* tests on the three coefficients representing the independent variables and the probabilities of those *t* tests (cells M18:M20 and N18:N20, respectively) that only the coefficient for the interaction is different from 0. This essentially means that neither the continuous variable *LOS* nor the dummy variable *Inpatient* contributes in a statistically significant way to the prediction of charges.

	A	B	C	D	E
1	Obs	LOS	Inpatient	Inter	Charges
2	1	7	0	0	2900
3	2	5	0	0	2539
4	3	7	0	0	2427
5	4	7	0	0	2202
6	5	9	0	0	2682
7	6	8	0	0	2581
8	7	3	0	0	2862
9	8	5	0	0	2857
10	9	4	0	0	2257
11	10	11	0	0	3190
12	11	3	1	3	3317
13	12	2	1	2	2970
14	13	9	1	9	5443
15	14	9	1	9	5011
16	15	8	1	8	4717
17	16	10	1	10	5214
18	17	3	1	3	3955
19	18	9	1	9	4906
20	19	2	1	2	2544
21	20	3	1	3	3987
22					

Figure 13.10 Charge data showing an interaction effect

	J	K	L	M	N	
16		Coefficients	Standard Error	t Stat	P-value	Low
17	Intercept	2360.91221	338.1670817	6.981496	3.09E-06	1
18	LOS	43.7557252	48.40847693	0.903886	0.379464	-€
19	Inpatient	255.441953	407.1281721	0.627424	0.539233	-€
20	Inter	230.390108	59.2131279	3.890862	0.001299	1C

Figure 13.11 Coefficients for charge data showing an interaction effect

	J	K	L	M	N	
39		Coefficients	Standard Error	t Stat	P-value	Lov
40	Intercept	2643.26954	96.27864552	27.45437	3.83E-16	2·
41	Inter	270.613952	20.4801831	13.21345	1.05E-10	2

Figure 13.12 Coefficients for charge data showing only the interaction effect

The total proportion of the variance in charges accounted for by all three variables (R^2) is 0.91.

Because neither the coefficient on LOS nor that on Inpatient is statistically different from 0 in the analysis of the data in Figure 13.10, it is not unreasonable to consider dropping those from the analysis in order to predict charges.

Conceptually, this amounts to imputing a fixed fee to outpatient contacts with the hospital. This result is regardless of the amount of time over which they extend, and in turn predicting inpatient stays on the basis of the time in the institution. The result of this analysis is shown in Figure 13.12. Here, the coefficient for the interaction has changed from 230.39 (Figure 13.11) to 270.61, but the total proportion of the variation accounted for remains essentially at 0.91. In essence, either model is equally good at predicting hospital charges as represented by the data in Figure 13.10.

Graphing the actual data points and both predicted values for the data, those using the coefficients in Figure 13.11 and those using the coefficients in Figure 13.12, will show this. The result is shown in Figure 13.13.

Comparison of Models in Graphical Form

In Figure 13.13, the gray squares represent charges for actual hospital stays. The black diamonds represent charges for outpatient contacts with the hospital over the numbers of days indicated on the horizontal axis. Turn your attention to the sloping line from about 2360, when days of contact

Figure 13.13   Graph of charge data with predicted lines

with the hospital are zero, to about 2800, when days of contact with the hospital are 12. It represents the predicted charges for those who were treated on an outpatient basis when the predicted values are calculated using all three coefficients (refer to Figure 13.11).

The horizontal line at 2643 represents the predicted charges for those people who were treated on an outpatient basis, using only the coefficients given in Figure 13.12. The line is essentially the mean of the outpatient charges. This occurs because there is no separate term to represent the length of contact with the hospital for the outpatient group.

Focus next on the diagonal line sloping from about 2600, when length of stay is zero days, to about 5700, when length of stay is 12 days. This line represents the predicted value of charges for those people who actually had hospital stays, using either set of coefficients. The lines are so close together that they cannot be shown separately on the graph. (The predicted line given the coefficients in Figure 13.11 is Charges = 274.05 LOS + 2,616.35, whereas for the coefficients in Figure 13.12, it is Charges = 270.61 LOS + 2,643.27.)

In considering the preceding discussion, an important point should be noted. Dropping both the slope and intercept terms and predicting the charges values simply on the basis of the interaction assume automatically that the outpatient contacts (given as 0 in the dummy variable) actually have no relationship to number of days of contact with the hospital. If they did, the coefficients for days and the intercept would have had to be included in the analysis, even if they were not statistically different from zero. Otherwise, the predicted values for charges for outpatients would always be a flat line.

EXERCISES FOR SECTION 13.1

1. Use the data shown in Figure 13.1 (available on the Charges1 worksheet in Chpt 13-1.xls).

   a. Replicate the analysis given in Figure 13.2 by using the Data Analysis ≻ Regression add-in.

   b. Generate predicted values of TC on the basis of the regression coefficients.

   c. Write out the regression equations for TC when $Sex = 0$ and $Sex = 1$.

   d. Develop an xy graph with TC and the predicted values of TC as the y variable and LOS as the x variable, and confirm that the predicted values of TC form two parallel lines.

2. The data file on the Costs worksheet of Chpt 13-1.xls is the same data file as that given on the Costs worksheet of Chpt 10-1.xls, and it is discussed in Section 10.1. The only difference is that the variable length of stay (*LOS*) has been added to the worksheet in Chpt 13-1.xls. Use these data to do the following:

   a. Insert a new column at column C, and create a variable called *Catawba*—that is, 1 for *Catawba* and 0 for the other three hospitals.

   b. Develop the multiple regression analysis by using the Tools ≻ Data Analysis ≻ Regression add-in with both the variables *Catawba* and *LOS* as the independent variables and *Costs* as the dependent variable.

   c. Interpret the t values and probabilities for the coefficients to determine whether either or both independent variables are statistically significant (different from 0).

   d. Write out the regression equations for costs when $Catawba = 0$ (for any other hospital) and $Catawba = 1$.

   e. Generate predicted values of costs on the basis of the regression coefficients.

   f. Develop an xy graph with costs and the predicted values of costs as the y variable and LOS as the x variable, and decide if the predicted values of costs form two parallel lines.

3. Use the data shown in Figure 13.6 (or use the data given on the Charges2 worksheet, insert a column, and add an interaction term).

   a. Replicate the analysis given in Figure 13.8 by using the Tools ≻ Data Analysis ≻ Regression add-in.

   b. Generate predicted values of TC on the basis of the regression coefficients.

   c. Write out the regression equations for TC when $Sex = 0$ and $Sex = 1$.

   d. Develop an xy graph with TC and the predicted values of TC as the y variable and LOS as the x variable, and confirm that the predicted values of TC form two parallel lines.

4. Use the data file on the Costs worksheet of Chpt 13-1.xls with the addition of the variable for Catawba.

a. Insert a column next to the *Catawba* variable and label it *Inter* (interaction), and then create a new variable that is the multiplication of the variable *Catawba* by the LOS.

b. Carry out a regression analysis with *Costs* as the dependent variable and the three independent variables—*Catawba*, *Inter*, and *LOS*—as the independent variables.

c. On the basis of the results, decide whether *Inter* is a statistically significant predictor of costs.

d. On the basis of this analysis and that in Exercise 2, decide which of the two analyses seems best for costs.

13.2   The Best Regression Model

The discussion in Section 13.1 focused on dummy variables and their treatment in regression. In that discussion there exists the question of whether to include a dummy variable or an interaction term in a general regression model. The decision to include was based on whether either was not statistically significant (i.e., different from 0). The conclusion from the discussion was that it did not make much difference either way in the prediction of the dependent variable.

In general, that result holds. However, the question of whether it is appropriate to drop variables from a regression model if they are not statistically significant is one that is widely debated. There is no generally accepted agreement on which is correct.

Theory or Dust Bowl Empiricism?

The argument for dropping statistically nonsignificant variables from a regression model is based on two points. First, including statistically non-significant variables in a model will not improve the prediction of the dependent variable in any statistically significant way. Second, including statistically nonsignificant variables unnecessarily complicates the under-standing of the dependent variable with extraneous independent variables that have no predictive value.

The argument for not dropping statistically nonsignificant variables from a regression model is based primarily on a single point, but it is an important one. This point is that a regression equation implies a causal relationship in which the values of the dependent variable are actually caused by the values of the independent variable set.

This causal relationship in turn implies some underlying theoretical model that says a certain set of independent variables should be included in a regression model. The fact that in a particular instance under analysis this may not have been found to be true does not necessarily invalidate the theory. Neither does it allow the analyst to drop a variable from the predictor model. To do so is not only to abandon the theory but, as we have seen in regard to dummy variables, also to change the values of the coefficients.

The argument that a regression model represents a theory is further supported by the empirical evidence that one set of predictor variables may be as useful as another completely different set of predictor variables in predicting a dependent variable. In such a situation, only a theory, and not simply the regression analysis alone, can determine which variables to include in the regression equation.

To Drop Regression Variables or Not to Drop Regression Variables: An Exploration

To explore some of these issues, we will use data taken from *The State of the World's Children 1996* (1996). These data are for 75 countries in the world for which all the data to be examined were available. (It should be noted that UNICEF publishes these data every year, so more recent data are available. The data from 1996 demonstrate several points that are to be made in this section, whereas data from later years do not necessarily demonstrate the same points. One of the difficult things about regression analysis is that the data do not always behave in the same ways from one sample to another.)

A sample of the data under consideration is shown in Figure 13.14. The data represent eight independent variables and one dependent variable. The dependent variable is *U5Mort* in column K, the under-five mortality for each country for 1994. The eight independent variables include five variables related to the public health system.

The variable *SafeW* is the proportion of households with access to safe water. The variable *Sanit* is the proportion of households with access to sanitary facilities. The variable *HealthS* is the proportion of households within a specified travel distance of a health facility. The variable *DPT* is the proportion of children immunized for diphtheria, pertussis, and tetanus by age one. The variable *CPR* is the contraceptive prevalence rate.

Also included as independent variables are three that are not dimensions of the health care system. The variable *LogGNP* is the log of the gross national product per capita (the log is used because the actual value of GNP is not linearly related to under-five mortality, whereas the log is). The

	B	C	D	E	F	G	H	I	J	K
1		SafeW	Sanit	HealthS	DPT	CPR	LogGNP	FemLit	TFR	U5Mort
2	Niger	54	15	32	20	4	2.4314	5	7.3	320
3	Angola	32	16	30	27	1	2.8451	29	7	292
4	Sierra Leone	34	11	38	43	4	2.1761	14	6.4	284
5	Mozambique	33	20	39	55	4	1.9542	19	6.4	277
6	Guinea-Bissau	53	21	40	74	1	2.3802	37	5.7	231
7	Guinea	55	21	80	70	1	2.6990	18	6.9	223
8	Malawi	47	53	80	98	13	2.3010	37	7	221
9	Liberia	46	30	39	43	6	2.6532	18	6.7	217
10	Mali	37	31	30	39	5	2.4314	17	7	214
11	Somalia	37	18	27	23	1	2.0792	14	6.9	211
12	Zambia	50	37	75	85	15	2.5798	65	5.8	203
13	Ethiopia	25	19	46	37	2	2.0000	21	6.9	200
14	Nigeria	40	35	66	41	6	2.4771	39	6.3	191
15	Zaire	27	23	26	29	1	2.3424	61	6.6	186
16	Uganda	34	57	49	79	5	2.2553	44	7.1	185
17	Burundi	70	51	80	48	9	2.2553	19	6.6	176
18	Central African Rep.	18	45	45	31	15	2.6021	41	5.6	175
19	Burkina Faso	78	18	90	41	8	2.4771	7	6.4	169
20	Madagascar	29	3	65	66	17	2.3424	73	6	164
21	Tanzania, U. Rep. of	50	64	80	79	18	1.9542	50	5.8	159
22	Lesotho	52	28	90	58	23	2.8129	57	5.1	156

Figure 13.14 Data from *The State of the World's Children 1996*

	AG	AH	AI	AJ	AK	AL	AM
1		Coefficients	Standard Error	t Stat	P-value	Intercept	R Square
2	SafeW	-2.364	0.312	-7.567	9.14E-11	255.452	0.440
3	Sanit	-2.308	0.239	-9.640	1.19E-14	227.016	0.560
4	HealthS	-2.271	0.302	-7.532	1.06E-10	265.128	0.437
5	DPT	-2.479	0.291	-8.534	1.4E-12	284.451	0.499
6	CPR	-2.665	0.197	-13.557	1.26E-21	196.177	0.716
7	FemLit	-2.177	0.223	-9.764	6.97E-15	225.211	0.499
8	TFR	37.340	3.079	12.126	3.66E-19	-70.733	0.668
9	LogGNP	-116.564	12.628	-9.231	6.88E-14	438.092	0.539

Figure 13.15 Coefficients for each of the predictor variables for *U5Mort* independently

variable *FemLit* is the female literacy rate for the country. The variable *TFR* is the average number of births per woman.

Each one of the independent variables in Figure 13.14 is approximately linear in its relation to *U5Mort*. In addition, each is a statistically significant predictor of *U5Mort*. Figure 13.15 is a composite of eight separate regression analyses, one for each of the independent variables predicting *U5Mort* on its own.

As the *t* statistics and their probabilities indicate (columns AJ and AK, respectively), each of the independent variables, taken separately, is a statistically significant predictor of under-five mortality. Furthermore, take a look at the R^2 value, shown in column AM. R^2 indicates that the independent variables, taken alone, account for between 43.7 percent (for *HealthS*) and 71.6 percent (for *CPR*) of the variance in under-five mortality across the data set.

	M	N	O	P	Q	L(
16		Coefficients	Standard Error	t Stat	P-value	
17	Intercept	264.8972296	71.10592989	3.725389	0.000406	1
18	SafeW	0.030147374	0.332918971	0.090555	0.928121	·
19	Sanit	-0.733757198	0.279558794	-2.6247	0.010765	·
20	HealthS	-0.318333165	0.259903869	-1.22481	0.225	·
21	DPT	-0.523582754	0.286016159	-1.83061	0.071675	·
22	CPR	-0.605704804	0.494921411	-1.22384	0.225364	·
23	LogGNP	-21.91231273	14.69602134	-1.49104	0.140716	·
24	FemLit	-0.289953578	0.292665598	-0.99073	0.325434	·
25	TFR	7.640583579	6.954863453	1.098596	0.275936	·
26						

Figure 13.16 Multiple regression coefficients of predictors for *U5Mort*

Consider first the question of what to do about statistically nonsignificant variables in a multiple regression model. To do this, we will look at all eight of the independent variables shown in Figures 13.14 and 13.15, analyzed simultaneously. The result of this analysis is shown in Figure 13.16.

As Figure 13.16 shows, when all seven independent variables are included in the regression model, only one coefficient, that for *Sanit*, is different from 0 (i.e., a probability of less than 0.05). This is despite the fact that when each variable is examined separately in regard to under-five mortality, each of the eight has a nonzero coefficient. The total variance accounted for (R^2) by all eight variables in the regression model (even though only one is statistically different from 0) is 0.815.

Comparing Models with and without Variables: Stepwise Regression

Within the context of the view that holds that a theory must be the basis of the regression model analyzed, it would have been assumed that some theory specified that all eight variables should be included in the multiple regression model. Within this perspective, the fact that only one variable (*Sanit*) actually shows a statistically significant coefficient would not be sufficient cause to eliminate any of the variables used as a way to simplify the regression model. Within the context of the alternative view, which seeks the simplest regression model for predicting the dependent variable, it is clear that some variables in the model are not useful and should be dropped. One approach to this would be simply to fall back to the use of *Sanit* alone to predict *U5Mort*. But we already know that *Sanit* alone is not the best predictor of *U5Mort*, that distinction being held by *CPR* (see Figure 13.15). So, how should we proceed?

A common approach to seeking the best multiple regression model is what is often called *stepwise regression*, a term that denotes a number of different methods. These methods vary in their levels of complexity for seeking the best set of independent variables for simultaneously predicting the dependent variable of interest. In general, the various stepwise regression approaches can be characterized as either backward stepwise elimination or forward stepwise inclusion.

Backward Stepwise Elimination

The simplest example of backward stepwise elimination begins with the complete model, as shown in Figure 13.16. It then successively eliminates in a stepwise manner the predictor with the least significant coefficient. This process continues until only variables with statistically significant coefficients remain. If the backward elimination approach to stepwise regression is employed, the first variable to be eliminated is *SafeW*, with a *p* value of 0.928. Although the result of that analysis with six independent variables is not shown, the next variable to be eliminated would be *TFR*. The stepwise process would continue until only variables with statistically significant coefficients remain.

Figure 13.17 shows the results of the backward elimination process beginning with all variables shown in Figure 13.16. As Figure 13.17 shows, four variables—*LogGNP*, *Sanit*, *DPT*, and *CPR*—have coefficients that are statistically different from 0 after the stepwise procedure. The resulting R^2 is 0.798.

Forward Stepwise Inclusion

Forward stepwise inclusion begins with the single variable that accounts for the largest proportion of the variance and proceeds at each step by adding a next variable that accounts for as much of the unexplained variance as possible. This essentially means selecting the next variable that, with the two variables taken together, accounts for the largest proportion of variance (has the largest *R square*). From the forward inclusion approach,

	M	N	O	P	Q
114		Coefficients	Standard Error	t Stat	P-value	L
115	Intercept	321.9082	34.59634683	9.3047	7.3E-14
116	LogGNP	-29.967464	13.39720112	-2.237	0.02848
117	Sanit	-0.7018368	0.25167603	-2.789	0.00681
118	DPT	-0.6947679	0.275624748	-2.521	0.01399
119	CPR	-1.2991115	0.317337595	-4.094	0.00011

Figure 13.17 Multiple regression coefficients of best predictors for *U5Mort*: Backward elimination

	BA	BB	BC	BD	BE
16		Coefficients	Standard Error	t Stat	P-value
17	Intercept	109.91	34.18740328	3.2149	0.00196
18	TFR	21.65734	3.580406439	6.0488	6.2E-08
19	Sanit	-1.1491147	0.209352248	-5.4889	5.9E-07
20	DPT	-0.6447902	0.264066091	-2.4418	0.01711

Figure 13.18 Multiple regression coefficients of best predictors for *U5Mort*: Forward inclusion

the first variable into the model would be *CPR*. *CPR* accounts for the largest proportion of variance in under-five mortality when each variable is taken singly ($R^2 = 0.716$ in Figure 13.15). With *CPR* included, the next best predictor is *Sanit*. Together, *CPR* and *Sanit* account for 0.768 percent of the variance in *U5Mort*. With *CPR* and *Sanit* included, the next best predictor turns out to be *TFR*. When *TFR* is included with *CPR* and *Sanit*, they account for 0.789 percent of the variance in *U5Mort*.

But now a problem arises in the analysis. When *TFR* is included with *CPR* and *Sanit*, the coefficient for *CPR* is no longer different from 0 (i.e., the probability for the *t* statistic is greater than 0.05—actually, 0.068). This requires a decision that, in general, does not usually arise with backward elimination. We can continue with *CPR*, *Sanit*, and *TFR*, even though *CPR* is no longer statistically different from 0. On the other hand, we could drop *CPR*, replace it with *TFR*, and continue to develop the model on the basis of *TFR* and *Sanit*. In this case, we will elect the latter approach.

The results of the forward inclusion method (substituting *TFR* for *CPR* because when *TFR*, *CPR*, and *Sanit* are included in the same model, *CPR* no longer has a coefficient different from zero) are shown in Figure 13.18. Three variables—*TFR*, *Sanit*, and *DPT*—have coefficients different from zero. Adding any other variable to this set of three results in a probability greater than 0.05 for the coefficient of the added variable. This model, with three predictor variables, accounts for 79.6 percent of the variance in *U5Mort*.

Backward Elimination or Forward Inclusion: Which Method to Choose?

It is possible that with a more sophisticated approach to backward elimination, both approaches would have reached the same result as shown in Figure 13.18. But a more sophisticated approach to forward inclusion, regardless of how good any single one was, might have also resulted in a different set of predictor variables—for example, selecting the best three predictors simultaneously.

The bottom line is this: In general, stepwise regression, though it may result in a simplified model, is probably less desirable as an approach to regression analysis than analysis based on a clear understanding of which independent variables should be included in a given model. This can be determined only from a clear understanding of the process that actually produces the results in the dependent variable of interest. The best place to obtain this understanding is a good theory.

Stepwise Regression in Excel

Dedicated statistics packages often have a few commands that will allow the user to perform a host of forward, backward, and sideways regression analyses (the sideways regression analysis is problematic), producing vast reams of printout. Microsoft Excel, though an outstanding statistical tool, does not produce stepwise regression results quite so easily. It is necessary with Excel to do each regression separately. So, if one is to replicate the discussion in the previous (first) subsection of this section (13.2), as is suggested in Exercise 1 of this section, a little direction is probably useful.

Single-Variable Regression Using Excel

To replicate the results in the previous discussion, begin with the data on the U5Mort1 worksheet of Chpt 13-1.xls. The first task is to reproduce the single-variable regression results shown in Figure 13.15. Begin with the data on the U5Mort1 worksheet, which are those given in Figure 13.14. Using Data Analysis ➢ Regression, specify *U5Mort* as the dependent variable and *SafeW* as the independent variable. Specify the output cell as M1. This will produce the regression that will allow you to replicate row 2 in Figure 13.15. Now recall the Data Analysis ➢ Regression dialog box, and change the independent variable to *Sanit* and the output cell to M21. This will cause the result to replicate row 3 in Figure 13.15. Proceed this way with the remaining six variables, putting the results in M41, M61, M81, and so on. This allows you to produce all of the results shown in Figure 13.15.

Backward Elimination Using Excel

To replicate the results in Figure 13.16, the entire independent variable set from *SafeW* to *TFR* should be included in a single regression model. Because this is the first step to the backward elimination process, insert a new worksheet, label it *U5Mort1-b* for backward elimination, and copy the data in cells A1:K76 to the new worksheet. Now invoke Data Analysis ➢ Regression, and specify all the variables from *SafeW* to *TFR* as the independent variables. Put this result in cell M1. This replicates Figure 13.16 and also provides the starting point for backward elimination.

As the analysis in Figure 13.16 shows, *SafeW* has the smallest p value in the complete model. This is the first variable to be eliminated in the next step. Copy all the data from cells D1:J1 (i.e., all the independent variables except for *SafeW*), and paste the copy into cell W1. This now leaves seven independent variables in columns W through AC. Invoke Data Analysis ➤ Regression again, and change the variable fields to reflect the moved data set. (It is necessary only to change the reference for the independent variables, because the dependent variable remains in column K.) Put the result into cell AE. In this analysis you will discover that *TFR* has the largest p value (0.275) and is the next to be eliminated.

Copy the six independent variables (columns W to AB), and paste them into cell AO1. This eliminates *TFR*. Now invoke Data Analysis ➤ Regression, specify the new set of six independent variables, and specify the output cell as AV1. In this analysis you will discover that *HealthS* has the largest p value (0.137) and will be the next variable eliminated. The easiest way to do this is to copy all the columns AO through AT and paste them into cell BF1. Then click the BG at the top of the HealthS column, and eliminate the entire column. This will now put the five remaining independent variables into columns AO:BJ. Analysis proceeds in this fashion until all variables in the model have p values of 0.05 or less, at which time the regression analysis result should look exactly like that in Figure 13.17 (it will take two more steps, and the variables will not appear in the same order, but the coefficients, t tests, and p values will be the same).

Forward Stepwise Inclusion Using Excel

Replicating forward stepwise inclusion to produce the result shown in Figure 13.18 is a similar, but somewhat more complicated, process. To begin the process, return to the U5Mort1 worksheet on which the regressions with each independent variable as a predictor of *U5Mort* were carried out. Then select the variable with the largest R^2 value. This happens to be *CPR* (shown in Figure 13.15).

Copy the variable *CPR* to column W, beginning in cell W1. Now select the first of the other independent variables, *SafeW*, and copy it to column X, beginning in cell X1. Now invoke Data Analysis ➤ Regression, and specify the two variables *CPR* and *SafeW* in columns W and X, respectively, as the independent variables. Put the results into cell Z1. Now it is time to pair *CPR* with *Sanit*.

Recall that it is necessary for the entire independent variable set in regression to be in contiguous columns. So *Sanit* must be contiguous with *CPR*. The easiest way to do this is to click the X that heads the column containing *SafeW* and insert a new column at this point. This moves the variable *SafeW* to column Y and the output from the most recent regression to column AA. Now copy the data for *Sanit*, and put it into column X, beginning in cell X1. Using the variables *CPR* and *Sanit*, replicate the previous regression and put the output into cell AA21. In doing this, it will be necessary to change only the destination cell.

To continue with the two-variable regression, continue to add a new column at X for each new variable to be paired with CPR until all the other six variables have been analyzed this way. It should not ever be necessary to change the data references, but it will be necessary to change the output reference each time to ensure that all the output is in the same column. The cell into which the last regression output will go for this sequence (which will be the pairing of *CPR* with *TFR* if you are following this example) will be cell AF121.

After completing this sequence of two variables, you will see that *CPR* and *Sanit*, taken together, have the largest R^2 at 0.768. So these two variables will be those included at the next step. This next step will proceed just as the last did, except that now the two variables—*CPR* and *Sanit*—will be copied to the columns AP and AQ, beginning in the first cell in those columns. Now the first of the remaining variables, *SafeW*, will be copied to column AR, and a new regression analysis will be performed with these three variables as the predictors. It will be necessary to change the *x* input range to reflect the three variables being analyzed, and also the output range, which should be specified as cell AT1.

Just as in the previous sequence, we now insert a column at AR and copy the next variable, *HealthS*, to that column. Now that we've done this, regression is again performed, changing only the output destination to AU22. Another column is inserted at AR, and the process continues. The destination of the last regression analysis will be cell AY106.

Having completed this stage of the analysis, we will see that the largest R^2 (0.789) is associated with regression that includes *CPR*, *Sanit*, and *TFR*. But as noted previously, *CPR* no longer has a statistically significant coefficient ($p = 0.068$). So we will drop *CPR* in favor of *TFR* and replicate the two-variable analysis with *Sanit* and *TFR*.

In the repeat of the two-variable analysis with *Sanit* and *TFR*, it turns out that only one of the other six variables, *DPT*, has a coefficient different from 0, and that is the last variable to be included. This set of three variables accounts for 79.6 percent of the variance ($R^2 = 0.796$), and the analysis is complete.

An Alternative Look at the Importance of Theory

This concern with a theoretical approach to regression is also supported with a somewhat different analysis of these same data. Suppose we have one group of analysts who believe that the important determinant of under-five mortality is the health and health services environment of a country. With that in mind, they might reasonably decide to predict under-five mortality by using those available variables that are health-related, which, in this case, could include the variables *SafeW*, *Sanit*, *HServe*, *DPT*, and *CPR*. Another group of analysts might believe that the important determinant of under-five mortality is not the health environment of the country but, rather, the general cultural environment. Therefore, they might determine that they should predict under-five mortality by using the cultural variables *FemLit*, *LogGNP*, and *Fert*.

Taking the health approach, and using backward elimination of non-significant coefficients, the results of the analysis are shown in Figure 13.19. The three variables, *Sanit*, *DPT*, and *CPR*, together account for 78.3 percent of the variance in under-five mortality. If the general cultural environment approach is taken, the results of the analysis are shown in Figure 13.20. Here, all three variables had statistically significant coefficients on the first analysis. The three variables, *LogGNP*, *FemLit*, and *Fert*, taken together account for 73.6 percent of the variance in under-five mortality. It is possible to account for similar proportions of the variation in under-five mortality, approaching it as strictly a health issue, or as a cultural issue. The

	I	J	K	L	M
61		Coefficients	Standard Error	t Stat	P-value	L
62	Intercept	253.64387	16.74887038	15.1439	6.3E-24	:
63	Sanit	-0.9348755	0.235470915	-3.9702	0.00017
64	DPT	-0.6163626	0.280988904	-2.1935	0.03154
65	CPR	-1.6090868	0.293419628	-5.4839	6E-07
66					

Figure 13.19 Multiple regression coefficients of best predictors for *U5Mort*: Health predictors

	G	H	I	J	K
16		Coefficients	Standard Error	t Stat	P-value	I
17	Intercept	183.29635	61.75869844	2.9679	0.00408
18	LogGNP	-44.275924	14.03687157	-3.154	0.00236
19	FemLit	-0.7447152	0.286887575	-2.596	0.01146
20	TFR	18.90089	5.19210462	3.6403	0.00051

Figure 13.20 Multiple regression coefficients of best predictors for *U5Mort*: Cultural predictors

bottom line is that the statistical analysis alone is a weak tool for deciding which variables should or should not be included in the analysis.

Despite the problems of determining the correct regression model on the basis of the statistical analysis alone, there will continue to be those who use the stepwise method—either forward or backward or both—to uncover the "best" regression models. There will also continue to be many who say that the regression model can be determined only by a theoretical framework and confirmed or not confirmed by the analysis.

Perhaps the best that can be said about the two approaches is that the former is largely exploratory, whereas the latter is an attempt at the confirmation of theory. Short of that, the controversy is not likely to be resolved.

EXERCISES FOR SECTION 13.2

1. The U5Mort1 worksheet of Chpt 13-1.xls shows the entire data set shown in Figure 13.14. Use this data set to replicate the analysis discussed in this section.

   a. Use the Data Analysis ➣ Regression add-in to perform the eight single-variable regressions needed to replicate Figure 13.15 and replicate the figure.

   b. Use the Data Analysis ➣ Regression add-in to perform the multiple regression needed to replicate Figure 13.16 and replicate the figure.

   c. Beginning with the lowest probability value in the result of b, proceed with backward stepwise elimination of the least important variable to replicate the result shown in Figure 13.17. Remember that to use the Data Analysis ➣ Regression add-in, all independent variables must be in contiguous columns.

   d. Beginning with the highest probability value in the result in (a), carry out forward stepwise inclusion to arrive at the results shown in Figure 13.18.

   e. Use stepwise backward elimination to replicate the analysis shown in Figure 13.19 for the health predictor set: *SafeW*, *Sanit*, *HealthS*, *DPT*, and *CPR*.

   f. Use stepwise backward elimination to replicate the analysis shown in Figure 13.20 for the cultural variables: *LogGNP*, *FemLit*, and *TFR*.

2. The U5Mort2 worksheet in Chpt 13-1.xls shows the same data as those shown in Section 13.2. Use the data and replicate the analyses carried out in Section 13.2.

   a. Use the Data Analysis ➣ Regression add-in to perform the seven single-variable regressions needed to replicate Figure 13.15 and replicate the figure for these data.

   b. Use the Data Analysis ➣ Regression add-in to perform the multiple regression needed to replicate Figure 13.16 and replicate the figure for these data.

c. Beginning with the lowest probability value in the result of (b), proceed with backward stepwise elimination of the least important variable to replicate the result shown in Figure 13.17 for these data.

d. Beginning with the highest probability value in the result in (a), carry out forward stepwise inclusion to replicate the result shown in Figure 13.18 for these data.

e. Use stepwise backward elimination to replicate the analysis shown in Figure 13.19 for the health predictor set: *Sanit, HealthS, DPT*, and *CPR*.

f. Use stepwise backward elimination to replicate the analysis shown in Figure 13.20 for the cultural variables: *LogGNP, FemLit*, and *TFR*.

g. Decide what the consequences of these results are for understanding the relationship between the seven independent variables and *U5Mort*.

13.3   Correlation and Multicolinearity

How is it that different independent variables can produce similar results in predicting a dependent variable? Or how is it that two variables can each separately predict 50 percent or more of the variance in an independent variable but together cannot predict more than 70 percent? The answer is that the predictor variables themselves are related. This is frequently called *multicolinearity*. Multicolinearity has two effects in multiple regression analysis—one is of little consequence and the other is of some significant consequence. The first result is what we have already seen: the result that different variables can produce similar results as predictors of a dependent variable and that the proportion of variance attributable to two variables taken together will not generally be the sum of the variance attributable independently by each. The second result—that of some consequence—is that as colinearity increases, the standard errors of the coefficients that are multicolinear will increase. This can result, for example, in two variables that are both statistically significant predictors of a third variable when taken independently, with neither being statistically significant when examined together.

Examining Multicolinearity

To examine multicolinearity, consider first the relationship between the independent variables examined in Section 13.2, the eight variables taken from *The State of the World's Children 1996* (1996). Figure 13.21 shows the *correlation* between the eight predictors of *U5Mort*. This was generated

	SafeW	Sanit	HealthS	DPT	CPR	LogGNP	FemLit	TFR
SafeW	1							
Sanit	0.66827	1						
HealthS	0.58598	0.53536	1					
DPT	0.5708	0.53551	0.57861	1				
CPR	0.69504	0.68752	0.64122	0.72175	1			
LogGNP	0.66665	0.69559	0.50875	0.47242	0.71137	1		
FemLit	0.41646	0.60439	0.57115	0.63066	0.77748	0.6083	1	
TFR	-0.63155	-0.58507	-0.6523	-0.68206	-0.91374	-0.72151	-0.78688	1

Figure 13.21 Correlation among the predictors for *U5Mort*

using the Excel add-in for correlation in Data Analysis ➢ Correlation. A correlation is exactly the same as the value of Multiple R in regression analysis that would be generated if only one independent variable were considered at a time. You will recall that the Multiple R is just the square root of R square. So the correlations shown in Figure 13.21 are essentially the square roots of the amount of variance shared between each of the variables shown. For example, the correlation between *SafeW* and *Sanit* (cell M4) is 0.668. This means that *SafeW* and *Sanit* share about 44.7 percent of their variance ($0.668^2 = 0.447$).

Calculating the Correlation Coefficient

Thus far, the correlation between two variables has been computed either by using the correlation add-in in Data Analysis or as the Multiple R in regression. The correlation coefficient can be calculated directly by using the formula given in Equation 13.6, where x refers to one of the two variables and y refers to the other.

$$r = \frac{\sum_i^n (x_i - \bar{x})(y_i - \bar{y})}{\sqrt{\sum_i^n (x_i - \bar{x})^2 \times \sum_i^n (y_i - \bar{y})^2}} \tag{13.6}$$

If the correlation table in Figure 13.21 is examined closely, it is possible to see that the highest correlation is between *CPR* (contraceptive prevalence rate) and *TFR* (total fertility rate) (0.914 in cell Q10). There is every reason to expect that these two variables would be highly correlated. Therein is reason to believe that higher contraceptive prevalence rates will actually produce lower total fertility rates. If these two variables are examined independently with regard to *U5Mort*, *CPR* accounts for 71.6 percent of the variance in *U5Mort* and *TFR* accounts for 66.8 percent (Figure 13.15). Both variables have statistically significant coefficients ($p = 1.26E-21$ for *CPR* and 3.66E-19 for *TFR*).

Considering Variables Simultaneously: A Test for Standard Error Inflation

Now consider what happens if the two variables are considered simultaneously. The result of the simultaneous analysis of *CPR* and *TFR* produces the coefficients and *t* tests shown in Figure 13.22. Now, the two variables together account for 72.8 percent of the variance in *U5Mort*, but *TFR* is no longer statistically different from 0 ($p = 0.079$). Furthermore, the probability for *CPR* now reaches only 0.0002. Is there a better demonstration of the effect of multicolinearity as an inflator of standard errors? To find one, it is necessary to modify the data a little.

CPR and *TFR* are highly correlated—that is, 0.914, which means they share about 83 percent of their variance ($0.914^2 = 0.83$). But the effects of extreme multicolinearity do not arise at that level. To see the effects, it is necessary to increase the relationship between *CPR* and *TFR*. To do that, 31 countries that had the lowest correlations between *CPR* and *TFR* were removed from the data set, resulting in 44 countries for which *CPR* and *TFR* were correlated at 0.962. At that level of correlation, they share about 92 percent of their variance. When each of the variables is separately related to *U5Mort*, the results are quite like those in Figure 13.15. The probability of the coefficient for *CPR* is 2.76E-12, and the probability of the coefficient for *TFR* is 2.36E-12. Each of the variables independently accounts for about 69 percent of the variance in *U5Mort*. But when they are examined simultaneously, the results are as those shown in Figure 13.23.

	K	L	M	N	O	
21		Coefficient	Standard Et Stat		P-value	L
22	Intercept	111.753	48.17262	2.319845	0.023188	
23	TFR	12.29324	6.914236	1.777961	0.079633	
24	CPR	-1.89031	0.476815	-3.96445	0.000172	

Figure 13.22 *CPR* and *TFR* together as predictors for *U5Mort*

	K	L	M	N	O	
20		Coefficient	Standard Et Stat		P-value	
21	Intercept	59.73911	99.59955	0.599793	0.551945	
22	TFR	20.36392	14.20315	1.433761	0.159223	
23	CPR	-1.30266	0.987915	-1.3186	0.194621	

Figure 13.23 *CPR* and *TFR* together as predictors for *U5Mort*: Reduced sample

It can be seen there that neither coefficient (*CPR* or *TFR*) has a statistically significant probability. This is the consequence of extreme multicolinearity. It inflates the standard errors to the extent that variables no longer show statistical significance. But it is important to note that this happened at a correlation between *CPR* and *TFR* of 0.962.

In general, multicolinearity is not a problem to be concerned about unless the correlation between variables exceeds about 0.90.

EXERCISES FOR SECTION 13.3

1. Use the data on the U5Mort1 worksheet from Chpt 13-1.xls and the formula in Equation 13.6 to calculate the correlation between *FemLit* and *CPR* and between *TFR* and *CPR*.

2. Use the data on the U5Mort2 worksheet from Chpt 13-1.xls and the formula in Equation 13.6 to calculate the correlation between *FemLit* and *CPR* and between *TFR* and *CPR*.

13.4 Nonlinear Relationships

Up to this point, we have considered regression analysis in its classical context. We examined the linear relationships between independent and dependent variables. But regression analysis can also be used in certain cases to analyze nonlinear relationships. This section discusses some of the ways in which Excel can be used to perform nonlinear regression analysis.

Estimating a Nonlinear Relationship

In examining the relationship between the independent variables taken from *The State of the World's Children 1996* and *U5Mort*, *LogGNP*, rather than *GNP* itself, was used as a predictor, because it was indicated that *GNP* is not linearly related to *U5Mort*, whereas *LogGNP* is. This decision deserves somewhat more discussion and some observations on the analysis of nonlinear relationships. To begin the discussion it is useful actually to look at the relationship in an *xy* graph.

A graph of the relationship between *GNP* and *U5Mort* is shown in Figure 13.24. It is possible to see that the relationship is decidedly nonlinear. Below a *GNP* of about $5,000 per year, *U5Mort* falls precipitously from over 300 to below 50. For the four countries above $5,000 per year, the differences in *U5Mort* are comparatively small. Although a straight line might fit the data either below or above $5,000, a straight line does not fit both segments of the data simultaneously.

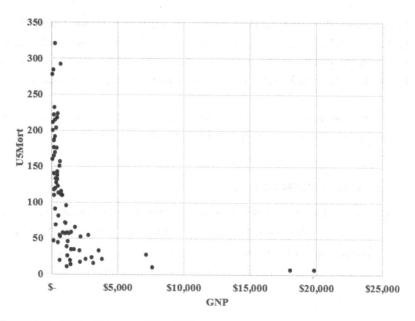

Figure 13.24 Relationship between *GNP* and *U5Mort*

Fitting Nonlinear Relationships Using Second-Degree Curves

There are a number of different ways to attempt to fit the data represented by the relation between *GNP* and *U5Mort*. Consider first the possibility of fitting the line with a second-degree curve. In general, a second-degree curve is any relationship between a dependent and an independent variable that is defined by the independent variable and a power of the independent variable. But, typically, a second-degree curve is defined by the original independent variable and its square.

A major characteristic of a second-degree curve is that it produces a graphed line that has one change of direction. In Figure 13.24, the data essentially change direction one time. This direction change occurs at about 25 deaths per 1,000 live births or at about $1,500 in *GNP* per capita. A third-degree curve would have two changes of direction, a fourth-degree curve would have three, and so on. In general, data that are encountered in health care–related applications will rarely benefit from going beyond a second-degree curve.

A sample of the data (for the first 10 countries) for analyzing the relationship in Figure 13.24 is shown in Figure 13.25. Column B is the actual value of *GNP* per capita, and column C is the square of *GNP* per capita. Column D is the actual value of *U5Mort*, and column E is the best-fitting second-degree curve through the data.

	A	B	C	D	E
1		GNP	GNP^2	U5Mort	U5MortP
2	Niger	270	72900	320	141.94
3	Angola	700	490000	292	122.26
4	Sierra Leone	150	22500	284	147.57
5	Mozambique	90	8100	277	150.41
6	Guinea-Bissau	240	57600	231	143.34
7	Guinea	500	250000	223	131.31
8	Malawi	200	40000	221	145.21
9	Liberia	450	202500	217	133.60
10	Mali	270	72900	214	141.94
11	Somalia	120	14400	211	148.99
12	Zambia	280	144400	203	136.83

Figure 13.25 Sample of data for second-degree curve analysis of *U5Mort*

The actual regression equation that predicts that curve (which was found by using Data Analysis ➤ Regression) is shown in Equation 13.7. This equation accounts for 39.6 percent of the variance in *U5Mort* ($R^2 = 0.396$), compared with only 17.5 percent of the variance accounted for when *GNP* alone (not the log of *GNP*) is used as a predictor. Clearly, from the point of view of the R square, the second-degree curve is a better fit for the data than the straight line (a first-degree curve). But let us see how well the second-degree curve, based on the square of *GNP*, actually fits the data. To see that, we will look at the predicted values of *U5Mort*, along with the actual values as graphed in Figure 13.26.

$$U5Mort = -0.048\ GNP + 0.00000214\ GNP^2 + 154.697 \qquad (13.7)$$

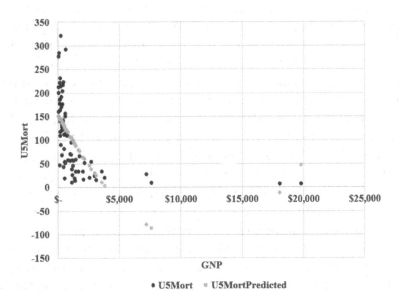

Figure 13.26 Relationship between *GNP* and *U5Mort* with *U5Mort* predicted: Second-degree curve

Figure 13.27   Relationship between *LogGNP* and *U5Mort*

Log Linear Relationships

As Figure 13.26 shows, the predicted values of *U5Mort* (shown as the gray squares) do not lie along a straight line. But at the same time, they do not fit the actual values of *U5Mort* as well as would be hoped. In particular, the predicted values of under-five mortality for three countries with *GNP* per capita above $5,000 are actually negative. Because this is clearly an impossibility, and because we already know that the log of *GNP* is a better predictor of *U5Mort* (*R* square = 0.539 from Figure 13.15), it is useful to look at that relationship more closely.

Figure 13.27 shows the actual values of *U5Mort* and the predicted values, based on *LogGNP* on the *LogGNP* scale. By using the log of *GNP* as the predictor, the distribution has become much more linear than when *GNP* itself is used. But the relationship is still not truly linear, as the figure shows. Furthermore, the predicted values of *U5Mort* are again below zero for some of the countries, particularly for those with *LogGNP* per capita in excess of about 3.8. You will recall that the coefficient for the log of *GNP* and the constant for this model were both given in Figure 13.15.

In an effort to come closer to a linear relationship, consider the possibility of taking the log of both *GNP* and of *U5Mort*. Figure 13.28 shows the relationship between *LogGNP* and *LogU5Mort*. As is evident in this figure, the relationship between the logs of these two variables is a very good approximation of a linear relationship. The figure also shows the predicted values for *LogU5Mort*. These are based on the regression equation in Equation 13.8, which was calculated by using Data Analysis ➢ Regression. Furthermore, *LogGNP* accounts for about 68 percent of the variance in *LogU5Mort*, which is right up in the range of the best predictors

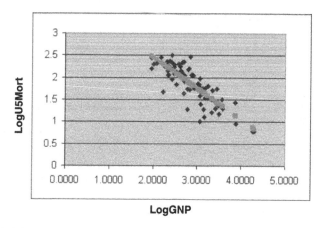

Figure 13.28 Relationship between *LogGNP* and *LogU5Mort*

of *U5Mort* itself: *CPR* and *TFR*.

$$LogU5Mort = -0.706LogGNP + 3.874 \qquad (13.8)$$

Fitting Nonlinear Relationships Using Dummy Variables

We will consider one last way of assessing the nonlinear relationship between *GNP* and *U5Mort*. The model is based on the use of a dummy variable. In this case, the dummy variable will simply be assigned as a 1 to countries with *GNP* greater than \$1,500 and 0 to other countries. So the regression equation that will be used to describe the relationship between *GNP* and *U5Mort* will contain *GNP* and a variable we will call *HiGNP*. In addition, there will be an interaction term, *GNP*HiGNP*.

Figure 13.29 shows the result of this analysis. As can be seen in the figure, the inclusion of a dummy variable representing high-income countries and an interaction produces predicted values along two separate regression lines. One line represents those countries with *GNP* per capita less than \$1,500. The other line represents countries with *GNP* per capita greater than \$1,500. The regression equation for this analysis is given in Equation 13.

$$U5Mort = -0.126\ GNP + (-163.833\ HiGNP) + 0.124\ GNP$$
$$\times\ HiGNP + 200.976 \qquad (13.9)$$

This model accounts for 59 percent of the variance in *U5Mort*. This is not as much as that accounted for when the log transformation of each variable was chosen. However, it is more than that accounted for by any

Figure 13.29   Relationship between *GNP* and *U5Mort* with *HIGNP* dummy

of the other models examined here. A question arises from this analysis: Why decide to use a dummy and why choose $1,500 as the cutoff point? The answer is simple. Look at the scatterplot (e.g., Figure 13.24) of the relationship between *GNP* and *U5Mort*. It appears from that graph that there is a discontinuity in the relationship between these two at about $1,500 (or $1,300, or $1,800). If we are seeking the best linear regression model to describe the relationship between *GNP* and *U5Mort*, it is a good idea not only to look at the data plots but also to benefit from them when specifying a model.

But is this not simply mining the data for anything we can find? Yes, but so is any other approach to regression analysis—for example, using stepwise regression, whether forward or backward, that does not begin with some type of theory. If all we hope to do is to get the best description that we can of the relationship, all of these tools are appropriate. However, if we wished to test the hypothesis that there is a discontinuity in the relationship between *GNP* and *U5Mort* at $1,500, then that is also a legitimate reason to include the dummy variable.

To conclude this section, there are a number of ways that nonlinear relationships might be examined using regression. They all involve some modification of the original data. When the second-degree equation was examined, the square of the original predictor, *GNP*, was employed, along with *GNP*. When the log values were examined, both the independent variable and the dependent variable were transformed into log values. The inclusion of a dummy variable is the addition of another transformation of the original variable—this time, a discontinuous transformation of 1 for values of *GNP* greater than some cutoff point, and 0 otherwise. All are reasonable strategies to employ (and there are others as well) if the purpose is to try to find the best-fitting line for a nonlinear relationship. Excel provides a shortcut for some of this activity, which is discussed in the next section.

Excel's Automatic Curve Fitter

Excel has the built-in capability to examine some of the possible alternative ways for fitting regression lines with data. To look at this capability, we will stay with the example of the relationship between *GNP* and *U5Mort*. And because we already know that the relationship between the log of GNP and the log of *U5Mort* is virtually linear, we will look at that relationship first. Figure 13.30 shows the first step in accessing Excel's built-in capability to examine relationships between two variables. If the cursor is placed over a point in the data series and right-clicked, a pop-up menu including the item Format Data Series appears. There are several options here, but we will concentrate on only one: Format Trendline.

The Format Trendline Option in Excel

If we select the Add Trendline option in the Format Data Series menu, the Format Trendline dialog box, shown in Figure 13.31, comes up. In this dialog box it is possible to select from six different options: exponential, linear, logarithmic, polynomial, power, and moving average.

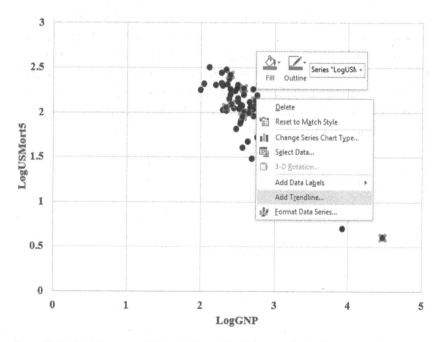

Figure 13.30 *LogGNP* versus *Log U5Mort* with Format Data Series menu displayed

Figure 13.31 Format Trendline dialog box

The linear option, which we will examine first, is essentially a simple linear regression model that relates a single independent variable (the variable that defines the horizontal axis) to the dependent variable (the variable that defines the vertical axis). Having selected the linear option, we can ask Excel to calculate the regression equation and the R square and display both on the graph. The selection of the regression equation and the R square is shown in Figure 13.32. Notice in that figure that there are check marks in both the boxes that precede Display equation on chart and Display R-squared value on chart.

Figure 13.32 Selections in the Format Trendline dialog box

Figure 13.33 Best-fitting line for LogGNP and LogU5Mort: Linear model

With the linear model selected and both the equation and R square values checked, the result is the best-fitting straight line shown on the chart with the original data. The regression equation and the R square value, as seen in Figure 13.33, are also shown. (It may be necessary to grab the regression formula and the R square with the cursor and drag these to a spot on the chart where they will be fully visible, as they tend to pop up right in the midst of the data.) Now it should be clear that the results shown in Figure 13.33 are exactly the same as the results shown in Figure 13.28. The regression formula and R square are the same as those produced for the latter figure. So, essentially, the charting capability of Excel has reproduced exactly what is produced by the regression add-in (albeit, with not nearly as much information; there are no significance tests, for example).

Other Trendline Options in Excel

Now that we have introduced the capabilities of the Format Trendline dialog box, it is necessary to say a little about each of the other trendline options. The Logarithmic option produces a curve that is based on conversion of the x-axis variable (GNP, in this case) to its natural logarithm. Ordinary least squares are then performed to generate the regression coefficients and R square. In turn, the resulting predicted values are graphed on the chart with the actual values of GNP. This produces the curve, the regression equation, and the R square shown in Figure 13.34.

It is useful to note that the regression constant of 438.09 and the R square of 0.5386 are the same, as they were generated for the relationship shown in Figure 13.27 and detailed in row 9 of Figure 13.15. The only difference is between the equation shown in Figure 13.34, and that indicated in row 9

Figure 13.34 Best-fitting line for GNP and U5Mort: Logarithmic model

of Figure 13.15. The value of the coefficient on LogGNP is −116.56 rather than −50.52.

The reason for this difference is that the data used to generate the values in Figure 13.15 were the log of GNP to the base 10. Excel uses the natural logarithm (base 2.71828) for the regression equation shown in Figure 13.34. However, there is a constant relationship between the log to the base 10 and the natural log. Therefore, the coefficient of logGNP in Figure 13.15 can be generated from the coefficient in Figure 13.34 by multiplying by the constant value 2.30585. Thus, the *logarithmic model* in the Format Trendline dialog box is simply the model generated by taking the log of the independent variable and relating it—using ordinary least squares regression—to the actual value of the dependent variable.

The Polynomial Option in Excel

The fourth option in the Format Trendline window is the *Polynomial option*. If the Polynomial option is selected, it is possible to select 2 through 6 from the scroll arrows beside the Polynomial option. If you select 2, you produce a second-degree curve with one change of direction. Selecting 3 produces a third-degree curve with two changes of direction, and so on. Selection of 2 produces exactly the same result in terms of predicted values and the same regression equation and R square as were produced for Figure 13.26 and given in Equation 13.7. If the Polynomial option is selected, it is important to realize that there will be as many predictors in the model as the number selected plus a constant. In other words, if 2 is selected, the model will contain the x-axis variable plus its square and a

Figure 13.35 Best-fitting line for GNP and U5Mort: Power model

constant. If 3 is selected, the model will contain the x-axis variable plus its square, its cube, and a constant, and so on.

The Power Option in Excel

The fifth option available in the Format Trendline dialog box is the *Power option*, the result of which is shown in Figure 13.35. The equation for the Power option, given in the figure, is the most complex yet encountered. But look at the R square for the power option. At 0.6812, it looks suspiciously like the R square for the model in which both GNP and U5Mort are converted to their log values (Figure 13.33). Furthermore, the −0.7063 power to which x is raised in Figure 13.35 looks very much like the −0.7063 by which x is multiplied in Figure 13.33.

Moreover, if we take the 3.8736 in Figure 13.33 and raise 10 to that power, we get 7,475.5, which is the multiplier of x in Figure 13.35. Thus, the formula for the Power model can be found by using ordinary least squares. First, convert both the independent and dependent variables to their log values (base 10), and calculate the regression coefficients. The next step is to set up an equation in which the actual value of the dependent variable is predicted by using the actual value of the independent variable. This is accomplished by raising the independent variable to the power of the coefficient on the log of the dependent variable and multiplying by 10, then raising it to the power of the intercept. The result is the Power model.

The Exponential Option in Excel

The first option in the Format Trendline dialog box is the *Exponential model*. The line, equation, and R square for the exponential model are

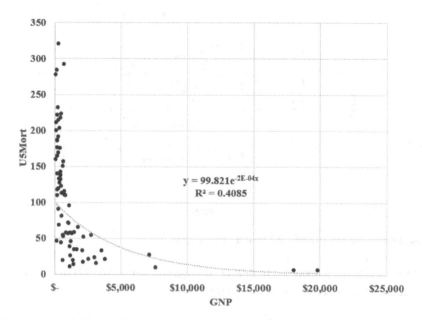

Figure 13.36   Best-fitting line for *GNP* and *U5Mort*: Exponential model

shown in Figure 13.36. The coefficients of the Exponential model can be found, using ordinary least squares, by first converting the dependent variable to its natural logarithm. The next step is to calculate the ordinary least square coefficients. This is accomplished by using the actual value of the independent variable and the natural log of the dependent variable. In the case of the *GNP* and *U5Mort* data, this produces the result shown in Equation 13.10. To get the values of *U5Mort* as expressed in the formula given in Figure 13.36, a few calculations must be completed. First, it is necessary to raise *e* (2.718282) to the power of the coefficient of *GNP* shown in Equation 13.10 and 10 times the actual value of *GNP*. Second, multiply that result by *e* raised to the power of the intercept term in Equation 13.10. This produces the result shown in Figure 13.36.

$$LnU5Mort = -0.0002GNP + 4.603 \qquad (13.10)$$

The last option shown in the Format Trendline dialog box is the *Moving Average model.* The Moving Average model applies specifically to time-related data, data where there is one measure for each of a string of time intervals. Because this book does not deal with time-related data, the Moving Average model will not be discussed.

EXERCISES FOR SECTION 13.4

1. The worksheet GNP1 in Chpt 13-1.xls contains the *GNP* per capita, the log of *GNP* per capita, and *U5Mort* for 75 countries of the world from *The State of the World's Children 1996* (1996).

   a. Use the *GNP* data along with *GNP* squared as independent variables to generate a regression analysis to predict *U5Mort*.

   b. Generate the predicted values of *U5Mort*, based on this analysis.

   c. Graph the actual and predicted values of *U5Mort* against *GNP* to replicate Figure 13.26.

   d. Use the Add Trendline option in the Format Data Series menu and the options tab to add a second-degree polynomial to the graph for the values of *GNP* and *U5Mort*, along with the regression equation and the *R* square, and compare this with the predicted values generated in (b) (preceding).

2. Use the worksheet GNP1 in Chpt 13-1.xls, and do the following:

   a. Use the log of *GNP* to generate a regression analysis to predict *U5Mort*.

   b. Generate the predicted values of *U5Mort*, based on this analysis.

   c. Graph the actual and predicted values of *U5Mort* against *logGNP* to replicate Figure 13.27.

   d. Graph the actual values of *U5Mort* against *GNP*, and use the Add Trendline option in the Format Data Series menu and the options tab to add the Logarithmic model with the regression equation and the *R* square to the graph.

   e. Confirm that the proportion of variance accounted for and the intercept are the same in both (a) and (d) and that the regression coefficient for *LogGNP* in (a) is 2.302585 times larger than the coefficient in (d) (the ratio of the natural log to the log base 10).

3. Use the worksheet GNP1 in Chpt 13-1.xls, and do the following:

   a. Generate a new variable *LogU5Mort* by using the =LOG () function.

   b. Use the log of *GNP* to generate a regression analysis to predict *LogU5Mort*.

   c. Generate the predicted values of *LogU5Mort*, based on this analysis.

   d. Graph the actual and predicted values of *LogU5Mort* against *logGNP* to replicate Figure 13.28.

   e. Graph the actual values of *U5Mort* against *GNP*, and use the Add Trendline option in the Format Data Series menu and the options tab to add the Power model with the regression equation and the *R* square to the graph.

f. Confirm that the proportion of variance accounted for are the same in both (b) and (e). Also, confirm that the power regression equation as given in (e) can be replicated by raising the actual value of *GNP* to the power of the regression coefficient on *LogGNP* (2.70633) and multiplying by 10 raised to the power of the intercept term (3.8736).

4. The data on worksheet BirthW in Chpt 13-1.xls represent constructed data for the mother's age and the child's birth weight for a sample of 200 mothers and children. Use the graphing capability of Excel and alternative curvilinear models to find the best-fitting nonstraight line for these data.

5. The data on worksheet Wait in Chpt 13-1.xls represent constructed data for length of time in quarter hours and time from scheduled appointment to admission to the physician's office in a clinic for a sample of 220 people selected randomly from clinic records. Use the graphing capability of Excel and alternative curvilinear models to find the best-fitting nonstraight line for these data.

6. The data on worksheet Size in Chpt 13-1.xls represent constructed data for hospital size measured in the number of beds and the hospital occupancy rate. Use the graphing capability of Excel and alternative curvilinear models to find the best-fitting nonstraight line for these data.

KEY TERMS

correlation	polynomial option
dependent variable	power option
dummy variable	*R* square
exponential model	regression analysis
independent variable	regression coefficient
interaction effect	stepwise regression
logarithmic model	*x*-axis
moving average model	*x* variable
multicolinearity	*y*-axis
multiple regression	*y* variable

CHAPTER 14

ANALYSIS WITH A DICHOTOMOUS CATEGORICAL DEPENDENT VARIABLE

We are just statistics, born to consume resources.

—Horace

The chi-square statistic deals with categorical data in both the independent and the dependent variables. However, the general limitation is that only two variables—one independent and one dependent, or, occasionally, two independent and one dependent—can be analyzed at one time. Furthermore, the chi-square is limited by the need to retain relatively large values (at least five or more) in all the cells of the tables in the analysis. The *t* test and *analysis of variance* (ANOVA) deal with categorical data in the *independent variable* but require a numerical variable in the dependent variable. Again, though, *t* tests are limited to a single independent variable that can take on only two values, whereas ANOVA is usually limited to no more than one or two independent variables. Regression analysis, the topic of the three previous chapters, is more flexible than any of the other three analysis methods. Regression can deal simultaneously with a large number of independent variables, and these can be either numerical or categorical. In addition, regression has no particular cell size requirements. But like *t* tests and ANOVA, regression as discussed thus far is limited to numerical data in the dependent variable. Frequently, though, there may arise a need to deal with categorical data in the dependent variable, and the desire may be to examine several (or many) independent variables simultaneously. This chapter addresses some alternative approaches to this problem—when the dependent variable is a dichotomous *categorical variable*.

14.1   Introduction to the Dichotomous Dependent Variable

As has been discussed, a dichotomous categorical variable is one that takes on only two values. *Gender, emergency or non-emergency*, and *Medicare or non-Medicare patients* are all examples of dichotomous categorical variables—also referred to as "dummy" variables especially when used as predictor or independent variables in regression analyses. They are universally coded 1 and 0, 1 designating one of the two alternatives and 0 designating the other. But it is also possible to consider a dichotomous categorical variable as a dependent variable. When this is done, the variable is again universally coded 1 or 0 to designate the two levels of the variable.

In early treatments of dichotomous dependent variables, it was common to use *ordinary least squares* regression. This is essentially what has been presented in the previous three chapters. In this form, regression has commonly been referred to as a *linear probability model*. This is because the predicted value of the dependent variable, based on the analysis, was considered the probability that an observation *would be* a 1 or a 0, not whether it actually *was* a 1 or a 0. As with any other regression model, there is a direct mathematical solution to the problem of finding regression coefficients with dichotomous categorical dependent or dummy variables. But there are also some clear problems with using regression with dummy variables. These problems will be discussed in more detail as we proceed.

In recent years, two things have led to the abandonment of ordinary least squares regression to analyze dummy dependent variables. The first has been the recognition of the problems in using ordinary least squares regression to deal with dummy dependent variables. The second has been the increasing availability of statistics software to carry out complex and time-consuming calculations. Especially because of the latter, there has been a universal shift to what is called *maximum likelihood* estimators, to derive the relationship between one or more independent variables and a dichotomous dependent variable. Two maximum likelihood estimators have gained the most favor in dealing with dichotomous categorical dependent variables—*Logit* and *Probit*. These two estimation procedures produce nearly identical results in practice. Because the Logit approach is substantially less complex, it is discussed in this chapter. But before turning to Logit, we will examine the ways in which dichotomous dependent variables have been analyzed in the past as a way of demonstrating the problems attendant with these treatments.

14.2 An Example with a Dichotomous Dependent Variable: Traditional Treatments

The staff at a well-baby clinic is concerned about the immunization levels of children being treated there. The clinic staff hopes to achieve full immunization levels for all children seen at the clinic. The staff also knows that some mothers are more likely than others to seek full immunization for their children and thus will need little or no push from the clinic. The question before the clinic staff is whether it is possible to predict which mothers are likely not to seek full immunization for their children so that they can concentrate their effort on those women in promoting full immunization.

The clinic staff has also observed that younger mothers, mothers with less education, and mothers with a low socioeconomic status (SES) are less likely to have their children fully immunized. The clinic staff are hopeful that knowing this will allow them to better concentrate their effort on education and the promotion of immunization. They have also observed that if a child is a second, third, or higher-birth-order child, it is more likely that the mother will seek full immunization on her own. The clinic has collected data on 32 mothers who are coming to the clinic. Each of these mothers has a child between one and two years of age. The data available to the health department include the mother's age, her years of formal education, the birth order of the child, and whether the child is fully immunized for one year of age. The data (which are wholly fabricated for this example) are shown in Figure 14.1. As the figure shows, the mothers

	A	B	C	D	E	F	G	H	I	J	K
1	Mother	Age	Educ	Order	Immun		Mother	Age	Educ	Order	Immun
2	1	21	7	3	0		17	21	12	1	1
3	2	19	12	2	1		18	21	8	4	0
4	3	23	10	3	0		19	22	6	3	0
5	4	25	8	2	1		20	21	8	3	0
6	5	25	7	2	1		21	21	10	3	1
7	6	26	15	4	1		22	21	10	1	1
8	7	17	6	1	0		23	25	10	3	1
9	8	21	6	3	0		24	22	10	3	1
10	9	25	13	6	1		25	22	7	3	0
11	10	19	11	3	1		26	21	8	3	0
12	11	20	13	4	1		27	27	7	2	1
13	12	18	10	1	1		28	24	12	3	1
14	13	17	6	2	0		29	28	14	5	1
15	14	20	12	4	1		30	20	7	2	1
16	15	21	7	1	1		31	26	13	2	1
17	16	17	5	3	0		32	18	10	1	1

Figure 14.1 Data for 32 mothers

range in age from 17 to 28 years. They have between 5 and 15 years of formal education, and they have one to six children. Of the children, 21 are fully immunized (those coded 1 in the column labeled Immun); the other 11 children are not fully immunized. The question is whether the clinic can gain any information from these data to help them better target their education efforts about immunization.

A Chi-Square Analysis

One way to approach the problem of deciding where to put education efforts is to use contingency table analysis and the chi-square statistic. Contingency tables and chi-square analysis are well suited to dealing with categorical dependent variables. However, contingency tables and the chi-square statistic approach basically require some observations in every cell. It is really not feasible to use this approach without collapsing the independent variable data—age, education, and parity—into some smaller set of categories. One way to collapse the independent variable data would be simply to split them into high and low at the mean. If we do that, the resulting data for the 32 mothers would be as those shown in Figure 14.2, where a 1 designates a value of the original variable that is greater than the mean and 0 represents a value of the original variable less than the mean. This is referred to as one-zero conversion and is displayed in Figure 14.2.

The data in Figure 14.2 can be used to generate two-by-two contingency tables and chi-square values. In turn, the immunization status of the child can be determined if it is dependent on any of the three variables: age, education, or parity. The analysis for age is shown in Figure 14.3. That

	A	B	C	D	E	F	G	H	I	J	K
20	Mother	Age	Educ	Order	Immun		Mother	Age	Educ	Order	Immun
21	1	0	0	1	0		17	0	1	0	1
22	2	0	1	0	1		18	0	0	1	0
23	3	1	1	1	0		19	1	0	1	0
24	4	1	0	0	1		20	0	0	1	0
25	5	1	0	0	1		21	0	1	1	1
26	6	1	1	1	1		22	0	1	0	1
27	7	0	0	0	0		23	1	1	1	1
28	8	0	0	1	0		24	1	1	1	1
29	9	1	1	1	1		25	1	0	1	0
30	10	0	1	1	1		26	0	0	1	0
31	11	0	1	1	1		27	1	0	0	1
32	12	0	1	0	1		28	1	1	1	1
33	13	0	0	0	0		29	1	1	1	1
34	14	0	1	1	1		30	0	0	0	1
35	15	0	0	0	1		31	1	1	0	1
36	16	0	0	1	0		32	0	1	0	1

Figure 14.2 One-zero conversion of data for 32 mothers

	O17	▼	=	=((ABS(O11-O5)-0.5)^2)/O11	
	N	O	P	Q	R
3	Count of Immun	Age ▼			
4	Immun ▼	0	1	Grand Total	
5	0	8	3	11	
6	1	11	10	21	
7	Grand Total	19	13	32	
8					
9	Count of Immun	Age	0	0	
10	Immun	0	1	Grand Total	
11	0	6.531	4.469	11	
12	1	12.47	8.531	21	
13	Grand Total	19	13	32	
14					
15	Count of Immun	Age	0	0	
16	Immun	0	1	Grand Total	
17	0	0.144	0.21	11	
18	1	0.075	0.11	21	
19	Grand Total	19	13	32	
20					
21			chi sq	0.5389698	
22			p	0.46286	

Figure 14.3 Chi-square analysis of immunization by age of mother

figure shows the pivot table results of crossing immunization with age in cells N3:Q7. In cells N9:Q13, the expected values for the cells in the original pivot table are given.

Issues with Chi-Square Analysis

One problem with using chi-square analysis for these data is immediately obvious from either the original data table or the expected value table. That problem is the small cell sizes, especially for the older age–no immunization category. In consequence, the chi-square is computed by using the *Yates's correction*. The formula for the contribution to the chi-square of cell O17 is shown in the formula bar. Note the absolute value of the difference between the observed and expected values and the 2.5 of the Yates's correction are shown there.

With or without the Yates's correction, the chi-square value produced by the analysis of full immunization by the mother's age suggests that the two variables are statistically independent. The chi-square is given in cell Q21, and its probability is given in cell Q22. Given that the probability of finding a chi-square value as large as 0.539 (if a mother's age and immunization status are independent of one another) is 0.46, we will conclude that they are, in fact, independent. The bottom line is that you can't predict a child's immunization status from the age of its mother.

We can carry out a similar analysis for both a mother's education and the birth order of the child. If we do so, the results are a chi-square of 10.49, with a probability of 0.001 for the mother's education, and a chi-square of 2.24, with a probability of 0.136 for the birth order of the child. The conclusion that we would draw, based on these data, is that of the three things about which the clinic has information, only the mother's education is related to the child's immunization status. Consequently, it would not be unreasonable for clinic staff to conclude that if they hope to have an effect with a targeted information program, they should target women with lower education.

There are a couple of problems with these analyses, though. First, because we have collapsed the data regarding the mother's education and the birth order of the child from multiple levels to just two, we have lost information. It is generally better, if possible, to select an analysis that uses all the available data. Second, we have looked at only one variable at a time. It is also generally better, if possible, to select an analysis that treats all variables of interest simultaneously. Although contingency tables and chi-square analysis can, in certain circumstances, be used to examine more than one independent variable at a time, in this case, the cell sizes would be too small to make it practical.

We have seen in Chapters 12 and 13 that multiple regression uses the full range of data available in the analysis. Multiple regression can also deal simultaneously with a number of independent variables (16 for the Microsoft Excel add-in). Theoretically, the number of independent variables is limited to one fewer than the number of observations. So can we use multiple regression—in this case, ordinary least squares, or OLS—to analyze these data? The answer turns out to be *yes* and *no*. To help us see why, the next section discusses the use of OLS with the data on immunization.

Ordinary Least Squares (OLS) with a Dichotomous Dependent Variable

Let us consider the data on children's immunization status, using OLS. Figure 14.4 shows the results of the regression analysis for the data shown in Figure 14.1. The data have been rearranged to carry out the analysis, and only the data for the first 20 women and their children are shown. The results of the analysis, using the Excel regression add-in, are given in cells G1:L20. The analysis indicates that 58 percent of the variance in immunization rates has been accounted for (cell H5). It also indicates a significant overall F test (cells K12 and L12). Furthermore, it confirms the conclusions about the age and education of the mother. Even with the additional data, the age of the mother is not a statistically significant predictor of immunization status (cells H18:K18). The additional data confirm also that a mother's

	A	B	C	D	E	F	G	H	I	J	K	L
1	Mother	Age	Educ	Order	Immun		SUMMARY OUTPUT					
2	1	21	7	3	0							
3	2	19	12	2	1		*Regression Statistics*					
4	3	23	10	3	0		Multiple R	0.759847				
5	4	25	8	2	1		R Square	0.577368				
6	5	25	7	2	1		Adjusted R Squ	0.532085				
7	6	26	15	4	1		Standard Error	0.330091				
8	7	17	6	1	0		Observations	32				
9	8	21	6	3	0							
10	9	25	13	6	1		ANOVA					
11	10	19	11	3	1							
12	11	20	13	4	1			df	SS	MS	F	ignificance F
							Regression	3	4.167872	1.389291	12.75047	1.96E-05
13	12	18	10	1	1		Residual	28	3.050878	0.10896		
14	13	17	6	2	0		Total	31	7.21875			
15	14	20	12	4	1							
16	15	21	7	1	1			*Coefficient*	*andard Err*	*t Stat*	*P-value*	*Lower 95% Uppe*
17	16	17	5	3	0		Intercept	-0.90395	0.439026	-2.05899	0.048905	-1.80326	-0.0
18	17	21	12	1	1		Age	0.039752	0.022498	1.766921	0.098142	-0.00633	0.08
19	18	21	8	4	0		Educ	0.125969	0.024454	5.151268	1.83E-05	0.075878	0.17
20	19	22	6	3	0		Order	-0.17968	0.055634	-3.22959	0.003159	-0.29364	-0.0
21	20	21	8	3	0							

Figure 14.4   Results of OLS for immunization data

education is a statistically significant predictor of immunization status (cells H19:K19). With the additional data provided by the OLS analysis for birth order of the child, that variable too appears to be a statistically significant predictor of immunization status. So the use of OLS instead of contingency tables and chi-square would lead clinic personnel to conclude that they might effectively concentrate their education effort not only on low-education women but also on low-parity women.

Problems with Ordinary Least Squares with a Dichotomous Dependent Variable

But there are also problems with this analysis. The problems have to do with the restriction of the dependent variable to two values: 1 and 0. In this situation the predicted regression values will not be actually 1 or 0. Rather, the values will be some number that must be interpreted as the probability that the true value will be 1 or 0. For this reason, OLS used in this manner is called a *linear probability model* (LPM). The fact that the actual values of the dependent variable take on only the values of 1 and 0 is not a problem for the regression coefficients themselves. They remain unbiased. The problem lies with the error terms, and thus with statistical tests based on the error terms. A basic assumption of the statistical tests (*F* tests and *t* tests) in regression is that the error terms are uncorrelated with the independent variables and have a constant variance and an expected value of 0. Aldrich and Nelson (1984) have provided a clear discussion of why these assumptions cannot be maintained when the dependent variable is restricted to 1 and 0. The basic problem is that the variance of the error terms turns out to be correlated systematically with the independent variables. In this situation the statistical tests based on OLS regression are invalid, even in large samples.

But there is a relatively simple fix for this situation in regard to the statistical test, which was originally proposed by Goldberger (1964) and clearly laid out by Aldrich and Nelson. This is a *weighted least squares* (WLS) procedure for estimating the linear probability model.

Weighted Least Squares (WLS) for Estimating Linear Probability Models

The weighted least squares procedure for the linear probability model is carried out in two steps. The first step is to estimate the regression model by using OLS. The second step is to use the results of OLS to create weights by which the original variables—both the independent variables x_i and the dependent variable y—are transformed. In turn, estimate the regression model a second time, on the basis of the transformed variables.

The weights for the transformation are as those given in Equation 14.1, which says that a weight for each observation is created by first calculating the predicted values of the dependent variable, using the OLS estimates of the coefficients. Then the predicted value of the dependent variable is multiplied by 1 minus the predicted value, and the square root of that number is taken. Finally, 1 is divided by the resulting value to obtain the appropriate weight. As Aldrich and Nelson point out, this is just the reciprocal of the estimated standard errors of the error term.

$$w_i = \frac{1}{\left[\hat{y}_i\left(1 - \hat{y}_i\right)\right]^{1/2}} \tag{14.1}$$

Issues with Generating Weights Greater than 1 or Less than 0

There is, however, a basic problem with this procedure for generating weights. Even though the predicted values of the dependent variable are appropriately interpreted as the probability that the dependent variable will be 1 or 0, it is likely that at least some of the predicted values will be either greater than 1 or less than 0. When a number greater than 1 or less than 0 is multiplied by 1 minus itself, it produces a negative result. The square root of a negative number is an imaginary number, and Excel will generate a #NUM! result in the cell that includes the square root of a negative number. Aldrich and Nelson suggest a relatively simple solution to this problem, which is to use some large number less than 1, such as 0.999, in place of the true predicted value when it is greater than 1 and some small number greater than 0, such as 0.001, when the predicted value is less than 0.

Example of Weighted Least Squares Weight Calculation

Figure 14.5 shows the original OLS data for the 32 mothers (only the first 20 are shown), along with the calculation of the weights for WLS. As it is possible to see, the actual OLS regression analysis has been moved to the right and three new columns have been inserted. The first of the new columns (column F) is the predicted value of the dependent variable *Immun* (which is $\hat{y}$ in Equation 14.1) and is called *Ipred* for *Immun* predicted. The values of *Ipred* were calculated using the regression formula with the original independent data in columns B, C, and D and the coefficients in cells K17:K21. By inspection of column F, it is possible to see that 3 of the first 20 predicted values of immunization are outside the range 0 to 1. Cells F3, F7, and F18 have values greater than 1, and cell F17 has a value less than 0. To accommodate that problem in the calculation of weights, a new column, Ipredadj—or Immun predicted adjusted—was included as column G. In column G, the Excel =IF() function is used to adjust the predicted values to ensure that they are all in the range 0 to 1. The =IF() statement as it appears in cell G2, for example, is =IF(F2>1, 0.999, IF(F2<0, 0.001, F2). That =IF() statement is then copied to each cell in column G.

The final new column in Figure 14.5 is the actual weight calculated from the adjusted predicted value of *Immun*. The formula for the calculation of the weights is given, for cell H2, in the formula bar above the spreadsheet. These are the values by which the independent variable set is modified for WLS.

	H2	▼	=	=1/(G2*(1-G2))^0.5						
	A	B	C	D	E	F	G	H	I	J	K
1	Mother	Age	Educ	Order	Immun	Ipred	Ipredadj	w		SUMMARY OUTPUT	
2	1	21	7	3	0	0.27359	0.27359	2.24314			
3	2	19	12	2	1	1.00361	0.999	31.6386		Regression Statistics	
4	3	23	10	3	0	0.73101	0.73101	2.25511		Multiple R	0.759847
5	4	25	8	2	1	0.73825	0.73825	2.27485		R Square	0.577368
6	5	25	7	2	1	0.61228	0.61228	2.05242		Adjusted R Squ	0.532085
7	6	26	15	4	1	1.30043	0.999	31.6386		Standard Error	0.330091
8	7	17	6	1	0	0.34797	0.34797	2.0994		Observations	32
9	8	21	6	3	0	0.14763	0.14763	2.81906			
10	9	25	13	6	1	0.64939	0.64939	2.09573		ANOVA	
11	10	19	11	3	1	0.69797	0.69797	2.17799			df
12	11	20	13	4	1	0.80998	0.80998	2.54898		Regression	3 4.1
13	12	18	10	1	1	0.8916	0.8916	3.2166		Residual	28 3.0
14	13	17	6	2	0	0.16829	0.16829	2.67289		Total	31 7.
15	14	20	12	4	1	0.68402	0.68402	2.15097			
16	15	21	7	1	1	0.63295	0.63295	2.07468		Coefficients and	
17	16	17	5	3	0	-0.13735	0.001	31.6386		Intercept	-0.90395 0.4
18	17	21	12	1	1	1.26279	0.999	31.6386		Age	0.039752 0.0
19	18	21	8	4	0	0.21989	0.21989	2.41446		Educ	0.125969 0.0
20	19	22	6	3	0	0.18738	0.18738	2.5627		Order	-0.17968 0.0
21	20	21	8	3	0	0.39956	0.39956	2.04161			
22	21	21	10	3	1	0.6515	0.6515	2.0896			

Figure 14.5 Calculation of weights for WLS

G37   = =$J$53+B2*$J$54+C2*$J$55+D2*$J$56

	A	B	C	D	E	F	G	H	I	J	K	L	M
36	Mother	Const	Age	Educ	Order	Immun	Ipred		SUMMARY OUTPUT				
37	1	2.243	47.11	15.7	6.729	0	0.32768						
38	2	31.64	601.1	379.7	63.28	31.6386	0.94838		Regression Statistics				
39	3	2.255	51.87	22.55	6.765	0	0.66463		Multiple R	0.990383			
40	4	2.275	56.87	18.2	4.55	2.27485	0.5817		R Square	0.980859			
41	5	2.052	51.31	14.37	4.105	2.05242	0.47573		Adjusted R Sq	0.943094			
42	6	31.64	822.6	474.6	126.6	31.6386	1.11311		Standard Error	1.860843			
43	7	2.099	35.69	12.6	2.099	0	0.40346		Observations	32			
44	8	2.819	59.2	16.91	8.457	0	0.22171						
45	9	2.096	52.39	27.24	12.57	2.09573	0.67177		ANOVA				
46	10	2.178	41.38	23.96	6.534	2.17799	0.73247			df	SS	MS	F	igni
47	11	2.549	60.98	33.14	10.2	2.54898	0.844		Regression	4	4968.374	1242.094	358.7027	5.
48	12	3.217	57.9	32.17	3.217	3.2166	0.83685		Residual	28	96.95666	3.462738	
49	13	2.673	45.44	16.04	5.346	0	0.29353		Total	32	5065.331		
50	14	2.151	43.02	25.81	8.604	2.15097	0.73803						
51	15	2.075	43.57	14.52	2.075	2.07468	0.54755			Coefficient	andard Err	t Stat	P-value	Low
52	16	31.64	537.9	158.2	94.92	0	0.07762		Intercept	0	#N/A	#N/A	#N/A	'
53	17	31.64	664.4	379.7	31.64	31.6386	1.07737		Const	-0.2844	0.147475	-1.92849	0.063989	-C
54	18	2.414	50.7	19.32	9.658	0	0.3237		Age	0.00953	0.011832	0.80545	0.427347	-C
55	19	2.563	56.38	15.38	7.688	0	0.23124		Educ	0.105965	0.012779	8.291955	5.05E-09	0.1
56	20	2.042	42.87	16.33	6.125	0	0.43364		Order	-0.10994	0.019975	-5.50364	7.01E-06	-C
57	21	2.099	44.07	20.99	6.296	2.09866	0.64557						

Figure 14.6   Weighted least squares results

The regression analysis based on the weighted values of the variables is shown in Figure 14.6, which again shows the first 20 mothers in the data set in column A. Column B, labeled *Const* for constant, is simply the weight calculated in Figure 14.5, but it can be thought of as the constant term in regression (1) multiplied by the weight. Each column—C, D, E, and F—is the original value of each variable—*Age, Educ, Order,* and *Immun*—multiplied by the weight from Figure 14.5.

Setting Up the Weighted Least Squares Analysis in Excel's Regression Package

The WLS analysis can be carried out on these data by using the regression package in Excel. But it must be employed somewhat differently from the way it is in most regression situations. The WLS procedure requires that each variable, including the dependent variable and the constant term (the value that will determine the intercept), be multiplied by the weight before we proceed with the regression analysis. This means that the variable *Const* (column B) becomes the set of values that will determine the intercept. In order to carry out the regression analysis with the variable *Const* as the determinant of the intercept, it is necessary to specify that the intercept is 0 in the regression window.

Recall the Regression analysis dialog box, which is shown again in Figure 14.7. The Input X Range now includes columns B through E. Column B, which represents the intercept term, is now part of the analysis, unlike the previous situations in which Excel was simply assumed to

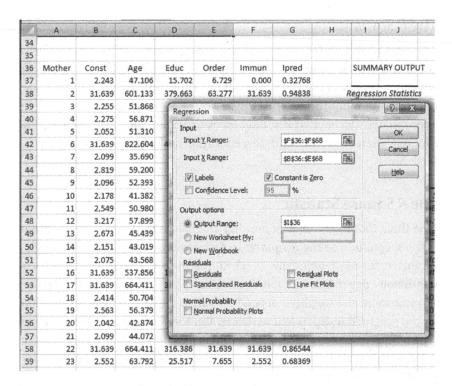

Figure 14.7 Regression setup for weighted least squares analysis

provide the constant for the calculation of the intercept term. At the same time, the box Constant is Zero is now checked. This means that Excel will calculate the regression results without including the column of ones for the intercept. Everything else in the Regression dialog box remains the same.

Interpreting the Output from the Weighted Least Squares Regression

The results of the WLS analysis are shown beginning in column I in Figure 14.6. A major difference between the regression results using OLS (Figure 14.4) and those using WLS is that the place in the regression output where the intercept usually appears (cell J52) is simply a zero, indicating that, in fact, the intercept is being considered 0 by the analysis. The value in cell J53 now represents the intercept term and has the same sign and is of the same order of magnitude as the intercept term in the OLS analysis. Similarly, whereas the other regression coefficients have changed somewhat, these have the same sign and are of the same order of magnitude as the coefficients calculated by using OLS.

The *F* Statistic

The statistical tests (*F* and *t* tests) are now unbiased, but they essentially confirm what was determined by using OLS, which is that both a mother's education level and the birth order of her child, but not the mother's age, influence immunization. On the basis of these results, the clinic might appropriately decide that it should focus education efforts to improve full immunization on women with low education and whose child is low in the birth order.

The *R* Square Statistic

One thing that might seem somewhat anomalous in the regression output is the magnitude of the *R square*. In fact, the *R* square is not meaningful in this case, as it generally is when regression is carried out with a continuous dependent variable. In this case, it represents the proportion of variance in the weighted dependent variable that can be accounted for by the weighted independent variables. But the *R* square of interest is that which represents the proportion of variance in the original 1, 0 dependent variable that is accounted for by the original independent variables, using the WLS coefficients.

There is some argument about whether an *R* square with a 1, 0 variable is even meaningful. Let's assume that it is desirable to have some measure comparable to the *R* square for the WLS analysis. In turn, it is possible to construct a pseudo *R* square by the formula in Equation 14.2. Equation 14.2 is probably the least conservative (i.e., it will create the largest *R* square value) of several possible ways in which a pseudo *R* square might be calculated. The initial step in generating this *R* square value is to calculate predicted values based on the regression weights given by the WLS analysis, but using the original unweighted data. These predicted values are shown, for the first 20 women, in column G of Figure 14.6. The Excel formula used to create the predicted values is given in the formula bar. Cells B2, C2, and D2 contain the original variables as shown in Figure 14.5. (It should be noted that the original data are in rows 2 through 33.) Now that we have calculated the predicted values based on the original data and the WLS coefficients, it is then possible to calculate error terms for each variable, as shown in Figure 14.8.

Figure 14.8 shows the predicted values of *Immun* based on the WLS coefficients, as given originally in Figure 14.6, for the first 20 women (column G). Column H shows the error as calculated from the predicted values in column G and the original values of *Immun*. The equation in the formula bar shows that the first error term is based on the value of *Immun*

	H37	▼	= =E2-G37		
	G	H	I	J	K
36	Ipred	Error	SSerror		
37	0.32768	-0.3277	0.10737	SSE	3.482462
38	0.94838	0.05162	0.00267	SST	7.21875
39	0.66463	-0.6646	0.44173	R^2	0.517581
40	0.5817	0.4183	0.17498		
41	0.47573	0.52427	0.27485		
42	1.11311	-0.1131	0.01279		
43	0.40346	-0.4035	0.16278		
44	0.22171	-0.2217	0.04916		
45	0.67177	0.32823	0.10773		
46	0.73247	0.26753	0.07157		
47	0.844	0.156	0.02434		
48	0.83685	0.16315	0.02662		
49	0.29353	-0.2935	0.08616		
50	0.73803	0.26197	0.06863		
51	0.54755	0.45245	0.20471		
52	0.07762	-0.0776	0.00603		
53	1.07737	-0.0774	0.00599		
54	0.3237	-0.3237	0.10478		
55	0.23124	-0.2312	0.05347		
56	0.43364	-0.4336	0.18804		

Figure 14.8 Calculation of pseudo R square for WLS

in E2, as shown in Figure 14.5. Column I is the square of column H, and the sum of the squared errors (SS_E) is given in cell K37. The total of the sum of squares (SS_T) is taken from cell I14 in Figure 14.4 but could be calculated as given in Equation 14.2. The pseudo R square, calculated as $(SS_T–SS_E)/SS_T$, is given in cell K39 as 0.518. In general, the pseudo R square calculated this way (or in any other manner) will always be less than the original R square from the OLS analysis.

$$pseudo\ R^2 = (SS_T - SS_E)/SST \tag{14.2}$$

where SS_T is the familiar $\sum_{i=1}^{n}(y_i - \bar{y})^2$ and SS_E is $\sum_{i=1}^{n}\left(y_i - \left(\sum_{j=1}^{m}\breve{b}_j x_{ij}\right)\right)^2$ with the values of y_i and x_{ij} being from the original data and $\breve{b}_j$ being the coefficients from the WLS analysis.

Moving from Weighted Least Squares to Logit Models

Up to this point the WLS results provide a statistically acceptable analysis of the data. The coefficients are unbiased, and the statistical tests are appropriate. But the predicted values of y remain problematic for most serious statisticians. It was mentioned earlier that OLS or WLS employed with a dichotomous dependent variable is referred to as a linear probability model. This is because the predicted values of the dependent variable are essentially equivalent to the probability that the dependent variable will be 1 or 0, depending on the values of the independent variable. All probabilities must be in the range 0 to 1; either a negative probability (less than 0) or a probability greater than 1 is meaningless. But, as can be seen in Figures 14.5 and 14.6, some of the predicted values using either OLS or WLS are greater than 1 or less than 0. The desire on the part of statisticians to remedy this situation in predicting values of dichotomous categorical dependent variables has led to the ascendance of Logit analysis.

EXERCISES FOR SECTION 14.2

1. Use the data on the Immun worksheet of Chpt 14-1.xls.

    a. Convert each of the variables *Age*, *Educ*, and *Order* to 1, 0 variables at their mean, and carry out the three chi-square analyses that relate these three variables to *FI* (full immunization).

    b. Generate the OLS regression analysis of *FI*, with *Age*, *Educ*, and *Order* as independent variables, and confirm that the results are as shown in Figure 14.4.

    c. Calculate the appropriate weights for weighted least squares (WLS) analysis of the Immun data, and carry out the weighted least squares analysis, following the discussion in the third subsection of Section 14.2, including Figures 14.5 and 14.7, to replicate the results given in Figure 14.6.

    d. Calculate a pseudo *R* square, using the approach given by the formula in Equation 14.2.

2. The data on the ChildF (child-friendly) worksheet of Chpt 14–1.xls was taken from *The State of the World's Children 1996* (1996). Use these data to relate safe water (*SafeW*), the log of GNP per capita (*LogGNP*), and female literacy (*FemLit*) to child friendliness (*ChildF*) for the 95 countries of the world. (Child-friendly countries are those with under-five mortality of 45 per 1,000 live births or less.)

    a. Convert each of the variables *SafeW*, *LogGNP*, and *FemLit* to 1, 0 variables at their mean, and carry out the three chi-square analyses that relate these three variables to *U5Mort*. What would you conclude from these analyses?

    b. Generate the OLS regression analysis of *U5Mort* with *SafeW*, *LogGNP*, and *FemLit* as independent variables. What would you conclude from this analysis?

    c. Calculate the appropriate weights for weighted least squares (WLS) analysis of the *U5Mort* data, and carry out the weighted least squares analysis, following the discussion in the third subsection of Section 14.2. What would you conclude from this analysis?

    d. Calculate a pseudo *R* square, using the approach given by the formula in Equation 14.2.

14.3   Logit for Estimating Dichotomous Dependent Variables

The previous sections of this chapter have considered chi-square and both ordinary least squares and weighted least squares as ways of dealing with dichotomous dependent variables. This section now takes up the discussion of *Logit* as a means of analyzing dichotomous dependent variables.

Setting up the Logit Model

The coefficients from a linear probability model, whether calculated using OLS or WLS, will produce a linear relationship between the independent and the dependent variables. If there is only one independent variable x, as well as a dichotomous dependent variable y, the predicted values of the dependent variable (the probabilities of the dependent variable being 0 or 1) will lie along a straight line—for example, as shown by the black diagonal line in Figure 14.9. The diagonal line in Figure 14.9 is actually generated by the linear equation $y = 0.09x - 0.04$. The diagonal line could be interpreted as a true probability as long as the value of the independent variable x is between about 5 and 15. If x is less than 5, y is less than 0 and thus cannot be interpreted as a probability. If x is greater than 15, y is greater than 1 and similarly cannot be interpreted as a probability. Because, in general, there is nothing to constrain x to a range from 5 to 15, it would be desirable to be able to specify a relationship—clearly a nonlinear one—that would constrain y to the range 0 to 1 for any values of x.

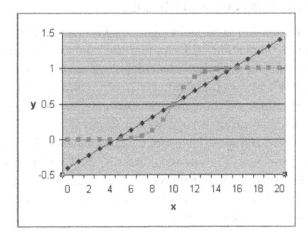

Figure 14.9   Graph of two relationships between independent and dependent variables

Introduction to Nonlinear Relationships

A number of *nonlinear relationships* allow the x to vary across any range while confining y to the range 0 to 1. Aldrich and Nelson describe several of these. Of these several alternatives, two have found favor among statisticians—what have come to be called the Logit relationship and the Probit relationship. As the Logit relationship is the simpler of the two, and as they produce almost identical results in the dichotomous dependent variable case, the remainder of this chapter focuses on the Logit relationship.

Introduction to Logit Models

The Logit relationship can be characterized by the gray curved line in Figure 14.9. It might also be called an *S curve* because it takes on that shape. For the particular Logit relationship pictured, the value of y when x is 10 is 0.5, exactly the same as it is for the linear relationship pictured by the black line. But the Logit relationship approaches both 1 and 0 much more rapidly than does the linear relationship, right to the point where the linear relationship crosses the 1, 0 boundary. When x is 14, for example, the value of y in the linear relationship is 0.86, but for the Logit relationship it is 0.98. However, the Logit relationship never allows the value of y to exceed 1. In fact, it never actually reaches 1 but only approaches it from below. Similarly, the Logit relationship never reaches 0 but only approaches it from above.

The Equation of the Logit Model

The Logit relationship pictured in Figure 14.9 is described by the formula in Equation 14.3. Equation 14.3 says that the values of the probability p_i (which represents the predicted values of y_i) are given by the value 1 divided by the quantity 1 plus e (approximately 2.718), raised to the power of the regression equation as characterized in OLS or WLS. But the coefficients of the regression equation in Logit are not simply the coefficients derived from OLS or WLS and substituted into the Logit equation. It is necessary to find a whole new set of coefficients to describe the Logit relationship. For example, the actual equation that produced the graph shown in Figure 14.9 was as that shown in Equation 14.4. This can be compared with the equation for the straight line given earlier.

$$p_i = \frac{1}{1 + e^{-b_x x_{ij}}} \tag{14.3}$$

where e is the natural log value of approximately 2.718, and p_i is considered to be a probability of any value of y_i.

$$p_i = \frac{1}{1 + e^{-(-10+1^*x)}}$$ (14.4)

The graph in Figure 14.9 was actually created in Excel. The formula for the Logit relationship as expressed in Excel was =1/(1+ EXP(-(-10+1*x))), where x refers to each value of the independent variable.

Finding the Logit Models Coefficients

If the coefficients for the Logit relationship are not found simply by substituting OLS or WLS coefficients, how then are they found? With OLS and WLS, there is a set of linear equations, derived through calculus, that can be solved to find the regression coefficients directly. With the Logit relationship, there is no such set of equations. The Logit relationship is found by a process known as maximum likelihood. The least squares process, including both OLS and WLS, attempts to minimize the sum of squared error terms through the best selection of coefficients. The maximum likelihood process attempts to maximize the fit between the observed data and a specified model of the data through the best selection of coefficients. The fit is based on the product of all values in the data set times the probability that the values will or will not occur. But products are mathematically difficult to deal with. Therefore, the common solution is to convert the probabilities to logarithms and maximize the fit between the observed data and the log of the specified model. Because of this, the actual value to be maximized in maximum likelihood is referred to as the log-likelihood.

Finding Log-Likelihoods Using Excel

How will this work in the case of Logit and in the specific case of the data on immunization of children? The first step is to set up the relationship for the log-likelihood to be maximized. The log-likelihood function to be maximized is as that given in Equation 14.5. Equation 14.5 is somewhat intimidating, so we will look at the construction of the log-likelihood function to be maximized using Excel.

$$\log L = \sum_{i=1}^{n} [\log(p_i)y_i + \log(1 - p_i)(1 - y_i)]$$ (14.5)

Figure 14.10 shows the initial step in constructing the log-likelihood function to be maximized. This step is to set up the Logit relationship

	F3	▼			=	=1/(1+EXP(-($A$1+$B$1*B3+$C$1*C3+$D$1*D3)))			
	A	B	C	D	E	F	G	H	I
1	1	0	0	0					
2	Mother	Age	Educ	Order	Immun	p	(1-p)		
3	1	21	7	3	0	0.7311	0.2689		
4	2	19	12	2	1	0.7311	0.2689		
5	3	23	10	3	0	0.7311	0.2689		
6	4	25	8	2	1	0.7311	0.2689		
7	5	25	7	2	1	0.7311	0.2689		
8	6	26	15	4	1	0.7311	0.2689		
9	7	17	6	1	0	0.7311	0.2689		
10	8	21	6	3	0	0.7311	0.2689		
11	9	25	13	6	1	0.7311	0.2689		
12	10	19	11	3	1	0.7311	0.2689		
13	11	20	13	4	1	0.7311	0.2689		
14	12	18	10	1	1	0.7311	0.2689		
15	13	17	6	2	0	0.7311	0.2689		
16	14	20	12	4	1	0.7311	0.2689		
17	15	21	7	1	1	0.7311	0.2689		
18	16	17	5	3	0	0.7311	0.2689		
19	17	21	12	1	1	0.7311	0.2689		
20	18	21	8	4	0	0.7311	0.2689		
21	19	22	6	3	0	0.7311	0.2689		
22	20	21	8	3	0	0.7311	0.2689		
23	21	21	10	3	1	0.7311	0.2689		

Figure 14.10 First step in finding logL

that defines the probability in Equation 14.3. In column A of Figure 14.10 is shown the identifier for each mother in the study, up to mother 20. Columns B, C, D, and E show the three independent variables—*Age*, *Educ*, and *Order*—and the dependent variable *Immun* for the first 20 mothers as well. Column F contains the initial calculation of the probability as given in Equation 14.3, and as expressed in Excel. The actual formula for cell F3 is given in the formula bar. In examining the formula for F3 in the formula bar, it is clear that the probability in cell F3 includes the values in cells A1, B1, C1, and D1. These values, 1, 0, 0, and 0, respectively, are initial values of the true coefficients to be found by maximizing the log-likelihood. The first of these, 1, represents the coefficient of the constant. Each of the 0 values represents the coefficient of the variable in the column in which they are located. When the maximization process is finished, these values will have changed to those that maximize logL, as is given in Equation 14.5. It can also be seen that column G contains the value $(1 - p)$, which also enters into the calculation of logL. The Excel formula for cell G3, for example, is simply $=1-F3$.

Spreadsheet Layout for Maximizing Log-Likelihoods in Excel

The complete layout for maximizing logL is given in Figure 14.11. Columns A through G remain the same as in Figure 14.10. Column H simply repeats

	J		=	=LN(F3)*H3								
	A	B	C	D	E	F	G	H	I	J	K	L
1	1	0	0	0	-21						log(1-p)	
2	Mother	Age	Educ	Order	Immun	p	(1-p)	y	(1-y)	logp*y	*(1-y)	logL
3	1	21	7	3	0	0.7311	0.2689	0	1	0	-1.3133	-1.3133
4	2	19	12	2	1	0.7311	0.2689	1	0	-0.3133	0	-0.3133
5	3	23	10	3	0	0.7311	0.2689	0	1	0	-1.3133	-1.3133
6	4	25	8	2	1	0.7311	0.2689	1	0	-0.3133	0	-0.3133
7	5	25	7	2	1	0.7311	0.2689	1	0	-0.3133	0	-0.3133
8	6	26	15	4	1	0.7311	0.2689	1	0	-0.3133	0	-0.3133
9	7	17	6	1	0	0.7311	0.2689	0	1	0	-1.3133	-1.3133
10	8	21	6	3	0	0.7311	0.2689	0	1	0	-1.3133	-1.3133
11	9	25	13	6	1	0.7311	0.2689	1	0	-0.3133	0	-0.3133
12	10	19	11	3	1	0.7311	0.2689	1	0	-0.3133	0	-0.3133
13	11	20	13	4	1	0.7311	0.2689	1	0	-0.3133	0	-0.3133
14	12	18	10	1	1	0.7311	0.2689	1	0	-0.3133	0	-0.3133
15	13	17	6	2	0	0.7311	0.2689	0	1	0	-1.3133	-1.3133
16	14	20	12	4	1	0.7311	0.2689	1	0	-0.3133	0	-0.3133
17	15	21	7	1	1	0.7311	0.2689	1	0	-0.3133	0	-0.3133
18	16	17	5	3	0	0.7311	0.2689	0	1	0	-1.3133	-1.3133
19	17	21	12	1	1	0.7311	0.2689	1	0	-0.3133	0	-0.3133
20	18	21	8	4	0	0.7311	0.2689	0	1	0	-1.3133	-1.3133
21	19	22	6	3	0	0.7311	0.2689	0	1	0	-1.3133	-1.3133
22	20	21	8	3	0	0.7311	0.2689	0	1	0	-1.3133	-1.3133
23	21	24	10	3	1	0.7311	0.2689	1	0	-0.3133	0	-0.3133

Figure 14.11 Complete layout for maximizing logL

the data in column E but is now designated y to conform to Equation 14.5. Column I is 1 minus column H. Columns J and K represent the calculation of log $p_i y_i$ and log$(1 - p_i)(1 - y_i)$, respectively. The Excel formula for cell J3 is given in the formula bar. =LN is the Excel function for the natural logarithm. Column L is the sum of columns J and K. It should be clear that when y is 1, column L will be log $p_i y_i$. When y is 0, column L will be log$(1 - p_i)(1 - y_i)$. There is also a new number, -21, in cell E1. This is the sum of the numbers in column L. It is the log-likelihood, the number to be maximized. It is no accident that the number in E1 is -21. When the coefficient of the constant (cell A1) is 1 and all other coefficients are 0, the log-likelihood for the Logit will always be the negative of the number of ones in the dependent variable. Table 14.1 contains the Excel formulas for Figure 14.11.

Solving for the Log-Likelihood Coefficients Using Excel's Solver

We have now laid out the spreadsheet for the maximization of the log-likelihood function. How do we find the maximum value of cell E1? Unfortunately, no single set of equations (as with least squares) can be solved for the answer. Basically, the maximization of the log-likelihood function is a trial-and-error process. But there are better and worse methods of going about the process of trial and error to find the set

Table 14.1   Formulas for Figure 14.11

Cell or Column	Formula	Action
A1	1	
B1	0	
C1	0	
D1	0	
E1	=SUM(L3:L35)	
F3	=1/(1+EXP(-($A$1+$B$1*B3+$C$1*C3+$D$1*D3)))	Copy down through cell F34
G3	=1-F3	Copy down through cell G34
H3	=E3	Copy down through cell H34
I3	=(1-H3)	Copy down through cell I34
J3	=LN(F3)*H3	Copy down through cell J34
K3	=LN(G3)*(I3)	Copy down through cell K34
L3	=(J3+K3)	Copy down through cell L34

of coefficients that maximize the log-likelihood function. Maddala (1983) provides a detailed description of the best process for finding the maximum of the log-likelihood function for the Logit model. However, that discussion is complex enough that for our purposes here, it is bypassed, and we will rely on an add-in capability of Excel to maximize the log-likelihood function.

The Solver Add-In

Excel includes an add-in called *Solver*. It is accessed within Excel in the same way as the Data Analysis add-in (refer to Chapter 2)—go to the Data ribbon, then to the Analysis menu, and click on Solver (see Figure 2.25). Solver is a general maximization routine that works on a wide variety of applications. In this chapter it is discussed only as it applies to the maximization of the log-likelihood function in Logit.

Setting Up Solver for the Logit Problem

The Solver Parameters dialog box is shown in Figure 14.12. The value to be maximized, in this case, cell E1, is shown in the field next to Set Target Cell. Solver provides several options for what to do with the value in cell E1. It can be maximized, minimized, or set equal to some specified value as determined by the Equal To row. The cells that are to be changed to seek the solution desired (in this case, a maximum) are specified in the field below By Changing Cells. Solver will guess which cells to modify if you wish, and it usually guesses right. Finally, a number of constraints can be set

Figure 14.12 Solver Parameters dialog box for maximizing logL

Figure 14.13 Solver solution for Logit model

on the solution Solver reaches in the field below Subject to the Constraints. In general, no constraints are required to reach a solution for the Logit model. Click Solve to invoke the add-in after you have made your choices.

The solution to the Logit model arrived at by Solver is shown in Figure 14.13. The value of logL produced by Solver is −6.24 (cell E1). The coefficients of the model that produce this value are given in cells

A1:D1. Cell A1 represents the intercept or constant value, and cells B1:D1 represent the coefficients of the three independent variables. Click OK to accept the solution reached by Solver.

Limitations to Solver when Solving the Logit Problem

There are clear limitations to Solver. The solution reached can depend on the initial values of the coefficients. In general, beginning with the value 1 for the constant and 0 for the independent variables will lead to a solution that represents the best fit between the model and the data. But beginning with other initial values can result in logL's increasing infinitely, so that the result would be a #NUM! in cell E1. If this were to happen, it would be best to begin again with 1 for the intercept and 0 for the other coefficients.

Overall Significance Test with Logit

Having found the coefficients developed by Solver, what is our next step? In least squares regression, one next step would be an overall F test to determine if any of the coefficients of the independent variables are different from 0. With Logit, there is no F test as such, but there is a chi-square test that accomplishes essentially the same thing. The formula for the appropriate chi-square is shown in Equation 14.6. The value of $logL_1$ is given in cell E1 in Figure 14.13. The value of $logL_0$ can be found by recalculating the Solver solution but restricting the cells to be changed (in the By Changing Cells fields; see Figure 14.12) to A1 (the intercept term) only. However, the value of $logL_0$ can also be found, as is given in Equation 14.7. (NOTE: logL is synonymous with LNL that is being used in Equations 14.6 and 14.7.)

$$X^2 = -2(LNL_0 - LNL_1) \qquad (14.6)$$

where $logL_0$ is the value of logL when all coefficients except the intercept are 0 and $logL_1$ is the value of logL for the best model.

$$LNL_0 = n_0 (LN (n_0/n)) + n_1 (LN (n_1/n)) \qquad (14.7)$$

where n is the total sample size, n_0 is the number of observations where y equals 0, and n_1 is the number of observations where y equals 1.

Figure 14.14 shows the calculation of the chi-square value for the Logit solution shown in Figure 14.13. The value of n, given in cell B1, is 32. The values of n_0 and n_1, in cells B2 and B3, respectively, are 11 and 21. The value 21.06784 in cell C2 was calculated with the Excel function =LN(B2/B1). Similarly, the value 20.4212 in cell C3 was calculated with the Excel function =LN(B3/B1). L_1 in cell B5 was taken from cell E1 in Figure 14.13. Cell B6 was calculated by the Excel statement =B2*C2+B3*C3. The formula

Figure 14.14 Calculation of chi-square for Logit

for the chi-square value in cell B8 is given in the formula bar. The degrees of freedom for this chi-square are equal to the number of regressors, not counting the intercept, or, in this case, three. The probability of the chi-square value was found with the Excel function =CHIDIST(B8,B9). The chi-square is 28.71 and the p value is < 0.0001. Therefore, the conclusion of this chi-square test, as with the OLS and WLS F tests, is that at least one of the regression coefficients other than the intercept coefficient is statistically different from 0.

Significance of Individual Coefficients

Of course, this now leads to the question of how to determine which of the coefficients can be considered different from 0. The test of this is the same as that with OLS or WLS—that is, it is the coefficient divided by its standard error. Unfortunately, though Solver can give us the coefficients, it cannot directly give us the standard errors of those coefficients. To find the standard errors, we must use the coefficients to produce something called the *information matrix*. The information matrix can most easily be produced using the matrix multiplication capabilities of Excel. To demonstrate the calculation of the information matrix, we must begin with the predicted values of the dependent variable *Immun*.

Maddala (1983) calls the information matrix, based on the best-fit coefficients for the Logit model, $I(\hat{\beta})$. The standard errors of the coefficients will be the square root of the main diagonal elements in $[I(\hat{\beta})]^{-1}$, the inverse of the information matrix. To find the information matrix and, hence, its inverse, we need first to find q_i for each value of the dependent variable. The value q_i can be found as shown in Equation 14.8. The calculation of q_i for the data on immunization is shown in Figure 14.15.

$$q_i = \frac{e_i^{bx_j}}{\left[1 + e_i^{bx_j}\right]^2} \qquad (14.8)$$

where x_j includes all regressors and the intercept term.

G3   = =EXP($B$1+$C$1*C3+$D$1*D3+$E$1*E3)

	A	B	C	D	E	F	G	H	I
1		-17.691	0.520	1.655	-2.606	-6.237			
2	Mother	Const	Age	Educ	Order	Immun	exp(bxj)	(1+exp(bxj))^2	qi
3	1	1	21	7	3	0	0.050	1.102	0.045
4	2	1	19	12	2	1	932.977	872313.770	0.001
5	3	1	23	10	3	0	20.103	445.317	0.045
6	4	1	25	8	2	1	28.111	847.444	0.033
7	5	1	25	7	2	1	5.370	40.574	0.132
8	6	1	26	15	4	1	27749.932	770114252.750	0.000
9	7	1	17	6	1	0	0.217	1.481	0.147
10	8	1	21	6	3	0	0.009	1.019	0.009
11	9	1	25	13	6	1	3.280	18.317	0.179
12	10	1	19	11	3	1	13.154	200.334	0.066
13	11	1	20	13	4	1	44.747	2092.796	0.021
14	12	1	18	10	1	1	274.260	75767.916	0.004
15	13	1	17	6	2	0	0.016	1.032	0.016
16	14	1	20	12	4	1	8.548	91.159	0.094
17	15	1	21	7	1	1	9.094	101.886	0.089
18	16	1	17	5	3	0	0.000	1.000	0.000
19	17	1	21	12	1	1	35754.134	1278429621.959	0.000
20	18	1	21	8	4	0	0.019	1.039	0.018
21	19	1	22	6	3	0	0.016	1.032	0.015
22	20	1	21	8	3	0	0.259	1.586	0.164

Figure 14.15 First step in the calculation of the information matrix

Calculation of the Information Matrix

Figure 14.15 shows again the data for the first 20 mothers and the coefficients (in row 1) that were generated by Solver in Figure 14.13. A new column has been added as column B, into which has been inserted a column of ones to represent the intercept or constant term. We will use this later in the calculations. All other variables have been shifted one column to the right. Column G is the calculation for the numerator of q_i, and column H is the calculation of the denominator. The formula bar shows how cell G3 was calculated. The value q_i is shown in column I.

The next step in the calculation of the information matrix is to calculate $q_i \times x_{ij}$ for each x_j, including the intercept term. In the Immunization example, there are three independent variables—Age, Educ, and Order—in addition to the intercept. The construction of the $q_i \times x_{ij}$ for the intercept and the three independent variables is shown in Figure 14.16. The first five columns in Figure 14.16 are, again, the data for the first 20 mothers. Two columns that appear in Figure 14.15, G and H, have been hidden in Figure 14.16, simply to provide additional room to display the rest of the columns. Column I is q_i, as calculated in Figure 14.15. Columns J, K, L, and M represent the values of $q_i \times x_{ij}$, column J being the intercept, which simply repeats the value of q_i.

Using the =MMULT () and =TRANSPOSE () Functions

The next step in the formation of the information matrix is to prepare to use =MMULT () to multiply the matrix represented by the original data by

	K3		= =$I3*C3								
	A	B	C	D	E	F	I	J	K	L	M
1		-17.691	0.520	1.655	-2.606	-6.237					
2	Mother	Const	Age	Educ	Order	Immun	qi	qi*Const	qi*Age	qi*Educ	qi*Immun
3	1	1	21	7	3	0	0.045	0.045	0.9444	0.3148	0.1349
4	2	1	19	12	2	1	0.001	0.001	0.0203	0.0128	0.0021
5	3	1	23	10	3	0	0.045	0.045	1.0383	0.4514	0.1354
6	4	1	25	8	2	1	0.033	0.033	0.8293	0.2654	0.0663
7	5	1	25	7	2	1	0.132	0.132	3.3086	0.9264	0.2647
8	6	1	26	15	4	1	0.000	0.000	0.0009	0.0005	0.0001
9	7	1	17	6	1	0	0.147	0.147	2.4917	0.8794	0.1466
10	8	1	21	6	3	0	0.009	0.009	0.1950	0.0557	0.0279
11	9	1	25	13	6	1	0.179	0.179	4.4765	2.3278	1.0744
12	10	1	19	11	3	1	0.066	0.066	1.2475	0.7223	0.1970
13	11	1	20	13	4	1	0.021	0.021	0.4276	0.2780	0.0855
14	12	1	18	10	1	1	0.004	0.004	0.0652	0.0362	0.0036
15	13	1	17	6	2	0	0.016	0.016	0.2639	0.0931	0.0310
16	14	1	20	12	4	1	0.094	0.094	1.8753	1.1252	0.3751
17	15	1	21	7	1	1	0.089	0.089	1.8744	0.6248	0.0893
18	16	1	17	5	3	0	0.000	0.000	0.0038	0.0011	0.0007
19	17	1	21	12	1	1	0.000	0.000	0.0006	0.0003	0.0000
20	18	1	21	8	4	0	0.018	0.018	0.3870	0.1474	0.0737
21	19	1	22	6	3	0	0.015	0.015	0.3392	0.0925	0.0463
22	20	1	21	8	3	0	0.164	0.164	3.4340	1.3082	0.4906
23	21	1	21	10	3	1	0.109	0.109	2.7708	1.0913	0.3244

Figure 14.16 Calculation of $q_i \times x_{ij}$

the transpose of the values in columns J, K, L, and M. To generate the transpose, the best approach is to use the Excel function =TRANSPOSE() and put the result somewhere on the spreadsheet where it will not interfere with other data.

Figure 14.17 shows the first eight columns of the transpose matrix that will be used as the premultiplier for the information matrix. The formula bar shows the =TRANSPOSE() function that was used to create the transpose matrix. The labels were copied from the first row of columns K, J, L, and M to cells V2:V5. If you remember the use of Excel functions that put values into more than one cell (e.g., =FREQUENCY), you remember that the entire area in which the result is to appear must be highlighted before you press Ctrl+Shift+Enter. The easiest way to know exactly what to highlight as the set of target cells for the =TRANSPOSE() function is to use Edit ➤ Copy to copy the entire original matrix (in this case, cells J3:M34). In turn, in the place where you wish to put the transpose matrix, use Edit ➤ Paste Special ➤ Transpose. This will put values into the cells in which you wish

	W2		= {=TRANSPOSE(J3:M34)}						
	V	W	X	Y	Z	AA	AB	AC	AD
1									
2	qi*Const	0.045	0.001	0.045	0.033	0.132	0.000	0.147	0.009
3	qi*Age	0.9444	0.0203	1.0383	0.8293	3.3086	0.0009	2.4917	0.1950
4	qi*Educ	0.3148	0.0128	0.4514	0.2654	0.9264	0.0005	0.8794	0.0557
5	qi*Immun	0.1349	0.0021	0.1354	0.0663	0.2647	0.0001	0.1466	0.0279

Figure 14.17 Formation of the transpose matrix

O3		▾	= {=MMULT(W2:BB5,B3:E34)}	
	N	O	P	Q	R
1					
2		I(betahat)			
3		1.777573	38.25721	15.33456	5.073644
4		38.25721	834.406	333.1399	111.8517
5		15.33456	333.1399	141.1063	48.26349
6		5.073644	111.8517	48.26349	17.61185
7					
8		I(betahat)-1			
9		60.67729	-2.38825	-2.62688	4.886309
10		-2.38825	0.116771	0.034863	-0.14913
11		-2.62688	0.034863	0.433041	-0.65136
12		4.886309	-0.14913	-0.65136	1.381241
13					
14	bj	-17.691	0.520	1.655	-2.606
15	SEbj	7.790	0.342	0.658	1.175
16	t	-2.271	1.521	2.516	-2.218
17	p	0.031	0.139	0.018	0.035

Figure 14.18 Information matrix and *t* tests

the results of =TRANSPOSE() to go. Then you can highlight that entire area and invoke the =TRANSPOSE() function.

The information matrix $I(\hat{\beta})$ can now be found by premultiplying the original data matrix (cells B3:E34) by the transpose matrix. Because the transpose is 4 × 32 and the original data matrix is 32 × 4, the resulting information matrix will be 4 × 4. The information matrix, as calculated using the Excel function =MMULT(), is shown, beginning in cell O3 of Figure 14.18. At this point the reason for adding the column of ones representing the intercept should be clear. It is necessary to include this column in the calculation of the information matrix.

The Standard Errors for the Logit Coefficients

Figure 14.18 also shows the inverse of the information matrix that is calculated using the =MINVERSE function, which begins in cell O9. The standard errors of the Logit coefficients are found by taking the square root of the values on the main diagonal of the inverse of the information matrix. The Logit coefficients themselves are shown in cells O14:R14. The standard errors for each coefficient are shown below them in cells O15:R15. The value in cell O15 (the standard error of the intercept) is the square root of the main diagonal element in the inverse of the information matrix at cell O9. The standard error of the coefficient on Age (cell P15) is the square root of the main diagonal element at cell P10. The standard error of the coefficient on Educ (cell Q15) is the square root of the value in cell Q11. Finally, the standard error of the coefficient for Order (cell R15) is the square root of the value in cell R12.

The t tests are shown in cells O16:R16, and their probabilities are shown in cells O17:R17. The conclusion reached with Logit is exactly the same as that reached with WLS. Both a mother's education level and the birth order of her child influence whether the child is fully immunized, while age does not. So, based on this analysis, if the clinic wishes to increase the proportion of children fully immunized, the staff should concentrate on children whose birth order is low and whose mothers' level of education is low.

Pseudo R Square Statistic

As a final topic in the solution of the Logit problem, it seems reasonable to consider a pseudo R square that can be calculated for the Logit. Aldrich and Nelson suggest as a pseudo R square the value shown in Equation 14.9. Using the formula in Equation 14.9 and the chi-square value from Figure 14.14, the pseudo R square for the Logit analysis is 0.4729. This contrasts with 0.5774 for the OLS analysis and 0.5176 for the WLS analysis.

$$pseudo\ R^2 = X^2/(n + X^2) \qquad (14.9)$$

where X^2 is taken from Equation 14.6.

EXERCISES FOR SECTION 14.3

1. Use the data on the Immun worksheet of Chpt 14–1.xls.

   a. Set up the spreadsheet for maximizing LogL for these data, following the example in Figures 14.10 and 14.11.

   b. Use the Solver add-in to find the values of the coefficients of *Age*, *Educ*, and *Order* to replicate Figure 14.13.

   c. Calculate the overall chi-square value for this analysis, using Equations 14.6 and 14.7 to replicate Figure 14.14.

   d. Set up the worksheet for calculating the information matrix $I(\hat{\beta})$ as given in Figures 14.15, 14.16, and 14.17, and complete the t tests of the individual coefficients, as shown in Figure 14.18.

   e. Confirm that all your results are the same as those given in the figures.

2. Use the data on the ChildF (child-friendly) worksheet of Chpt 14–1.xls.

   a. Set up the spreadsheet for maximizing LogL for these data, following the example in Figures 14.10 and 14.11.

   b. Use the Solver add-in to find the values of the coefficients of *SafeW*, *LogGNP*, and *FemLit* to replicate Figure 14.13.

c. Calculate the overall chi-square value for this analysis, using Equations 14.6 and 14.7 to replicate Figure 14.14.

d. Set up the worksheet for calculating the information matrix $I(\hat{\beta})$, as given in Figures 14.15, 14.16, and 14.17, and complete the t tests of the individual coefficients, as shown in Figure 14.18.

e. Decide if your conclusions are the same or different, based on this analysis, as compared with ordinary or weighted least squares.

14.4   A Comparison of Ordinary Least Squares, Weighted Least Squares, and Logit

Perhaps the last thing to do in this chapter should be to compare the OLS, WLS, and Logit results in terms of the prediction of whether a child will be fully immunized. How well do these three analyses actually predict which children will be immunized, and how do they compare with one another? The predicted value of the dependent variable *Immun* is a probability that the true value of *Immun* will be either 1 or 0; therefore, it seems reasonable to assign a 1 to those observations in which the predicted value of *Immun* is greater than 0.5 and a 0 to those observations where the predicted value is less than 0.5. (Because none of the predicted values is exactly 0.5, we do not have to worry about what we would do in that case.)

Comparison of the Three Estimates of the Dependent Variable

Figure 14.19 shows a comparison of the three estimates of the dependent variable *Immun*. The first column in Figure 14.19 represents the mothers in the sample, again, through mother number 20. Column B is the actual value of *Immun*. Column C is a 1 or 0 value of *Immun* as predicted by OLS. The =IF statement (as shown in the formula bar) was used to create this as well as columns D and E. Column D is a 1 or 0 value of *Immun* as predicted by WLS, and column D is a 1 or 0 value as predicted by Logit. Simply looking at the three columns C, D, and E reveals that they are very similar.

   Beginning in column G are three pivot tables created from the data in columns B:E. The first pivot table compares the actual values of Immun with the predictions based on OLS. The second compares the actual values with the predictions based on WLS. The third compares the actual values with the predictions based on Logit. For both OLS and Logit, there are two errors. One true 0 is predicted to be a 1, and one true 1 is

C2 ▼ = =IF('14-4,5,6'!F2>0.5,1,0)

	A	B	C	D	E	F	G	H	I	J
1	Mother	Immun	Pols	Pwls	Plog		Count of Pols	Immun ▼		
2	1	0	0	0	0		Pols ▼	0	1	Grand Total
3	2	1	1	1	1		0	10	1	11
4	3	0	1	1	1		1	1	20	21
5	4	1	1	1	1		Grand Total	11	21	32
6	5	1	1	0	1					
7	6	1	1	1	1		Count of Pwls	Immun ▼		
8	7	0	0	0	0		Pwls ▼	0	1	Grand Total
9	8	0	0	0	0		0	10	3	13
10	9	1	1	1	1		1	1	18	19
11	10	1	1	1	1		Grand Total	11	21	32
12	11	1	1	1	1					
13	12	1	1	1	1		Count of Plog	Immun ▼		
14	13	0	0	0	0		Plog ▼	0	1	Grand Total
15	14	1	1	1	1		0	10	1	11
16	15	1	1	1	1		1	1	20	21
17	16	0	0	0	0		Grand Total	11	21	32
18	17	1	1	1	1					
19	18	0	0	0	0					
20	19	0	0	0	0					
21	20	0	0	0	0					
22	21	1	1	1	1					

Figure 14.19 Comparison of OLS-, WLS-, and Logit-predicted values

predicted to be a 0 by both methods. For WLS there are four errors. One true 0 is predicted to be a 1, and the three records that had true values of '1' are predicted to be 0. Though Figure 14.19 does not show this, the match between OLS and Logit predictions is perfect, whereas WLS predicts two observations to be 0, which are predicted to be 1 by OLS and Logit.

It is important to note that this is only one example in a number of comparisons between OLS, WLS, and Logit. However, it appears that OLS and Logit seem to perform about equally in predicting the actual values of a dichotomous dependent variable, and WLS performs slightly less well. In consequence, if the desire is only to predict which observations will be 1 and which will be 0, it seems that OLS, which is relatively simple, compared with Logit, might be satisfactory. However, in this case, OLS did not reveal that birth order was a statistically significant predictor of Immun, whereas both WLS and Logit did. But, in general, if the dependent variable is dichotomous, you cannot go far wrong assuming the Logit relationship and using the techniques described in the Logit section of this chapter.

Note on Interpretation of Logistic Regression Results/Coefficients

Estimated coefficients of a logistic regression model must be interpreted with care. Although the logistic regression coefficients are akin to slope coefficients in a linear regression model their meaning is much different.

Slope coefficients in a linear regression model are interpreted as the rate of change in y (the dependent variable) as x's (the independent variables) change. In contrast, the logistic regression coefficient is interpreted as the rate of change in the "log odds" as x changes. This comparison is not very intuitive. However, if we compute the more intuitive "marginal effect" of a continuous independent variable on the probability, the relation is clarified. The marginal effect can be written as:

$$dp/dB = f(BX)B$$

where $f()$ is the density function of the cumulative probability distribution function ($F(BX)$, which ranges from 0 to 1). In turn, the marginal effects depend on the values of the independent variables. It is often the case that we evaluate the marginal effects of the variables at their means.

The marginal effects can be investigated using the "odds ratio." The odds ratio is the probability of the event divided by the probability of the nonevent. This interpretation of the logistic coefficient is usually more intuitive where $expB$ is the effect of the independent variable on the "odds ratio." For example, if $expB3 = 3$, then a one-unit change in $X3$ would make the event three times as likely (0.75/0.25) to occur. Odds ratios equal to 1 mean that there is a 50/50 chance that the event will occur with a small change in the independent variable. Negative coefficients lead to odds ratios less than one: if $expB2 = 0.5$, then a one-unit change in $X2$ leads to the event being less likely (0.33/0.67) to occur. Just take caution in interpreting negative coefficients as they are harder to interpret than positive coefficients.

Survival Analysis: A Brief Discussion

Survival analysis is widely used in health care to quantify "survivorship" in a population being studied. It is termed "survival analysis" because it is indicative of the time elapsed from treatment to death. However, survival analysis is applicable to many areas other than mortality. In short, investigators are concerned with the time from a treatment until an event of interest occurs (i.e., time for a leg fracture to heal after casting).

Survival models can also be viewed as ordinary regression models in which the response variable is time. The three main characteristics of survival models are as follows:

- The dependent variable or response is the waiting time until the occurrence of a well-defined event.

Table 14.2   Comparing linear regression, logic regression, and survival analysis

Technique	Predictor Variables	Outcome Variable	Mathematical Model	Yields
Linear regression	Categorical or continuous	Normally distributed	$Y = B_1X + B_0$ (Linear)	Linear changes
Logistic regression	Categorical or continuous	Binary (except in polytomous logistic regression)	$Ln(P/1\text{-}P) = B_1X + B_0$ (sigmoidal prob.)	Odds ratios
Survival analyses	Time and categorical or continuous	Binary	$h(t) = h_0(t)exp(B_1X + B_0)$	Hazard rates

- Observations are censored (i.e., for some units the event of interest has not occurred at the time the data are analyzed).

- Predictors or explanatory variables exist whose effect on waiting time we wish to assess or control.

Table 14.2 juxtaposes the techniques of linear regression, logistic regression, and survival analysis with respect to predictor variables, outcome variable, basic mathematical model, and final model yield.

Other reasons survival analysis is preferred to other models are:

- It quantifies time to a single, dichotomous event.
- It handles censored data well.
- It results in a dichotomous (binary) outcome.
- It analyzes the time to an event.

As was previously mentioned, survival analysis is common to health care; however, a more in-depth discussion of the topic is outside the scope of this textbook. Please refer to the following works on survival analysis to obtain a deeper understanding:

Fleming, T. R., and Harrington, D. P. 2013. *Counting Processes and Survival Analysis.* Hoboken, NJ: John Wiley & Sons.

Kleinbaum, D. G. 2011. *Survival Analysis: A Self-Learning Text.* 3rd ed. New York: Springer.

Lee, E. T., and Want, J. W. 2013. *Statistical Methods for Survival Data Analysis.* 4th ed. Hoboken, NJ: John Wiley & Sons.

Liu, X. 2012. *Survival Analysis: Models and Applications.* Hoboken, NJ: John Wiley & Sons.

EXERCISES FOR SECTION 14.4

1. Use the previous analyses of the data on the Immun worksheet of Chpt 14-1.xls.

   a. Convert the predicted values of Immun to a 1, 0 variable at 0.05 for each of the prediction methods—OLS, WLS, and Logit.

   b. Generate the comparison table as shown in Figure 14.19.

2. Use the previous analyses of the data on the ChildF worksheet of Chpt 14-1.xls.

   a. Convert the predicted values of ChildF to a 1, 0 variable at 0.05 for each of the prediction methods—OLS, WLS, and Logit.

   b. Generate the comparison table, following Figure 14.19.

   c. What conclusions do you draw from these comparisons?

KEY TERMS

#NUM!	Logit
=MINVERSE()	maximum likelihood
=MMULT	nonlinear relationship
=TRANSPOSE()	ordinary least squares
analysis of variance	Probit
categorical variable	Solver
independent variable	weighted least squares
information matrix	Yates's correction
linear probability model	

MULTIPLE REGRESSION AND MATRICES

In order to understand how the computer carries out regression analysis—which automatically leads to a better understanding of regression—it is necessary to understand something about matrix math. This section provides a brief introduction to matrix math.

> Matrices are used to describe linear equations by tracking the coefficients of linear transformations and to record data that depend on multiple parameters.

An Introduction to Matrix Math

A *matrix* is a set of numbers in a two-dimensional space. Matrices are almost always designated with capital letters in boldface type. In general, a matrix $\mathbf{X}$ has n rows and m columns, as shown in Equation A.1, where the first subscript denotes the row and the second denotes the column.

$$\mathbf{X} = \begin{bmatrix} x_{11} & x_{12} & \cdots & x_{1m} \\ x_{21} & x_{22} & \cdots & x_{2m} \\ \cdot & \cdot & & \cdot \\ \cdot & \cdot & & \cdot \\ x_{n1} & x_{n2} & \cdots & x_{nm} \end{bmatrix} \tag{A.1}$$

A matrix is said to have dimensions equal to n and m so that the matrix $\mathbf{X}$ has dimensions $n \times m$ (rows first, columns second). The following is a typical example of a 2×3 matrix.

$$\begin{bmatrix} 2 & 5 & 7 \\ 1 & 14 & 11 \end{bmatrix}$$

A vector is a matrix with dimensions $n \times 1$ or $1 \times m$, as shown in Equation A.2.

$$\mathbf{x} = \begin{bmatrix} x_1 \\ x_2 \\ \cdot \\ \cdot \\ x_n \end{bmatrix}, \quad \mathbf{y} = [y_1 \ y_2 \cdots y_m] \tag{A.2}$$

The following are typical examples of a 3×1 vector and a 1×3 vector.

$$\begin{bmatrix} 3 \\ 15 \\ 6 \end{bmatrix}, [9 \ 27 \ 52].$$

A *scalar* can be considered a matrix of dimensions 1×1. The individual entries of any matrix or vector are scalars, but scalars can stand alone. A scalar is simply a number.

The transpose of a matrix $\mathbf{X}$, designated $\mathbf{X'}$, is a matrix in which the first row of $\mathbf{X}$ becomes the first column of $\mathbf{X'}$, the second row of $\mathbf{X}$ the second column of $\mathbf{X'}$, and so on, so that if

$$\mathbf{X} = \begin{bmatrix} x_{11} & x_{12} & x_{13} \\ x_{21} & x_{22} & x_{23} \end{bmatrix}, \quad \text{then} \quad \mathbf{X'} = \begin{bmatrix} x_{11} & x_{21} \\ x_{12} & x_{22} \\ x_{13} & x_{23} \end{bmatrix};$$

or if

$$\mathbf{X} = \begin{bmatrix} 7 & 3 & 2 \\ 1 & 9 & 5 \end{bmatrix}, \quad \text{then} \quad \mathbf{X'} = \begin{bmatrix} 7 & 1 \\ 3 & 9 \\ 2 & 5 \end{bmatrix}$$

Addition and Subtraction of Matrices

Addition and subtraction may be performed on matrices if each has equal rows and equal columns. The two matrices $\mathbf{X}$ and $\mathbf{Y}$ may be added, as shown in Equation A.3.

$$\mathbf{X} \quad + \quad \mathbf{Y} \quad = \quad (\mathbf{X}+\mathbf{Y})$$

$$\begin{bmatrix} x_{11} & x_{12} \\ x_{21} & x_{22} \\ x_{31} & x_{32} \end{bmatrix} + \begin{bmatrix} y_{11} & y_{12} \\ y_{21} & y_{22} \\ y_{31} & y_{32} \end{bmatrix} = \begin{bmatrix} x_{11}+y_{11} & x_{12}+y_{12} \\ x_{21}+y_{21} & x_{22}+y_{22} \\ x_{31}+y_{31} & x_{32}+y_{32} \end{bmatrix};$$

or

$$\begin{bmatrix} 7 & 1 \\ 3 & 9 \\ 2 & 5 \end{bmatrix} + \begin{bmatrix} 6 & 2 \\ 2 & 4 \\ 4 & 3 \end{bmatrix} = \begin{bmatrix} 13 & 3 \\ 5 & 13 \\ 6 & 8 \end{bmatrix} \tag{A.3}$$

The matrix Y can also be subtracted from X, as shown in Equation A.4.

$$\mathbf{X} \quad - \quad \mathbf{Y} \quad = \quad (\mathbf{X}-\mathbf{Y})$$

$$\begin{bmatrix} x_{11} & x_{12} \\ x_{21} & x_{22} \\ x_{31} & x_{32} \end{bmatrix} - \begin{bmatrix} y_{11} & y_{12} \\ y_{21} & y_{22} \\ y_{31} & y_{32} \end{bmatrix} = \begin{bmatrix} x_{11}-y_{11} & x_{12}-y_{12} \\ x_{21}-y_{21} & x_{22}-y_{22} \\ x_{31}-y_{31} & x_{32}-y_{32} \end{bmatrix};$$

or

$$\begin{bmatrix} 7 & 1 \\ 3 & 9 \\ 2 & 5 \end{bmatrix} - \begin{bmatrix} 6 & 2 \\ 2 & 4 \\ 4 & 3 \end{bmatrix} = \begin{bmatrix} 1 & -1 \\ 1 & 5 \\ -2 & 2 \end{bmatrix} \tag{A.4}$$

Multiplication of Matrices

Multiplication can be performed on matrices if the number of columns in the first matrix is equal to the number of rows in the second. Such matrices will be said to conform for multiplication. The two matrices $\mathbf{X}'(2 \times 3)$ and $\mathbf{Y}(3 \times 2)$ can be multiplied, and the resulting matrix $\mathbf{X}'\mathbf{Y}$ will be of dimension 2×2, as shown in Equation A.5. Although $ab = ba$ when a and b are both scalars, in general, $\mathbf{X}'\mathbf{Y}(2 \times 2)$ does not equal $\mathbf{Y}\mathbf{X}'(3 \times 3)$ and will not have the same dimensions. When the operation $\mathbf{X}'\mathbf{Y}$ is carried out, $\mathbf{Y}$ may be said to be premultiplied by $\mathbf{X}'$. When $\mathbf{Y}\mathbf{X}'$ is carried out, $\mathbf{Y}$ is postmultiplied by $\mathbf{X}'$. A particularly useful matrix product is $\mathbf{X}\mathbf{X}'$, which provides the sum of squares and cross products for **X**.

$$\mathbf{X'} \quad \cdot \quad \mathbf{Y} \quad = \quad \mathbf{X'Y}$$

$$\begin{bmatrix} x_{11} & x_{21} & x_{31} \\ x_{12} & x_{22} & x_{32} \end{bmatrix} \cdot \begin{bmatrix} y_{11} & y_{12} \\ y_{21} & y_{22} \\ y_{31} & y_{32} \end{bmatrix}$$

$$= \begin{bmatrix} x_{11}y_{11} + x_{21}y_{21} + x_{31}y_{31} & x_{11}y_{12} + x_{21}y_{22} + x_{31}y_{32} \\ x_{21}y_{11} + x_{22}y_{21} + x_{32}y_{31} & x_{12}y_{12} + x_{22}y_{22} + x_{32}y_{32} \end{bmatrix}$$

or

$$\begin{bmatrix} 7 & 3 & 2 \\ 1 & 9 & 5 \end{bmatrix} \cdot \begin{bmatrix} 6 & 2 \\ 2 & 4 \\ 4 & 3 \end{bmatrix} = \begin{bmatrix} 56 & 32 \\ 44 & 53 \end{bmatrix} \tag{A.5}$$

Matrix Multiplication and Scalars

Any matrices or vectors that are to be multiplied must conform for multiplication, with one exception: Any matrix or vector of any dimension can be pre- or postmultiplied by a scalar, as shown in Equation A.6.

$$a \cdot \mathbf{X} = a \cdot \begin{bmatrix} x_{11} & x_{12} \\ x_{21} & x_{22} \\ x_{31} & x_{32} \end{bmatrix} = \begin{bmatrix} ax_{11} & ax_{12} \\ ax_{21} & ax_{22} \\ ax_{31} & ax_{32} \end{bmatrix} = \mathbf{X} \cdot a$$

or

$$5 \cdot \begin{bmatrix} 7 & 1 \\ 3 & 9 \\ 2 & 5 \end{bmatrix} = \begin{bmatrix} 35 & 5 \\ 15 & 45 \\ 10 & 25 \end{bmatrix} \tag{A.6}$$

Finding the Determinant of a Matrix

Division is, in general, undefined for matrices. With matrices in which rows equal columns and the *determinant* of the matrix does not equal 0, multiplication of a matrix by its *inverse* produces the same result as division. The determinant of a matrix is a scalar defined only for matrices in which rows equal columns. For the 2×2 matrix **W**, the determinant of **W** may be written as shown in Equation A.7.

$$|\mathbf{W}| = \begin{bmatrix} w_{11} & w_{12} \\ w_{21} & w_{22} \end{bmatrix} = w_{11}w_{22} - w_{21}w_{12}$$

or

$$|\mathbf{W}| = \begin{bmatrix} 6 & 3 \\ 4 & 7 \end{bmatrix} = (6 \cdot 7) - (4 \cdot 3) = 30 \qquad (A.7)$$

If any column of a matrix is a linear transformation of one or more other columns, the determinant will be 0. If, for example, the matrix $\mathbf{V}$ is as shown in Equation A.8, the determinant of $\mathbf{V}$ will be 0 and the inverse of $\mathbf{V}$ (written $\mathbf{V}^{-1}$) will not exist.

$$|\mathbf{V}| = \begin{bmatrix} v_{11} & 2v_{11} \\ v_{21} & 2v_{21} \end{bmatrix} = \begin{bmatrix} 6 & 12 \\ 4 & 8 \end{bmatrix}; \text{ then } |\mathbf{V}| = (6 \cdot 8) - (4 \cdot 12) = 0 \quad (A.8)$$

In scalar arithmetic, $a/a = a \times 1/a = aa^{-1} = 1$. If the inverse of a matrix $\mathbf{W}$ exists (see Equations A.7 and A.8), then $\mathbf{WW}^{-1} = \mathbf{I}$, where I is a matrix with 1 in each entry on the main diagonal and 0 everywhere else. For example, suppose $\mathbf{W}$ is as defined in Equation A.9 (the matrix whose determinant is shown in Equation A.7).

$$|\mathbf{W}| = \begin{bmatrix} w_{11} & w_{12} \\ w_{21} & w_{22} \end{bmatrix} \qquad (A.9)$$

Then, $\mathbf{W}^{-1}$ is as defined in Equation A.10, where $w_{11}w_{22} - w_{12}w_{21}$ is $|\mathbf{W}|$, as defined in Equation A.7.

$$\mathbf{W}^{-1} = \begin{bmatrix} \dfrac{w_{22}}{w_{11}w_{22} - w_{12}w_{21}} & \dfrac{-w_{12}}{w_{11}w_{22} - w_{12}w_{21}} \\ \dfrac{-w_{21}}{w_{11}w_{22} - w_{12}w_{21}} & \dfrac{w_{11}}{w_{11}w_{22} - w_{12}w_{21}} \end{bmatrix} \qquad (A.10)$$

Finally, $\mathbf{WW}^{-1} = \mathbf{I}$, as shown in Equation A.11.

$$\mathbf{WW}^{-1} = \begin{bmatrix} w_{11} & w_{12} \\ w_{21} & w_{22} \end{bmatrix} \begin{bmatrix} \dfrac{w_{22}}{w_{11}w_{22} - w_{12}w_{21}} & \dfrac{-w_{12}}{w_{11}w_{22} - w_{12}w_{21}} \\ \dfrac{-w_{21}}{w_{11}w_{22} - w_{12}w_{21}} & \dfrac{w_{11}}{w_{11}w_{22} - w_{12}w_{21}} \end{bmatrix}$$

$$= \begin{bmatrix} \dfrac{w_{11}w_{22} - w_{12}w_{21}}{w_{11}w_{22} - w_{12}w_{21}} & \dfrac{-w_{11}w_{12} + w_{12}w_{11}}{w_{11}w_{22} - w_{12}w_{21}} \\ \dfrac{w_{21}w_{22} - w_{22}w_{21}}{w_{11}w_{22} - w_{12}w_{21}} & \dfrac{-w_{12}w_{21} - w_{11}w_{22}}{w_{11}w_{22} - w_{12}w_{21}} \end{bmatrix} = \begin{bmatrix} 1 & 0 \\ 0 & 1 \end{bmatrix} = \mathbf{I}$$

$$\begin{bmatrix} 6 & 3 \\ 4 & 7 \end{bmatrix} \begin{bmatrix} 7/30 & -3/30 \\ -4/30 & 6/30 \end{bmatrix} = \begin{bmatrix} 1 & 0 \\ 0 & 1 \end{bmatrix} \qquad (A.11)$$

Whereas it is relatively easy to find the inverse of a 2×2 matrix, finding the inverse of a 3×3 or larger matrix becomes increasingly difficult. One method developed early on in linear algebra is the square root method—described, for example, in Harmon (1960). Today it is easier to rely on computer programs that have the capability to produce the matrix inverse in order to obtain it. Fortunately, Excel is one such computer program. In the next section, we look at this capability of Excel's and how it works to solve the simultaneous equation problem of multiple regression.

Matrix Capabilities of Excel

Excel provides several functions that are specifically matrix functions and that are particularly useful in regard to the solution of the multiple regression problem. (Interestingly, Excel refers to matrices as *arrays*, and that term will be used to refer to a matrix during much of this discussion. But it is often confusing to try to stay with one or the other, so if you see "matrix" and "array" used interchangeably here, just remember that they are basically the same things.) Excel provides four functions that are specifically designed to manipulate arrays (or matrices). These are =MMULT, =MINVERSE, =MDETERM, and =TRANSPOSE.

Excel's Array Functions: =MMULT, =MINVERSE, =MDETERM, and =TRANSPOSE

The first of these functions, =MMULT, multiplies any two arrays together as long as the two conform for multiplication. The second, =MINVERSE, finds the inverse of any square array that has a nonzero determinant. If the determinant of the array is 0, Excel will return NUM# in the cells selected. Excel returns the determinant of the array for =MDETERM and the transpose of the array for =TRANSPOSE. To see how these operate and the results obtained, let us look again at the data in Figure 12.1. We will also use the intercept variable (constant), as shown in Figure 12.4, and this is reproduced in Figure A.1. In Figure A.1, the area that is highlighted in black will be referred to with matrix notation as **X** (matrices other than those that are $m \times 1$ or $1 \times m$ are always designated with bold roman capitals). The cost column (not highlighted) will be designated with matrix notation as **y** (matrices that are $m \times 1$ or $1 \times m$ are called *vectors* and are always referred to with bold roman lowercase letters).

Manipulating a Matrix with Excel

Figure A.2 shows the data given in Figure A.2, but with several modifications. Now, the independent variable array is designated as simply **y**, the

Figure A.1 Hospital data

Figure A.2 Arrays y, X, and X′

independent variable array is designated as **X**, and a new array, designated as **X′**, is shown in cells G2:P4. In the formula line in Figure A.2 is the expression $\{$=TRANSPOSE(C2:E11)$\}$. This is the *transpose* function, and the resulting array **X9** is the transpose of **X**. It should be noted that the braces surrounding the =TRANSPOSE function mean that it is one of those functions that enter data into more than one cell and must be invoked by holding down Ctrl+Shift and then pressing Enter.

Important

In invoking any of the functions that produce results in more than one cell of the spreadsheet, such as the array functions discussed here or the =FREQUENCY function discussed earlier in the book, it is necessary to highlight the entire area into which the results are to go before typing the function. In Figure A.2 the area G2:P4 was highlighted before the =TRANSPOSE function was typed.

Using the MMULT Function in Excel

The =MMULT array function can be used to produce two new arrays, $\mathbf{X'X}$ and $\mathbf{X'y}$, which are shown in Figure A.3. The array $\mathbf{X'X}$ is highlighted, and the formula for that array is shown in the formula bar. It can be seen there that the array is produced with {=MMULT(G2:P4,C2:E11)}. The braces again indicate that the function was completed with Ctrl+Shift+Enter. The array $\mathbf{X'y}$ is produced with the array function {=MMULT(G2:P4,A2:A11)}.

There is something else to note about Figure A.3 and its comparison with the data in cells G3:G11 of Figure 12.4. The array $\mathbf{X'X}$ includes all the values in cells G3 to G8, and the array $\mathbf{X'y}$ includes the values in cells G9 to G11. The calculation of the $\mathbf{X'X}$ and the $\mathbf{X'y}$ arrays using the matrix capabilities of Excel produces all the values needed for the calculation of the coefficients b_j. It is important to note that the results shown in $\mathbf{X'X}$ (3 × 3) would not be the same as the results for $\mathbf{X'X}$, which would be 10 × 10. Moreover, $y\mathbf{X'}$ does not even exist, because the two arrays in that format, (10 × 1) and (3 × 10), cannot be multiplied.

Solving the Regression Equations in Excel

Using the data in $\mathbf{X'X}$ and $\mathbf{X'y}$ from Figure A.3, it is possible to rewrite the second three expressions in Equation 12.7, as shown in Equation A.12. We have already seen that these three equations can be solved for the coefficients b_j with successive elimination. But with our understanding of matrix math, it can also be seen that Equation A.12 can be rewritten in matrix format, as shown in Equation A.13.

$$b_1 794,375 + b_2 55,825 + b_0 2725 = 6,896,750$$

$$b_1 55,825 + b_2 4833 + b_0 201 = 497,750 \tag{A.12}$$

$$b_1 2725 + b_2 201 + b_0 10 = 26,140$$

	G7		▼		=	{=MMULT(G2:P4,C2:E11)}									
	A	B	C	D	E	F	G	H	I	J	K	L	M	N	O	P
1	y		X				X'									
2	2750		225	6	1		225	200	300	350	200	250	175	400	350	275
3	2400		200	37	1		6	37	14	33	11	21	21	22	20	16
4	2920		300	14	1		1	1	1	1	1	1	1	1	1	1
5	1800		350	33	1											
6	3520		200	11	1		X'X				X'y					
7	2270		250	21	1		794375	55825	2725		6896750					
8	3100		175	21	1		55825	4833	201		497750					
9	1980		400	22	1		2725	201	10		26140					
10	2680		350	20	1											
11	2720		275	16	1											
12																

Figure A.3   Arrays $\mathbf{X'X}$ and $\mathbf{X'y}$

$$\begin{bmatrix} 794,375 & 55,825 & 2,735 \\ 55,825 & 4,833 & 201 \\ 2,755 & 201 & 10 \end{bmatrix} \cdot \begin{bmatrix} b_0 \\ b_1 \\ b_3 \end{bmatrix} = \begin{bmatrix} 6,896,750 \\ 497,750 \\ 26,140 \end{bmatrix} \qquad (A.13)$$

In matrix notation, the formulation in Equation A.13 is $X'Xb = X'y$. Now, how can matrix math be used to solve this equation for b? If we were dealing strictly with scalar arithmetic and we had an equation such as $xb = y$, and x and y were known, we could solve for b by $b = y/x$. But this formulation is the same as $1/x \times xb = 1/x \times y$. The expression $1/x$ is the inverse of x and can also be written as x^{-1}. Similarly, in matrix terms, it turns out that if we can find the inverse of $X'X$, we can solve the equation $X'Xb = X'y$ with the equation $X'X^{-1} X'Xb = X'X^{-1} Xy$, which turns out to be $X'X^{-1} Xy = b$. Happily, Excel provides the ability to find $X'X^{-1}$. To see how Excel provides the inverse, we can look at Figure A.4. In Figure A.4, the inverse of $X'X$ is shown in the highlighted area, cells M7:O9. The {=MINVERSE()} function used to produce the inverse array is shown on the formula bar. Note again that it is enclosed in braces to denote that it was completed with Ctrl+Shift+Enter. Also, it is important to remember that the entire area consisting of cells M7:O9 was highlighted before the {=MINVERSE()} function was typed.

Explanation of Excel Output Displayed with Scientific Notation

A further point that should be made about the inverse array is that the numbers, particularly in cells M7, N7, and M8, may appear a little strange. The way these numbers are shown is known as scientific notation. In more familiar terms, the number 1.98E-05 is actually the number 0.0000198. The E-05 means that there are five decimal places before the decimal place in 1.98E-05. It should be recognized that any number that is followed by E with a minus sign and a number is a very small number. Excel uses the E

Figure A.4 Inverse of X'X

Figure A.5 The b coefficients

convention to put numbers into cells that otherwise would be two narrow to display the string of decimal places before the actual values begin.

The E convention is also used for very large numbers. For example, a number that would be shown in Excel as 1.98E+11 would actually be 198,000,000,000. This is a relatively economical way for Excel to display very large numbers.

Now that we have found the inverse of $X'X$, it is possible to solve for the vector b. This solution is shown in Figure A.5. The coefficients b_j (found by the =MMULT function, as shown in the formula line of Figure A.5) are exactly the same (except for order and decimal places) as the b_j values found by using the built-in Excel package under Data Analysis &cmdarr; Regression. Refer to Figure 12.3 for the Data Analysis results.

Using the *b* Coefficients to Generate Regression Results

In general, the calculation of all the important results relative to multiple regression can all be developed, once the **b** coefficients are available. These include the predicted value of $y(\hat{y})$, the total sum of squares (SS_T), regression sum of squares (SS_R) and error sum of squares (SS_E), the value of R^2 and the correlation coefficient (R), the standard error of estimate (Syx), and the F tests. These follow the same development as that described for simple linear regression in Chapter 11. There is one place in which the remaining calculations diverge from that shown for simple linear regression, in the calculation of the standard errors for the coefficients b_j. The calculation of the standard errors of the coefficients for multiple regression relies on values that appear only in the matrix $X'X^{-1}$.

Recall that the standard error of estimate, Syx, the standard error of the predicted values of y, is found by dividing the error sum of squares, SS_E, by $n - 2$ and taking the square root of the result. In simple linear regression,

	M	N	O	P
	X'X⁻¹			
	1.98E-05	-2.6E-05	-0.00488	
	-2.6E-05	0.0013	-0.01888	
	-0.00488	-0.01888	1.808118	
	323.9537			
	1.442784	#NUM!	#NUM!	
	#NUM!	11.663	#NUM!	
	#NUM!	#NUM!	435.6084	

Formula bar: `= =$M$11*SQRT(M7)`

Figure A.6 Calculation of standard errors of b

the standard error of b_j is found by dividing Syx by the square root of the sum of squares in x (SS_X). This is essentially the same as multiplying Syx by the square root of $1/SS_X$. In multiple regression, the equivalent result is obtained by multiplying Syx by the square root of each of the main diagonal elements of $X'X^{-1}$.

To see the calculation of the standard errors for the coefficients b_j, consider Figure A.6. Here the value of Syx has been copied from Figure 12.3. The formula bar shows that the cell highlighted in white is calculated by multiplying the value in cell $M\$11$ (Syx) by the square root of the value in cell M7 (here 1.98E-05). Because cell $M\$11$ is fixed, the formula can then be copied into the other cells in row M and in rows N and O to produce, on the main diagonal, the standard errors for all the values of the coefficients b. The expression #NUM! that appears in the off-diagonal cells indicates, in this case, that we tried to take the square root of a negative number. In any case, it is the main diagonal elements that are of interest. It can be seen that except for ordering, they match the values found for the standard errors of the coefficients b in Figure 12.3. These standard error values can be used directly to perform the t test that determines whether the appropriate coefficients are different from 0.

Calculation of All Multiple Regression Results

Figure A.7 shows the analysis as given in Figure A.5 and Figure A.6. In addition, it shows all the other important results of multiple regression, as shown originally in Figure 12.3. The section of column A labeled $\hat{y}$ was calculated using the matrix function =MMULT(C2:E11,G13:G15), which is essentially the formula for the prediction of the y values cast in matrix form. The values in column C labeled $y - \bar{y}$ represent the difference between the actual values of y and the mean of y. The value in cell C14

	A	B	C	D	E	F	G	H	I	J	K	L	M	N	O	P
1	y	X					X'									
2	2750	225	6	1		225	200	300	350	200	250	175	400	350	275	
3	2400	200	37	1		6	37	14	33	11	21	21	22	20	16	
4	2920	300	14	1		1	1	1	1	1	1	1	1	1	1	
5	1800	350	33	1												
6	3520	200	11	1		X'X				X'y		X'x⁻¹				
7	2270	250	21	1		794375	55825	2725		6896750		1.98E-05	-2.6E-05	-0.00488		
8	3100	175	21	1		55825	4833	201		497750		-2.6E-05	0.0013	-0.01888		
9	1980	400	22	1		2725	201	10		26140		-0.00488	-0.01888	1.808118		
10	2680	350	20	1												
11	2720	275	16	1												
12						b	S.E.b	t	p				1.442784	#NUM!	#NUM!	
13	yhat	y-ybar	yh-yb	y-yh		-3.7623	1.44278	-2.61	0.03503				#NUM!	11.86298	#NUM!	
14	3214	136	600.2	-464		-29.896	11.663	-2.56	0.03737				#NUM!	#NUM!	435.6084	
15	2382	-214	-232.5	18.47		4240.13	435.608	9.734	2.6E-05							
16	2693	306	78.9	227.1												
17	1937	-814	-677.2	-137		SS	d.f.	MS	F	p						
18	3159	906	544.8	361.2	SST	2413440	9									
19	2672	-344	57.75	-402	SSR	1678818	2	839409	7.99849	0.016						
20	2954	486	339.9	146.1	SSE	734622	7	104946								
21	2078	-634	-536.5	-97.5												
22	2325	66	-288.6	354.6	R^2	0.69561										
23	2727	106	113.2	-7.17	S.E.	323.954										

Figure A.7 Calculation of all results from Figure 12.3

was calculated with the formula =A2-AVERAGE($A$2:$A$11). That formula can be copied all the way to C23 to produce all the $y - \bar{y}$ values. The value for the total sum of squares, SST, in cell H18, is calculated using the Excel function =SUMSQ(C14:C23).

The column labeled yh (for $\hat{y}$) $- yb$ (for $\bar{y}$) was calculated by subtracting the predicted values of y from the average values for y. The formula for cell D14 is =A14-AVERAGE($A$2:$A$11). That formula can be copied to all the cells from D14 to D23 to create all the values of $yh - yb$. The value of the sum of squares due to regression, SS_R, in cell H19 is calculated using =SUMSQ(D14:D23). The column labeled $y - yh$ was calculated by subtracting each value of $\hat{y}$ from y. The formula for cell E14 is =A2-A14. The sum of squares error, SS_E, in cell H20 was calculated using =SUMSQ(E14:E23).

Degrees of freedom in any multiple regression will always be $n - 1$ for SS_T, equal to m (the number of predictor variables) for SS_R, and $n - m - 1$ for SS_E. In the case of this analysis, these values are shown in cells I18:I20 as 9, 2, and 7, respectively. The mean square values in cells J19 and J20 are the sum of squares values divided by their degrees of freedom. The overall F test for the independence of y from the two variables x is calculated by dividing the mean square due to regression by the mean square error. The probability of the F value, p, is given by the Excel function =FDIST(K19,2,7).

The R^2 value in cell H22 is calculated by dividing SS_R by SS_T. The value of $S.E.$ (standard error of estimate) in cell H23 is obtained by dividing SS_E by its degrees of freedom and taking the square root of the result. This value was used to multiply by the square root of the values in cells M12, N13, and O14 to produce the standard error of each value of b_j in cells H13:H15. The t values for each of the b_j are calculated by dividing each value of b by its standard error. The probabilities of the t values are given by =TDIST(t,d.f.,2). The degrees of freedom for any value of b_j are equal to the degrees of freedom for SS_E. Because two of the b_j values are negative, the =TDIST function will produce only the result #NUM!. In order to produce the actual probability of the coefficients, it is necessary to include the Excel =ABS function to get the absolute value of t before getting the probability of the t value. So, for example, the probability in cell J13 was obtained with =TDIST(ABS(I13),7,2). Table A.1 displays the formulas for the calculation of the multiple regression output from Figure A.7.

Table A.1 Formulas for Figure A.7

Cell or Column	Formula	Notes
G2:P4	{=TRANSPOSE(C2:E11)}	Remember that the braces signify that you must press Crtl+Shift to invoke the function.
G7:I9	{=MMULT(G2:P4,C2:E11)}	This generates the X × X matrix.
K7:K9	{=MMULT(G2:P4,A2:A11)}	This generates the X × y matrix.
M7:O9	{=MINVERSE(G7:I9)}	This generates the X × X^{-1} matrix.
G13:G15	{=MMULT(M7:O9,K7:K9)}	This generates the b coefficients.
M12	=323.9537*SQRT(M7)	Copied from cell M12 through to cell M14 and over to cell O14
A14:A23	{=MMULT(C2:E11,G13:G15)}	This generates the ŷ values.
C14	=A2-AVERAGE($A$2:$A$11)	Copied down to cell C23
D14	=A14-AVERAGE($A$2:$A$11)	Copied down to cell D23
E14	=A2-A14	Copied down to cell E23
H18	=SUMSQ(C14:C23)	This generates the total sum of squares, SST.
H19	=SUMSQ(D14:D23)	This generates the sum of square error, SSR.
H20	=SUMSQ(E14:E23)	This generates the sum of square error, SSE.
I18	9	Equals $n - 1$ or $10 - 1 = 9$
I19	2	Equals m or 2
I20	7	Equals $n - m - 1$ or $10 - 2 - 1 = 7$
J19	=H19/I19	Copied down to cell J20
K19	=J19/J20	
L19	=FDIST(K19,2,7)	
H22	=H19/H18	
H23	=SQRT(H20/I20)	
H13	=M12	
H14	=N13	
H15	=O14	
I13	=G13/H13	Copied down to cell I15
J13	=TDIST(ABS(I13),I20,I19)	Copied down to cell J15

EXERCISES FOR APPENDIX A

1. Use the data on the Hospitals worksheet of Chpt 12-1.xls, and replicate the analysis shown in Figure A.7.

    a. Set up the data from the Hospitals worksheet, as shown in Figure A.7, with the variables X_1 and X_2 in cells C2:C11 and D2:D11, respectively, and supply a third independent variable, the constant, as shown in cells E2:E11.

    b. Generate the transpose of the matrix **X** in cells G2:P4 by using =TRANSPOSE(C2:E11). Remember that the entire area into which the transpose matrix will go must be highlighted prior to invoking the function and that the function must be invoked with Ctrl+Shift+Enter.

    c. Calculate the values of **X'X** in cells G7:I9 by using =MMULT (G2:P4,C2:E11). This function, too, requires highlighting of the entire three-by-three cell area and pressing Ctrl+Shift+Enter.

    d. Use =MMULT(G2:P4,A2:A11) to calculate the values of **X'y** in cells K7:K9.

    e. Use =MINVERSE(G7:I9) to obtain the inverse of the matrix **X'X** in cells M7:O9.

    f. Calculate the values of *b* in cells G13:G15, using =MMULT (M7:O9,K7:K9).

    g. Using the values of *b* and the original matrix **X**, generate the values of $\hat{y}$ in cells A14:A23 with =MMULT(C2:D11,G13:G15).

    h. Generate the values of $y - \bar{y}$ in cells C14:C23, using y-AVERAGE ($A$2:$A$11), and calculate the total sum of squares (SS_T) in cell H18, using =SUMSQ(C14:C23).

    i. Generate the values of $yh - yb$ in cells D14:D23, using yhat-AVERAGE ($A$2:$A$11), and calculate the regression sum of squares (SS_R) in cell H19, using =SUMSQ(D14:D23).

    j. Generate the values of $y - yh$ in cells E14:E23, and calculate the error sum of squares (SS_E) with =SUMSQ(E14:E23).

    k. Calculate the value of R^2 in cell H22 by dividing the regression sum of squares by the total sum of squares.

    l. Calculate the value of *S.E.* in cell H23 by taking the square root of $[SS_E/(n - m - 1)]$.

    m. Determine the degrees of freedom for SS_T $(n - 1)$, SS_R (m), and SS_E $(n - m - 1)$, and put these into cells H13:H15. Calculate the values of MS_R and MS_E in cells J19 and J20, and calculate the value of *F* in cell K19 to determine its probability in cell K19.

    n. Calculate the values of the *S.E. b* by multiplying the value of *S.E.* by the square root of each value in cells M7:O9 and by putting the answer in cells M12:O14. Copy the main diagonal cells (the standard error of the coefficients) to cells H13:H15.

    o. Calculate the values of t in cells I13:I15, and determine the probability of these values of t in cells J13:J15.

2. Give an interpretation of this analysis by briefly stating in words the following:

    a. The meaning of the three b coefficients in cells G13:G15

    b. The meaning of the three t tests and their probabilities

    c. The meaning of the values of SS_T, SS_R, and SS_E

    d. The meaning of the F test and its probability

    e. The meaning of R^2

    f. The meaning of $S.E.$

3. Use the data on the SWC worksheet of Chpt 12-1.xls, and carry out an analysis, as shown in Figure A.7.

    a. Supply a third independent variable—the constant.

    b. Generate the transpose of the matrix **X**, using the =TRANSPOSE function. Remember that the entire area into which the transpose matrix will go must be highlighted prior to invoking the function, and that the function must be invoked with Ctrl+Shift+Enter.

    c. Calculate the values of **X′X**, using the =MMULT function. This function, too, requires highlighting the entire three-by-three cell area and pressing Ctrl+Shift+Enter.

    d. Use =MMULT to calculate the values of **X′y**.

    e. Use =MINVERSE to obtain the inverse of the matrix **X′y**.

    f. Calculate the values of b, using the =MMULT function.

    g. Using the values of b and the original matrix **X**, generate the values of with =MMULT.

    h. Generate the values of $y - \bar{y}$, using y-AVERAGE, and calculate the total sum of squares (SS_T), using the =SUMSQ function.

    i. Generate the values of $yh - yb$, using $\hat{y} - AVERAGE()$, and calculate the regression sum of squares (SS_R), using the =SUMSQ function.

    j. Generate the values of $y - yh$, and calculate the error sum of squares (SS_E) with the =SUMSQ function.

    k. Calculate the value of R^2 by dividing the regression sum of squares by the total sum of squares.

    l. Calculate the value of $S.E.$ by taking the square root of $[SS_E/(n - m - 1)]$.

    m. Determine the degrees of freedom for SS_T $(n - 1)$, SS_R (m), and SS_E $(n - m - 1)$. Calculate the values of MS_R and MS_E and the value of F and determine its probability.

   n. Calculate the values of the *S.E. b* by multiplying the value of *S.E.* by the square root of each value in $\mathbf{X'X}^{-1}$.

   o. Calculate the values of *t*, and determine the probability of these values of *t*.

4. Give an interpretation of this analysis by briefly stating in words the following:

   a. The meaning of the three *b* coefficients in cells G13:G15

   b. The meaning of the three *t* tests and their probabilities

   c. The meaning of the values of SS_T, SS_R, and SS_E

   d. The meaning of the *F* test and its probability

   e. The meaning of R^2

   f. The meaning of *S.E.*

REFERENCES

Aldrich, J., and F. Nelson. 1984. "Linear Probability, Logit, and Probit Models." SAGE University Paper 45. Newbury Park, CA: SAGE.

Brook, R. H., and F. A. Appel. 1973. "Quality of Care Assessment: Choosing a Method for Peer Review." *The New England Journal of Medicine* 288 (June 21): 1323–1329.

Freund, J. E., and R. E. Walpole. 1987. *Mathematical Statistics.* 4th ed. Englewood Cliffs, NJ: Prentice-Hall.

Goldberger, A. S. 1964. *Econometric Theory.* New York: John Wiley & Sons.

Halpern, C. T., et al. 2001. "Partner Violence among Adolescents in Opposite-Sex Romantic Relationships: Findings from the National Longitudinal Study of Adolescent Health." *American Journal of Public Health* 91(10): 1679–1685.

Harmon, H. H. 1960. *Modern Factor Analysis.* Chicago: University of Chicago Press.

Kros, J. F. 2014. *Spreadsheet Modeling for Business Decisions.* 4th ed. Dubuque, IA: KendallHunt.

Levine, D. M., D. Stephan, and K. A. Szabat. 2007. *Statistics for Managers Using Microsoft Excel.* 5th ed. Upper Saddle River, NJ: Prentice-Hall.

———. 2013. *Statistics for Managers Using Microsoft Excel.* 7th ed. Englewood Cliffs, NJ: Prentice-Hall.

Maddala, G. S. 1983. *Limited-Dependent and Qualitative Variables in Econometrics.* New York: Cambridge University Press.

McDermott, R. E. 2001. "Using Multiple Regression to Establish Labor Rates." *Healthcare Financial Management* (September 2001): 49–60.

"Sudan 1989/1990: Results from the Demographic and Health Survey." *Studies in Family Planning,* 1992, 23(1): 66–70.

The State of the World's Children 1996. 1996. New York: UNICEF. https://www.unicef.org/reports/state-worlds-children-1996.

The State of the World's Children 2001. 2000 (December). New York: UNICEF. https://www.unicef.org/media/84781/file/SOWC-2001.pdf.

U.S. Census Bureau. 2001. *Statistical Abstract of the United States: 2000.* http://www.beardbooks.com/beardbooks/evaluation_and_decision_making_for_health_services.html.

Veney, J. E., and A. D. Kaluzny. 1998. *Evaluation and Decision Making for Health Services.* Chicago: Health Administration Press.

Winer, B. J. 1962. *Statistical Principles in Experimental Design.* New York: McGraw-Hill.

#DIV/0! An Excel error message caused by trying to divide by 0.

#NAME? An Excel error message generally denoting the misspelling of an Excel function name.

#NUM! An Excel error message generally caused by trying to perform an undefined mathematical procedure, such as taking the square root of a negative number, or by requesting a result that exceeds Excel's limits, such as =FACT(171).

#VALUE! An Excel error message generally caused by including a nonnumerical value in a mathematical operation.

=AND() Excel function that returns the result of two comparisons, TRUE if both comparisons are true and FALSE if either comparison is false.

=AVERAGE() Excel function that returns the mean of a series of data.

=BINOMDIST() Excel function that returns the probability for the appearance of any value from a binomial distribution, given the number of trials and the outcome probability for a single trial.

=CHIDIST() Excel function that returns the probability of a chi-square value, given degrees of freedom.

=CHIINV() Excel function that returns the chi-square value, given the probability of the chi-square value and degrees of freedom.

=CHITEST() Excel function that returns the probability of a chi-square value, given the observed and expected values.

=COUNT() Excel function that returns the number of values in a series of numerical data.

=COUNTIF() Excel function that returns the number of times a given value appears in a series of data.

=EXP() Excel function that returns the value of e (approximately 2.718282) raised to the power of the number in the parentheses.

=FACT() Excel function that returns the factorial of the number in parentheses. Limited to numbers less than 171.

=FDIST() Excel function that returns the probability of an F value, given degrees of freedom.

=FINV() Excel function that returns the F value, given the probability of the F value and degrees of freedom.

=FREQUENCY() Excel function that returns a frequency distribution for a series of data in terms of a series of categories.

=IF() Excel function that returns the result of an if–then decision.

=MAX() Excel function that returns the maximum value in a series of data.

=MDETERM() Excel function that returns the determinant for a square matrix.

=MEDIAN() Excel function that returns the median value for a series of data.

=MIN() Excel function that returns the minimum value in a series of data.

=MINVERSE() Excel function that returns the inverse of a matrix (array).

=MMULT() Excel function that returns the product of two matrices (arrays).

=MODE() Excel function that returns the modal value for a series of data. If the data have more than one mode, =MODE() will return the value of the numerically smallest mode.

=NORMDIST() Excel function that returns probability for any value from a normal distribution, given the mean and standard deviation of the distribution.

=OR() Excel function that returns TRUE if either or both of two comparisons are true and FALSE if both comparisons are false.

=POISSON() Excel function that returns the probability of a appearance of any value from a Poisson distribution, given the mean of the distribution.

=RAND() Excel function that returns a uniform random number between 0 and 1.

=RANDBETWEEN() Excel function that returns a uniform random number between two selected numbers.

=ROUND() Excel function that returns the selected number rounded to the number of decimal places specified.

=SQRT() Excel function that returns the square root of a number.

=STDEV() Excel function that returns the standard deviation of a series of data assumed to represent a sample.

=SUM() Excel function that returns the sum of a series of data.

=SUMPRODUCT() Excel function that returns the sum of the product of the values of two series of data.

=SUMSQ() Excel function that returns the sum of the squares of a series of data.

=TDIST() Excel function that returns the probability of a t value, given degrees of freedom and a one- or two-tailed test.

=TINV() Excel function that returns the t value, given the probability of the t value and degrees of freedom.

=TRANSPOSE() Excel function that returns the transpose of a matrix (array).

=TRUNC() Excel function that returns the integer portion of a number.

=TTEST() Excel function that returns the probability of a t value, given a data set with a numerical dependent variable and a two-level categorical independent variable.

=VAR() Excel function that returns the variance of a series of data assumed to represent a sample.

=VARP() Excel function that returns the variance of a series of data assumed to represent a population.

=YEARFRAC Excel function that returns the number of years between two calendar dates.

A priori probability Likelihood of the occurrence of an event that can be determined from the nature of the process that generates the event.

Alpha The level of Type I error, usually set by the researcher at 0.05 or 0.01. *See* Type I error.

Analysis of variance (ANOVA) A test used to determine whether a numerical variable is independent of one or more categorical variables that may take on more than two values.

Analysis tool pak Package of statistical procedures that can be added to Excel to perform such things as t tests, analysis of variance, random sampling, and regression.

Array A set of data in contiguous rows and columns. An Excel designation of a matrix. In Excel, it often refers to a set of cells that are linked so that no one cell can be changed independently of the others.

Bartlett test A test for homogeneity of within group variance between more than two groups.

Bell-shaped curve The shape of a normal distribution.

Bernoulli distribution A probability distribution that contains only values of 1 or 0, the number of which depend on the probability of 1.

Best-fitting line A line determined by an independent variable that passes closest to the values of a dependent variable in a two-dimensional graph. Usually defined as the line that minimizes the sum of squared differences between the line and the values of the dependent variable for all values of the independent variable.

Beta The level of Type II error, usually not known unless a specific value is stated for an alternative hypothesis. *See* Type II error.

Between group variance Variance that exists among the means of some value for two or more groups.

Binomial distribution A probability distribution that represents the accumulation of a Bernoulli distribution for any number of trials and any value of the probability of 1.

Bins Excel designation for the categories into which the =FREQUENCY () function accumulates a data series.

Categorical variable A variable whose values are logically classified by names (i.e., male, female), as opposed to numbers. May be coded as numbers, however.

Causal variable A variable whose values are assumed to influence the values of other variables in a given analysis but assumed not to be affected by these others.

Causality The concept that the value of one variable may be a cause of the value of another variable.

Central tendency A way of referring to the central or midpoint around which a data series clusters. Measured by the mean, median, or mode.

Chi-square statistic A statistical test that assesses whether a categorical variable is independent of one or more other categorical variables.

Cluster sample A sample drawn by first dividing the total population into several mutually exclusive and all-inclusive groups and then selecting some of the groups from which to take all members of the group or a sample of the group.

Conditional probability The probability of some outcome, given knowledge of some other event—for example, the likelihood that a person will arrive at an emergency room with a true emergency, given that the person arrives during the night.

Confidence interval Interval on the number scale within which a population value is expected to lie with some predetermined probability, such as 95 percent.

Constant A number or characteristic that is assigned to members of a sample and that is identical for every member of the sample.

Contingency table Simultaneous distribution of two usually categorical variables. *See* Cross-tabulation.

Continuous numerical variable A numerical variable that can, theoretically, be infinitely divided, such as blood pressure.

Control group Those persons in an experiment who do not receive the actual experimental intervention; they generally receive some placebo intervention that mimics the actual experimental intervention but is expected to have no effect.

Correlation A value derived from a statistic that describes the relationship between two variables. May range from −1 for a perfect negative relationship to 1 for a perfect positive relationship. Zero indicates no relationship.

Critical value The value of a test statistic (chi-square, t value, F), above which the hypothesis of interest is rejected.

Cross-tabulation (or Cross-tab) Simultaneous distribution of two usually categorical variables. *See* Contingency table.

Cumulative frequency Frequency distribution that shows the accumulation of values from the lowest category to the highest.

Data range A set of generally contiguous cells that represent data to be included in some Excel operation.

Degrees of freedom A value that designates the number of options that can be exercised before no others are available.

Delimited Refers to one of two ways that data may be stored in a .txt file. Each data element is followed by a common character that designates or delimits the end of that data element. *See* Fixed-length.

Dependent variable A variable whose values are assumed to be affected or modified by the value of other variables in a given analysis.

Determinant A single number that can be used to describe a square matrix. For a two-by-two matrix, equal to the product of the main diagonal elements minus the product of the off-diagonal elements.

Diagnostic-related group (DRG) A categorization of medical conditions used for determining payment by Medicare and Medicaid.

Discrete distribution An Excel option that allows the user to define the probability of the selection of any value from a predetermined set of values.

Discrete numerical variable A numerical variable that cannot be divided into units smaller than integers, such as the number of persons in a waiting room.

Dispersion A way of referring to the variability in a set of data. Measured by the variance or standard deviation.

Double-blind random clinical trial An experimental design in which neither the subjects under study, the persons administering the intervention of the study, nor the persons assessing the results of the study know which group or groups received which intervention.

Dummy variable A categorical variable that takes on two values and is coded 1 and 0. For example, the two colors blue and red could be coded 1 for blue and 0 for red. They would then represent a dummy variable.

Dust Bowl empiricism Term applied to the use of statistics to sift through data to find the best relationships, independent of theory.

Empirical probability The likelihood of the occurrence of an event that can be determined only on the basis of historical data about similar events that have already occurred.

Event The occurrence in a stochastic process to which a probability can be assigned.

Excel function A built-in Excel option that will produce the result of a formula or algorithm. Accessible on the Formatting toolbar.

Exponential model A regression model that is based on converting the dependent variable to its logarithmic value, either natural or base 10.

Factorial design Analysis that includes more than one independent variable. Usually used in reference to analysis of variance.

Finite population correction (fpc) A multiplier for reducing the standard error of a measure taken from a finite population when the sample is large relative to the size of the population.

Fisher exact test An alternative to chi-square for two-by-two tables with extremely small expected values (less than 5) in any cell.

Fixed-length Refers to one of two ways that data may be stored in a .txt file. Each data element is the same length. *See* Delimited.

Formula bar *See* Formula line.

Formula line The field at the top of an Excel spreadsheet that shows the content of the currently selected cell.

HDI (Human Development Index) A composite number ranging from 0 to 100, developed by the United Nations Development Programme (UNDP) for each country, from per capita income, literacy, and life expectancy.

Header row The row at the top of a column that contains the name of the data in that column.

Histogram A graph that shows data values as vertical columns.

Homogeneity of variance Equal within group variation across two or more groups.

Hypothesis A statement of belief about a population to be assessed, using data from a sample.

ICD-9 (International Classification of Diseases, ninth revision) A coding scheme maintained by the World Health Organization that provides a code for classifying mortality data from death certificates.

Identity matrix A square matrix with 1 in the main diagonal cells and 0 in all other cells.

Independence Formally, the understanding that conditional probabilities equal marginal probabilities; the recognition that two variables or two events are not dependent on each other.

Independent variable A variable whose values are assumed to be unaffected by other variables in a given analysis. *See also* Causal variable, Predictor variable.

Information matrix A matrix derived from Logit analysis that provides an intermediary step in the calculation of standard errors of coefficients derived using Logit.

Interaction effect The joint effect of two or more independent variables on a dependent variable. *See* Main effect.

Interval scale A numerical variable scale that has no real zero point, such as IQ or temperature measured in Celsius or Fahrenheit.

Inverse The value by which a number must be multiplied for the product to be 1 or by which a matrix must be multiplied for the product to be an identity matrix. For a scalar (single number), the inverse of x is $1/x$.

Joint probability The likelihood of two simultaneously occurring events—for example, the likelihood that a person will come to an emergency room during the day and will come for a true emergency.

Likert scale An ordinal scale that is usually constructed with categories such as "Strongly agree," "Agree," "Undecided," "Disagree," and "Strongly disagree."

Linear probability model A regression model derived by using ordinary least squares to estimate regression coefficients for a dichotomous dependent variable.

Linear regression A statistical technique for relating a dependent numerical variable to an independent numerical or two-level categorical variable that generally assumes a straight-line relationship.

Logarithmic model Regression analysis in which the x axis variable is converted to a logarithm, either natural or base 10.

Logit An analysis method that allows for the assessment of whether a two-level categorical variable is independent of one or more numerical or two-level categorical predictor variables. Based on maximum likelihood.

Main effect The direct effect of a single independent variable on an independent variable. *See* Interaction effect.

Marginal probability The probability of some outcome without regard to any other event; for example, the likelihood that a person who arrives at an emergency room will come for a true emergency versus a nonemergency condition is a marginal probability.

Matrix A set of data in contiguous rows and columns. *See* Array.

Maximum likelihood The estimation of regression coefficients based on the maximization of a likelihood function (rather than on the minimization of the sum of squared errors).

Mean The overall average of all values for a single variable. Calculated by summing all values and dividing by the total number of values.

Median The midpoint of the values of a single variable. Calculated by finding the value for which half the observations are larger and half the observations are smaller.

Medicare A program administered by the U.S. government that pays specified medical expenses, primarily for persons over the age of sixty-five.

Mode The most commonly occurring number in a series of data.

Monte Carlo technique A method of simulating the results of an analysis or process using randomly assigned values.

Moving average model A regression-like model that is generated based on the average of two or more previous time periods.

Multicolinearity A term descriptive of the relationship between two—usually independent or predictor—variables that vary together or are highly correlated with each other.

Multiple regression A technique for determining whether a single numerical variable is independent of two or more other numerical or two-level categorical variables.

Mutually exclusive Two or more outcomes of a stochastic process that cannot simultaneously occur.

Nested functions Two or more Excel functions in the same cell. Generally used for multiple decisions.

Nominal variable A categorical variable that is not ordered.

Nonlinear relationship A relationship between two variables that does not show evidence of a straight-line relationship.

Normal distribution A probability distribution in which values near the mean are more likely than values farther from the mean. Often referred to as a bell-shaped curve.

Numerical variable A variable that is measured on a number scale. May be continuous or discrete.

Ordinal variable A categorical variable that is ordered by magnitude or intensity (e.g., *good, better, best*).

Ordinary least squares (OLS) The least complex multiple regression technique.

Outcome The results of the events in a stochastic process.

Parameter Measure of a characteristic of a population.

Pareto chart A graph that shows actual frequencies as a histogram and cumulative frequencies as a line graph. Always ordered from the largest data category on the left of the graph to the smallest on the right.

Patterned distribution An Excel option that allows the user to generate a series of values in any pattern selected. Not a probability distribution.

Pivot table An Excel designation for a frequency distribution or cross-tabulation created by using the Pivot Table Tool.

Poisson distribution A probability distribution that represents the likelihood of a rare event.

Polynomial model A regression analysis in which a single independent variable is converted to its square, cube, fourth power, and so on to describe a dependent variable.

Population The group of persons or organizations about which there is an interest.

Power model Regression model in which both the independent and the dependent variables are converted to a logarithmic value, either natural or base 10.

Predictor variable A causal variable. A variable whose values are predictive of the values of other variables in a given analysis.

Probability The likelihood of an outcome of an event.

Probit An analysis method that allows for the assessment of whether a two-level categorical is independent of one or more numerical or two-level categorical predictor variables. Based on maximum likelihood.

Pseudorandom number A random number generated by a computer. Called pseudorandom because any computer-generation scheme inevitably incorporates some selection pattern.

R square (R^2) Proportion of variance in a dependent variable that can be accounted for or explained by knowledge of variation in an independent variable or variables.

Random number table A table of numbers arranged in rows and columns. Each number is randomly ordered with respect to all other numbers in the table. Used to select random samples before the advent of computers.

Random sample A subset of a larger population selected in such a way that every member of the larger population has a known and nonzero likelihood of being included.

Ratio variable A numerical variable that has a real zero point. May be continuous, such as weight, or discrete, such as the number of persons in a physician's waiting room.

Regression analysis A statistical analysis that seeks to determine whether a given numerical variable is independent of some set of other numerical variables or two-level categorical variables.

Regression coefficient A value by which an independent variable can be multiplied to predict the values of a dependent variable.

Repeated measures More than one measure of a variable on the same group of subject (persons, organizations).

Sample A subset of a population about which there is an interest. Selected to determine the values of interest for the population.

Sample space All possible outcomes of a stochastic process.

Sampled population The population that is actually sampled. May or may not be the same as the target population.

Scalar A way of referring to a single number when discussed in the context of matrices or arrays.

Scatterplot (or scatter graph) A graph that shows the simultaneous distribution of the data points for two variables. Also called an *XY* graph.

Simple random sample A sample drawn in such a way that every possible sample of a given size has an equal probability of being selected.

Skewed left A designation for a data distribution that has a median value greater than its mean and a "tail" of data to the left side of the distribution.

Skewed right A designation for a data distribution that has a median value less than its mean and a "tail" of data to the right side of the distribution.

Solver An Excel add-in that solves a wide variety of optimization problems.

Spreadsheet A computer-generated sheet of rows and columns. The area in Excel where work is done (a set of 1,048,576 numbered rows and 16,384 columns designated A through XFD).

Standard deviation A measure of overall variation in a set of data, the square root of the variance. *See* Variance.

Standard error A measure of the overall variation in the means from samples of a given size taken from a population. Equals the standard deviation divided by the square root of the sample size.

Statistic Measure of a characteristic of a sample. Estimates a parameter.

Statistical significance Refers to a statistical test result that leads to the rejection of the implicit or explicit hypothesis of independence between two or more variables.

Stepwise regression A technique for using regression analysis to find a model that accounts for the largest possible share of the variance in the independent variable while eliminating variables that do not contribute to the prediction. Can be forward inclusion or backward elimination.

Stochastic process A series of events, the outcome of any one being determined by some probability.

Stratified sample A sample drawn by first dividing the total population into two or more mutually exclusive and all-inclusive groups and then drawing samples from each of these groups.

Sums of squares The addition of the difference between all values for a particular data set and the mean value for the data. May be calculated.

Systematic sample A sample drawn by dividing the population into several ordered groups and then randomly selecting a first member of the sample from the first group and selecting each comparable member from all other groups.

***t* distribution** A probability distribution similar to the normal distribution but having fewer values near the mean and more in the tails, depending on degrees of freedom.

t test A test that compares an estimated value from a sample with the standard error for that value. Used to determine whether a numerical variable is independent of a two-level categorical variable.

Target population The population of interest from which a sample is desired.

Text Import Wizard A set of dialog boxes invoked by the attempt to load a non-Excel file into an Excel spreadsheet that provides step-by-step direction in converting the non-Excel file into an Excel file.

Transpose Operation by which the columns of an array (matrix) become rows and the rows become columns.

Trend line The single line through an XY scatterplot that provides the best linear or nonlinear fit to the data.

Type I error The likelihood of rejecting a hypothesis when it is true. Always set by the level of confidence selected.

Type II error The likelihood of not rejecting a hypothesis when it is false. Known only if a specific value of an alternative hypothesis is given.

Uniform distribution A probability distribution in which any number in a given range is equally likely. Often called a flat distribution.

Variable A measure of some attribute for a set of entities, persons, or organizations that takes on more than one value.

Variance A measure of overall variation in a set of data that represents the average squared difference between each value in the data set and the mean of all values.

Vector A matrix (array) made up of a single row or a single column.

Weighted least squares (WLS) A regression technique that takes account of possible unequal variation in the dependent variable at different levels of the predictor variables.

Within group variance Variance that exists among the values for a specified group.

Workbook An Excel computer file consisting of one or more spreadsheets.

x axis A horizontal axis in a graph or chart. Usually considered to be the independent variable.

x variable A variable generally considered to be the independent or causal variable.

y axis A vertical axis in a graph or chart. Usually considered to be the dependent variable.

y variable Variable generally considered to be the caused or dependent variable.

Yates's correction A modification of the chi-square formula for two-by-two tables with expected values less than 10.

Page references followed by *fig* and *t* indicate an illustrated figure and table, respectively.